MEDICINAL PLANTS :
ETHNOMEDICINE & BIOTECHNOLOGICAL POTENTIAL

MEDICINAL PLANTS :

ETHNOMEDICINE & BIOTECHNOLOGICAL POTENTIAL

S.D. ROUT
H.N. THATOI
North Orissa University
Sriramchandra Vihar, Takatpur
Baripada-757003, Mayurbhanj

BIOTECH

2011
BIOTECH BOOKS
NEW DELHI

ISBN : 978-81-7622-237-2

Published by : **BIOTECH BOOKS**
Head Office : 1123/74, Deva Ram Park, Tri Nagar, Delhi - 110035
Showroom : 4762-63/23, Ansari Road, Darya Ganj, New Delhi - 110 002
Phone : 23262132
email : biotechbooks@yahoo.co.in

PRINTED IN INDIA

CONTENTS

PREFACE

India is one of the twelve-mega biodiversity countries of the world having rich vegetation with a wide variety of plants having medicinal value. The use of medicinal plants plays an important role in the lives of rural people, especially in the developing countries of the world, which are poorly served with modern health facilities. Much of world's population depends upon traditional medicine to meet daily health requirements. At present about 65% of the Indian population is dependent on the traditional system of medicine.

Similipal Biosphere Reserve (SBR) is located in the central part of Mayurbhanj district of Orissa. Similipal has attracted the attention of global scientists for its amazing species diversity including both flora and fauna. It harbores 7% of flowering plants, 8% of the orchids, 7% reptiles, 20% birds, 11% mammals of India. Moreover, it is the home of melanistic tiger and black panther. Similipal is the treasure house of 1076 species of vascular plants including 93 species of orchids. Similipal is one of the richest forest with medicinal plant diversity in Orissa. Neither much study has been carried out earlier nor any book available for medicinal plants diversity of Similipal Biosphere Reserve. Several years of arduous effort and intensive first hand field observation and subsequently laboratory studies have helped us to come out with this unique book. This book embodies enumeration of medicinal plants, their ethnomedicinal uses by the tribals of Similipal, evaluation of biotechnological potentials of some medicinal plants. A large number colour photographs of medicinal plants have been provided.

The book is aimed to enumerate potential medicinal plants of Similipal Biosphere Reserve and document some traditional uses of these plants by the local people belonging to different tribal communities for curing various diseases. The traditional herbal practitioners efficiently treat various ailments with animals, plants, minerals etc. available in their surroundings. Apart from traditional herbal practitioners, the heads of the villages also use to give some folklore medicine. Ethnomedicine is the system of maintaining health and curing diseases based on folk beliefs and traditional knowledge, skills, methods and practices. The knowledge of ethnomedicine is carried out from generation to generation among ethnic people orally and the medicinal plants survived in their minds and souls. As the knowledge is disappearing because of rapid socioeconomic, environmental and technological changes, there is need to document and conserve the biodiversity through systematic studies, before it is lost forever.

The book presents medicinal plants on more than 200 species belonging to 105 families. Besides, ethnomedicinal spectrum of Similipal has been focused. A scope and application of biotechnological approaches of some medicinal plants has been highlighted. We are sure this book will be of immense help to foresters, students, researchers, ethnobiologists, biotechnologists, ecologists and plant lovers.

We acknowledge our thanks to various sources from where the text material, photographs, economic data and resources have been used. Readers perception in the form of constructive suggestions and valuable comments for improvement of the book will be highly appreciated.

MILESTONE

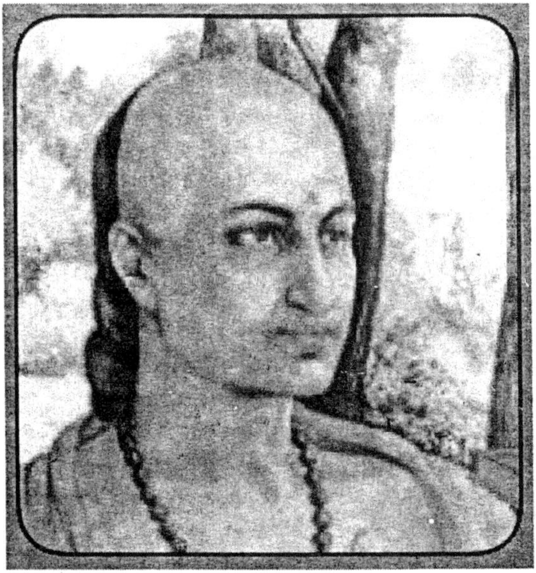

CHARAKA

Charaka, sometimes spelled Caraka, born c. 300 BC in a Maga Brahmin family was one of the principal contributors to Ayurveda, ancient system of medicine and lifestyle developed in India. Charaka was a selfless seer who bestowed great boons to alleviate the sufferings of human beings, to free them from the fear of death and diseases. Under the guidance of the ancient physician Atreya, Agnivesa had written an encyclopaedic treatise in the eighth century B.C. However, it was only when Charaka revised this treatise that it gained popularity and came to be known as Charaka Samhita describing medicinal properties and functions of 100,000 herbal plants. For two millennia it remained a standard work on the subject and was translated into many foreign languages, including Arabic and Latin.

Charaka was the first physician to present the concept of digestion, metabolism and immunity. According to him, a body functions because it contains three dosha *viz*. bile, phlegm and wind. He has described microorganisms as causative factors for leprosy, tuberculosis, influenza, dental caries and some types of fevers and also mentioned that microorganisms are present in the intestines, the whole of the alimentary tract and cardiovascular system, and diseases manifest when the immunity lowers. The contributions of Charaka in genetics are worth exploring. Manipulation to change the sex of the foetus has also been described. Charaka has explained many procedures like panchakarma, rasayana, sadvrtha, etc. which undoubtedly transform the genes to behave beneficially. Charaka stated that Alzheimer's disease is passed on to the off spring by the father's genes. Preventive aspects have been given much importance. Charaka was fully aware of the impact of the environment on the health of living beings so he advised how and why the environment should be maintained in perfect order. Statistical approach in Charaka Samhita is based on keen observation, scientific analysis conducted for many years on thousands of individuals, irrespective factors such as religion, time, age, stage of diseases, etc. This ancient seer encouraged unique methods of research, scientific outlook and critical observation before any theory could be accepted by a vaidya (clinician) who is essentially a researcher too and has also given guidelines as to how, when and why it is essential to develop a holistic scientific medical system.

Basic Principles of Traditional Indian Medicine (TIM)

Ayurveda, the traditional Indian medicine (TIM) remain the most ancient yet living traditions. This is one of the 'great traditions' with sound philosophical, experiential and experimental basis. Increased side effects, lack of curative treatment for several chronic diseases, high cost of new drugs, microbial resistance and emerging diseases are some reasons for renewed public interest in complementary and alternative medicines Ayurveda focus is on the patient rather than disease. The systems fundamentally aims to promote health and enhance the quality of life, with therapeutic strategies for treatment of specific diseases or symptoms in holistic fashion. Ayurveda considers that the universe is made up of combinations of the five elements (pancha mahabhutas). These are akasha (ether), vayu (air), teja (fire), aapa (water) and prithvi (earth). The five elements can be seen to exist in the material universe at all scales of life and in both organic and inorganic things. In biological system, such as humans, elements are coded into three forces, which govern all life processes. These three forces (kapha, pitta and vata) are known as the three doshas or simply the tridosha. Each of the doshas is composed of one or two elements. Vata is composed of space and air, Pitta of fire, and Kapha of water and earth. Vata dosha has the mobility and quickness of space and air; pitta dosha the metabolic qualities of fire; kapha dosha the stability and solidity of water and earth. The tridosha regulates every physiological and psychological process in the living organism. The interplay among them determines the qualities and conditions of the individual. A harmonious state of the three doshas creates balance and health; an imbalance, which might be an excess (vriddhi) or deficiency (kshaya), manifests as a sign or symptom of disease (24, 25) (Figs. 1 and 2).

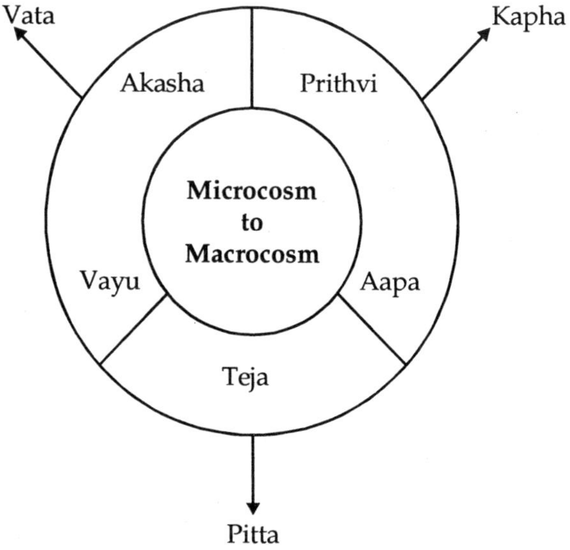

Basic principles of TIM : Relation of pancha mahabhutas and tridosha.

INTRODUCTION

People have been associated with plants since time immemorial and dependent for their various uses such as food, fodder and medicine. From the very earliest days of civilization, mankind has turned to plants for healing, a tradition that has survived till the arrival of modern medicine and found new strength at the end of 20th century. About 64% of the total global population remains dependent on traditional medicine for their health care system. The World Health Organization (WHO) lists over 21,000 plant species that have reported medicinal uses around the world, while a recent estimate by the International Union for Conservation of Nature and Natural Resources (IUCN) speaks of 25,000 species. India alone has a record of 7,000 species of medicinal plants, which are used by different indigenous tribes and systems of medicine. This knowledge on traditional medicine (ancestral experience) was used in the diagnosis, prevention and elimination of physical, mental or social imbalances, has practiced and handed down from generation to generation either verbally or in writing. Traditional healers and remedies made from plants play an important role of the health care of millions of people.

The traditional definition of medicinal plants is given in Ashtaanga Hrdaya (600AD), Sutra sthana Chapter 9 verse 10 as :

> *"Jagatyevam anoushadham na kinchit vidyate dravyam vasatnanartha yoga yoh."*

(There is nothing in this universe, which is non-medicinal, which can not be made use of for many purposes and by many modes).

Ancient Indian literature incorporates a remarkably broad definition of medicinal plants and considers 'all' plant entities to be potential sources of medicinal substances. While all plant entities are thus potentially medicinal, at a practical level, only those plants are considered 'medicinal' whose medicinal use has already been discovered for human or veterinary application. Such an application could either be in the western bio-medical system or homeopathy or any of the traditional systems of medicine like Ayurveda, Unani, Siddha and Swa-rigpa or the rich and diverse folk medical traditions. Medicinal plants have curative properties due to the presence of various complex chemical substances of different composition, which are found as secondary plant metabolites in one or more parts of these plants. These plant metabolites according to their composition are grouped as alkaloids, glycosides, corticosteroids, essential oil etc. However, our knowledge on phytological diversity of medicinal plants is poor and we know still less about the biosynthetic pathways leading to the formation of active constituents for which these crops are valued.

In India, earliest references of the curative properties of plants appeared in 'Rigveda'. In Rigveda (between 3500 and 1800 BC) which is one of the oldest repositories of human knowledge mention has been made of 'soma plants'. So much were the vedic worshipper ecstatic over the existing effect of the fermented juice expressed from it, that they regarded it (like Greek's Ambrosia) as the 'Amrit' and raised it to the dignity of God. Other plant herbs with potent and active properties were treated as Vanausadhi. Although references to the plants in 'Rigveda' are very brief, the identity of some plants referred in the Suktas of Rigveda can be determined with reasonable certainty, *e.g.* 'Simli', 'Palash', and 'Pipal' etc. More detailed accounts of Medicinal plants are available in Atharvaveda.

After the Vedas, there is no information on the development of this science in India for a period of about 1000 years. Then, came the two most important works on the Indian system of Medicines in the age of the Charak and Susruta (2500 B.C. to 600 B.C.) written to pre-Buddhistic period. Susruta Samhita deals with about 700 drugs, some of those were not indigenous to India. However, 'Susrutas' contain accounts on surgery. With the passing of time, more and more plants foundentry into native medicine. Innumerable drug plants are described in ancient sanskrit literatures and are included in Indian Materia Medica (1954). But a large number of such vegetable drugs used for different remedies are not found in literature although they have been used with in the treatment of diseases.

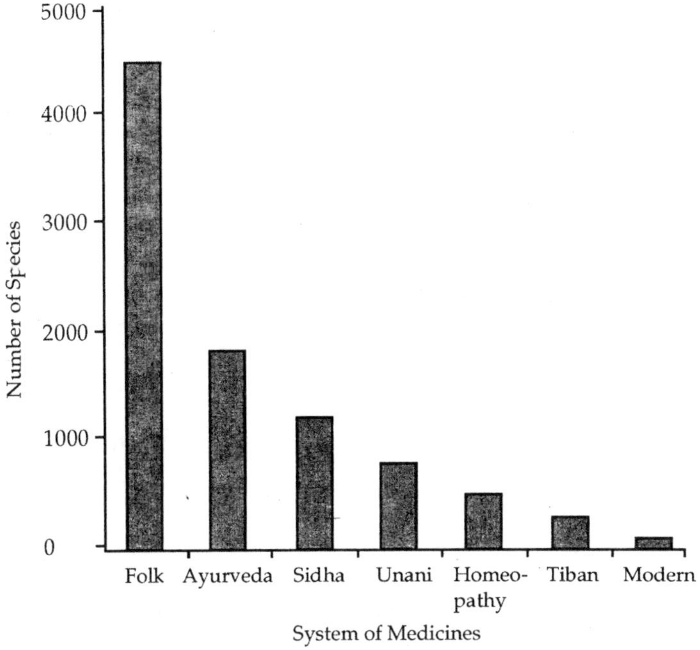

After a long time, the potentialities of the Indian Medicinal Plants were again realized during British period and since then many workers have attempted to find out the botanical sources of many drug plants through the help of Vaidyas, Kaviraj, Hakims and local people. The work of Sir William Jones (1799) is one of the earliest contributions in this direction. This is followed by John Fleming's 'Medicinal Plant & Drugs' (1810), Arristies 'Materia Medica of Hindustan' (1813), Roxburgh's 'Flora Indica' (1832) and subsequently the work of Royle (1837) on the 'Antiquity of Hindu Medicine'. 'Ayurveda', the science of health and healing which was practiced by the ancient Aryans, is now considered the medicinal science of Hindu culture. Even now, the Ayurvedic system is quite prevalent in the country. The rural and tribal people in India are more likely dependant on Ayrvedic medicines for their health related problems. In the history of modern medicine less importance was given to an ancient Ayurvedic literature of the Indian herbalists. Their contributions towards the medicinal usefulness of plants were neglected. Actually these Ayurvedic medicinal uses are based on their experiences and with no side effect on the physiology of human body (Sangai and Chavan, 2002).

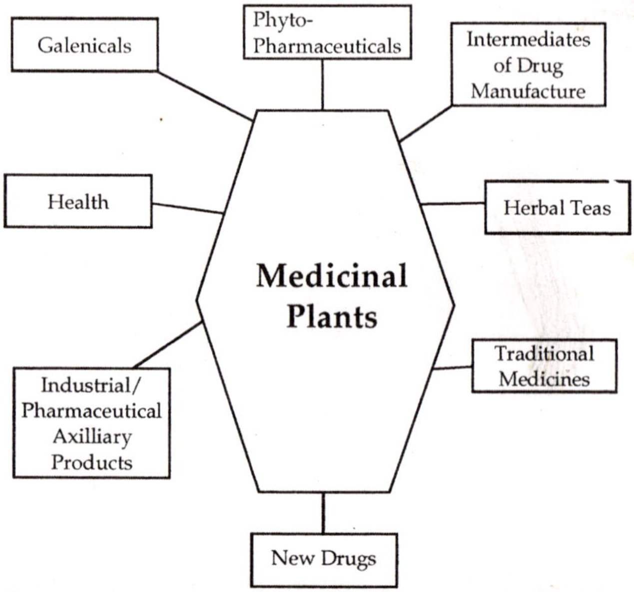

During the past one century there has been a rapid extension of the allopathic system of medical treatment in India. It generated commercial demand for pharmacopoeias drugs and their products in India. India has a wide range of soil and climatic conditions and has thus inherited an enormous wealth in diverse plant life (Pareek and Gupta, 1993). Efforts have been made to introduce many of these drug plants to farmers. Several research institutes have undertaken studies on the cultivation practices of medicinal plants, which were found suitable and remunerative for commercial cultivation. The agronomic practices for growing *poppy, isabgol, senna, cinchona, belladonna,*

ergot and few others have been developed and there is now localized cultivation of these medicinal plants commercially.

DIVERSITY, DISTRIBUTION AND STATUS

World Health Organization has listed over, 21,000 plant species used around the world for medicinal purposes. Although India possess about 7000 species of medicinal plants, yet in India about 2,500 plant species belonging to more than 1000 genera, are used in indigenous systems of medicines. The analysis of distribution shows that medicinal plants are distributed across diverse habitats. Around 70% of India's medicinal plants are found in tropical forests spread across the western and eastern Ghats, the Vindhyas, Chota Nagpur plateau, Aravalis, the Tarai region in the foot hills of the Himalayas and North East. Less than 30% of the medicinal plants are found in the temperate forests and at higher altitudes. A larger percentage of medicinal plants occur in the dry deciduous forests as compared to the evergreen of temperate forests. The Ministry of Environment and Forests has set up 12 biosphere reserves (out of 14 identified sites, 85 national parks and 448 sanctuaries under the wildlife (protection) Act, 1972, altogether covering the area of 180,000 km^2. These are not specifically aimed at medicinal species and those present in these ecosystems have not yet been critically investigated the distribution of medicinal plants in these areas need to be determined.

THREATS TO MEDICINAL PLANTS IN PARTICULAR

The major causes of the loss of biological diversity in India both in hills and plains are anthropogenic. However, eight major causes for the loss of biodiversity have been identified namely- (*i*) habitat loss and fragmentation, (*ii*) introduced exotic species, (*iii*) over exploitation of plant and animal species, (*iv*) pollution of soil, water and atmosphere, (*v*) global climate change, (*vi*) expansion of industry, agriculture and forestry, (*vii*) want of pollinating vectors and (*viii*) unisexual flowered species. Over-exploitation and indiscriminate use of wild resources in commercial demand play great role not only behind the quick decline of the species concerned, but also becomes a threat for the survival of other associated species, thus acting as the major factors disturbing the entire ecosystem. For medicinal plants, like other plant parts in commercial demand, premature exploitation is another factor which is additionally responsible for rapid destruction of wild stock. Whenever, a plant is in high demand, premature exploitation is expected to threaten next season's propagation and regeneration of the species.

Besides above, about 250 plant species are used in regular production of Ayurvedic, Unani, Siddha and tribal medicines which comprise about 75% plant species from tropical and 25% from temperate forests. In medicinal plants, 30% of materials are roots, 14% bark, 16% whole plants 5% flowers, 10% fruits, 6% leaves, 7% seeds, 2% wood, 4% rhizomes and 6% stems.

MEDICINAL PLANT RESOURCES OF ORISSA

The state of Orissa extending over an area of 1,55,842 km^2 lies on the east coast of India between 17°48′–23°34′ latitude and 81°24′–87°29′E longitude. It is surrounded in the north by Jharkhand and West Bengal on the west by Chhatishgarh, on the south by Andhra Pradesh and on the east by Bay of Bengal. Physiographically the entire area can be broadly divided into 4 distinct regions–the northern plateau, the central river basins, the eastern hills and the coastal plains. The northern plateau is undulating, often intersected by hill ranges that slope down from north to south. The central river basin is characterized by presence of Mahanadi, Brahmani and Baitarini rivers which gave rise to vast streches of fertile agricultural lands.The eastern hills extending for about 248 less in northeast and south west direction contain some of the potential high peaks which harbor diversified taxa. The coastal plains are very narrow along the Bay of Bengal but has given birth to 2 unique centers of biodiversity, Mangroves of Bhitarkanika and brakish water lake of Chilika. Based on the floristic surveys carried out in Orissa certain forest pockets have been identified as the potential centers of biodiversity. These are Similipal forests of Mayurbhanj District. Gandhamardan hill ranges of Bolangir and Bargarh Districts, Bhitarkanika of Kendrapara District, Mahendragiri hills of Gajapati District, Deiomali hills of Rayagada District and

Chilika lake. The total number of species of vascular plants of Orissa as given in Flora or Orissa is 2727 including 166 species of cultivated plants (Saxena & Brahman, 1994).

The climate and topography of Orissa is highly congenial for growth of a large number of medicinal plants and also for their cultivation. In the areas of Koraput, Phulbani and Mayurbhanj, large number of medicinal plants naturally occur. Different forest products, parts of the trees, and plants found in forests such as: roots, tubers, stems, barks, leaves, fruits, seeds and flowers of various medicinal plants are used as curative of different diseases. The important medicinal plants collected from different parts of Orissa are Amla, Baghanakha, Bahada, Baidanka, Banahaladi, Bana Kulthi, Bana tulsi, Chakunda, Charseeds, Chireita, Dhatukiflower, Gaba, Harida, Indrajaba, Kaincha, Kurchi, Kochila (Nuxvomica), Landa Baguli, Lodhra, Mankadakendu, Mahu (honey), Nageswar flower, Palash, Pita alu, Putrani, R.S Root, Sikakai etc. These products are immensely used by the indigenous people (tribals) in remote areas of forest owing to their exclusive dependence on such precious resource (having no alternative source). Also, the tribals are very keen in using those as medicines in which tribal ethos is involved. However, medicinal plants are in great demand in recent years for all the indigenous systems of medicines. Collection of medicinal plants is performed either by the specialised collectors, who know the plants or by the herbalists in the rural areas, who grow them in small plots in their gardens.

Evidently, a number of valuable recorded vegetable drugs are obtained from the forests of Orissa. Medicinal plants are by and large available on hill peaks and mountains like *'Megasan'* in Mayurbhanj, 'Gandhamardan' in Kendujhar, 'Malayagiri' in Angul, *'Nimragir'* in Koraput, 'Bankasham' in Kalahandi and 'Mahendragiri' in Ganjam. Drugs are prepared from fruits, flowers, leaves, roots, shrubs, creepers and herbs. Among the principal medicinal NTFPs, 'Myrobalan' is a trade name of Harida, Bahara and Amla. These fruits contain a good percentage of tannin, and are extremely useful for tanning. The other varieties of vegetable tanning materials are wattle bark, babul, besides, Dhawara leaves, and bark, Karada bark and Sunhari bark. Harida and Bahara have relatively greater importance because of their astringent, fermentative and acidic forming properties. However, a combination of Harida, Bahara and Amla has greater medicinal components. These are mainly exported to outside states, such as: Madhya Pradesh and Andhra Pradesh to feed tannin extraction factories. However, a small part of the forest potential is collected from the forests due to absence of suitable promoting agencies, though collection is not made from the remote as well as inaccessible areas at all.

The fruits of medicinal plants which are more useful for Ayurvedic formulations are plentily available in forests of Orissa. The life span of those medicinal plants varies according to species. These are collected by private persons, physicians and manufacturing industrial units. The tribals and local people living in and around forests have indeed greater access to these items. But, in the absence of suitable and extensive market network of co-operatives formed by tribals and forest dwellers, illicit trading activities of private businessmen are rampant in the tribal areas, who, by and large resort to 'distress sales' to private contractors and traders, and, very often, at a throw away prices.

For the compilation of medicinal tree of Orissa state, an extensive survey of literature was carried out. About 70 medicinal plants have been reported by Saxena & Brahmam (1989) for commercial exploitation from Similipal forest. Thatoi *et al.* (2008) reported about 40 medicinal plants having ethnomedicinal uses and antimicrobial properties from Similipal Biosphere Reserves, Orissa. Dhal (2004) reported about 145 plants having medicinal uses from Nabarangpur district. Thirty eight (38) plants species have been used by natives of Bhadrak District for treatment of skin diseases (Girach *et al.* 1999). Fourtyfive (45) medicinal plants have been reported by Satpathy and Panda (1992). Used by tribal of Sundaragarh District Mandal and Mukherjee (1992) reported 60 medicinal plants to be practiced by tribal of Keonjhar district. Sarangi and Sahoo (2004) reported about 32 plant species used in Gynecological and venereal disorders from Kalahandi district of Orissa. Sen and Behera (2003) has documented 78 ethnomedicinal plants belonging to 47 families for the treatment of skin diseases in Bargarh district of Orissa. As per enumeration by MSSR about 135 plant belong to medicinal plants have been documented for Kalahandi district. Out of 220 medicinal quase medicinal and economic plants found in Gadhamardan, Botanical Survey of India (BSI) reported 110 important medicinal plants. But local vaidyas also tribal doctors practicing traditional medicinal system to serve the tribal people claim that more than 500 species having medicinal values exist is this area. During this survey use of along 150 species has been documented. Pandey & Rout (2006) has documented an account of ethnomedicinal uses of 42 plant species known among the tribals of Similipal Biosphere Reserve. Even today in different areas of district Mayurbhanj, Orissa the important medicinal plants are found viz., *Acalypha indica, Adhatoda vasica, Andrographis paniculata, Argyreia nervosa, Bacopa monnieri, Baringtonia acutangula, Cassia fistula, Centella asiatica, Curculigo orchioides, Dioscorea alata, Emblica officinalis, Holorhena pubescens, Mentha spicata, Occimum grantissimum, Paederia foetida, Randia dumeratum, Rauvolfia serpentina, Terminalia chebula* and *Woodfordia fruticosa*. A perusal of literature reveals that study of threatened plants in Mayurbhanj district with special reference to Similipal Biosphere Reserve is lacking. Haines (1921-25), Mooney (1950), Bal (1942), Panigrahi *et al.* (1964) collected some species of vascular plants and useful plants of Similipal. Jain and Sastry (1983), Mishra (1989) and Saxena and Brahmam (1989) enumerated plants found in Similipal. Pandey (2000), Pandey *et al.* (2002) and Rout (2004) surveyed 34 compartments (out of 220 compartments) of Similipal Biosphere Reserve and collected more than 600 medicinal plant species, which shows that SBR is rich in medicinal plants. Kumar *et al.* (2006) presented a paper regarding 65 medicinal plants belonging to 34 families of flowering plants from Hatikote Reserve Forests of Mayurbhanj, Orissa. Ethno-medico biological use of 28 species of plants and animals of Similipal Biosphere Reserves has documented by Rout and Pandey, 2007.

Panda and Padhi (2008) published on ethnomedicinal plants used buy tribes of Kalahandi districts, Orissa covering 111 flowering plants of 60 families. Rout *et. al.* (2005) reported on conservation strategies of 89 medicinal plant species belonging to 38 families of vascular plants from Orissa. Panigrahi (1963) published some 250 species of medicinal/quasi medicinal species of Gandhamardan Parbat. Saxena & Brahmam (1994-96) published the flora of Orissa in four volume, they have reported 2561 indigenous/naturalized taxa belonging to 1062 genera and 228 families (including Pteridophytes). They do not mention occurrence of economic/medicinal properties of any taxon. Although, Saxena observes that 1230 species are medicinal plants of which 138 species are potential for commercial exploitation and 35 species widely used as medicinal plants found in Orissa (Saxena and Brahmam (1994-96)).

Several publications (Ahmedullah and Nayar, 1986; Jain and Rao, 1983; Jain and Sastry, 1980 and Nayar and Sastry, 1987-88) revealed many endemic and rare plants of Indian subcontinent. Nayar *et al.* (1984) and Saxena and Brahmam (1983) have done an assessment of the rare, endemic and endangered plants of Eastern Ghats and Orissa respectively.

Some preliminary reports dealing with the status of rare and threatened plants of Similipal Biosphere Reserve are available (Mishra, 1997; Rout, 2004). However, they do not highlight the rare and threatened plants of this region and is thus far from complete. Besides, there have been continuous biotic activities operating in the region, primarily due to human interferences.

TRADE IN MEDICINAL PLANT AND HERBAL EXPORT MARKET

The global market for medicinal plant materials and herbal medicines is estimated to be worth several billion dollars a year. International export trade in medicinal plants is dominated by China, which exports 1,21,900 tons of materials a year, and India exports 32,600 tons annually (Anonymous 1997b). India share in world herbal medicine market is mere 11% and the total market from Indian systems of medicine and Homeopathy is about US$ 1 billion. India is losing out on the herbal export front, while China earns US $5 billion annually from herbal trade which is five times more than India's export turnover. Intensive efforts are being made in India to boost its export of traditional medicines to match at least half of China's current export level by 2010. Recently, the WHO has also recommended to all the member countries to actively promote native medicines and also to initiate steps to conserve and cultivate medicinal plants.

The markets dealing with medicinal plant parts (herbs and crude drugs) in India is highly disorganized and less studied sector. So far little idea has been generated on the nature and quantum of trade in medicinal plant parts. The demand, supply and price structures are highly unstable. Even today, India lacks a total and updated inventory on which particular plant parts are being traded in the market. There are much confusion and controversy regarding names of the items in trade. Moreover, there exists practices of adulteration and also of selling totally different items as inferior substitutes. There is no definite system of quality control. There are items banned to be exported without cultivation certificate, but majority of the enforcement staff do not have any idea on identification of such items or even the existing law. The trade routes and source of most of the items are not exactly known. Transit formalities and tax structure is not uniform in different states and major wholesale markets. The overall situation demands immediate attention from the Central Government, respective State Governments, and other sectors dependent on the market. A commercial database on the market has to be prepared and carrying out a detailed analytical survey on the market economy is an urgent necessity.

MARKETING OF MEDICINAL PLANTS IN ORISSA

Forest Department of Orissa collects a small number medicinal plants and their parts. Patalgaruda, Noxvomica and Dhatuki flowers are considered as precious plants. Patalgaruda (*Rauvolfia serpentina*) is an adorous shrub that thrives under the shade of forest trees in its native habitat. Noxvomica (*Stryehnos nux-vomica*) is a native of India. There is wide demand for this product for preparation of homeopathic medicines. This is widely available in areas like Boudh, Baliguda, Rayagada,

Parlakhemundi, Kendujhar, Nayagarh, Dasapalla etc. Another shrub called 'Dhatuki' (*Woodfordia fruticosa*) is also available in the forests of Orissa, and its exploitation is too meagre despite huge potential. A large portion of these plants is collected by ayurvedic doctors, medicine manufacturers, forest dwellers and tribals. But, these are not computed in the States estimates. However, looking at the number of Ayurvedic Colleges (6), Homeopathic Colleges (4), Homeopathic Dispensaries (460), Ayurvedic Dispensaries (519) and large number of private practitioners on the one hand, and growing dependence of the people on Ayurvedic and homeopathic drugs on the other, the present process of quantity of collection, plantation and regeneration of these precious species are inadequate to meet the growing needs. It appears that no systematic attempt has been made so far for cultivation of such precious plants. Though 'Genduligum' is widely available in the fruits of Orissa, its meagre collection of 3029 quintals reflects on the follow up of unsystematic collection methods.

PROMOTION OF MEDICINAL PLANTS

Medicinal plants are precious and very useful for their life-saving contents. Therefore, regeneration of the species assumes crucial significance in the afforestation programme so as to ensure sustainable supply of these NTFPs in future. These products also need a great deal of protection from illicit collection, encroachment, fire damage, grazing and attacks of insects and diseases in order to save from extinctions. Its sustainable supply indeed requires successful implementation of reforestation programme with involvement of local people in plantation as well as protection of such plants.

Very recently, at the instance of the Government of India in the Ministry of Health and Family Welfare, a scheme called "Vanaspati Vana" is constituted at the State level. Accordingly, the Government of Orissa have constituted a special purpose society called "Orissa State Vanaspati Vana Society" under the Societies Registration Act (Government of Orissa Resolution 4315 F&E, March 08, 2001).

Among the aims and objectives of the society are (*a*) identification of natural habitats of medicinal plants; (*b*) conservation and development of the medicinal plant resources; (*c*) raising of important medicinal plants; (*d*) development of hi-tech plant resources for *ex-situ* conservation of medicinal plants; (*e*) research activities on nursery and plantation techniques; (*f*) documentation and dissemination of indigenous technical knowledge with respect to conservation, propagation, non-destructive extraction; (*g*) preparation of project programmes for conservation and use of medicinal plants required by Indian System of Medicine; (*h*) creation of awareness about the importance of medicinal plants; (*i*) development of link between the growers of medicinal plants and reputed pharmaceutical houses etc.

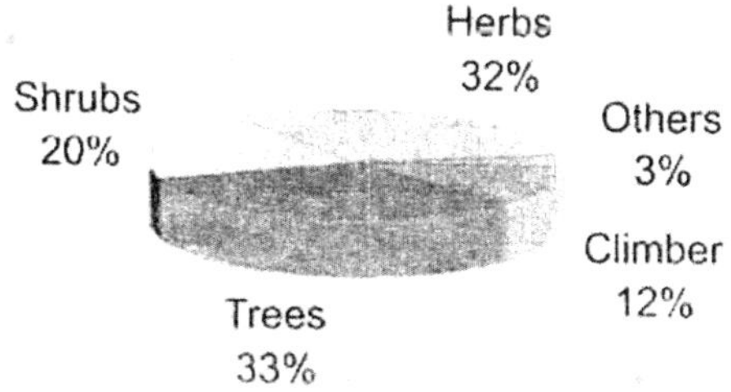

Distribution of medicinal plants by habits

Further, as per the Government of Orissa Resolution no-4328 it has been decided to constitute a Medicinal Plants Advisory Board with Minister, Forest and Environment as Chairman, and Minister of State, Health and Family Welfare as Vice-Chairman, besides 18 other members drawn from various departments; such as Agriculture, Forest, Health, S.C. and ST Development, Agriculture Production Commissioner, CMD, OFDC Ltd. Director, Institute of Minerals and Materials Technology, Director, Regional Plant Resources Center, Director Horticulture and so on.

The State Medicinal Plant Board have the following functions : (*a*) to co-ordinate formulation of appropriate policies and strategies for the development of Medicinal Plants Sector; (*b*) to advise the Government on identification, regeneration, protection, harvesting, cultivation etc. (*c*) to assign Government

Departments and Agencies about the specific tasks for developing infrastructure and support with respect to cultivation, collection, storage, marketing etc; (*d*) to identify suitable Government Departments/Agencies, research institutions/universities, NGOs to undertake research and promotional activities; (*e*) to provide market information, and marketing of medicinal products of the primary collectors and growers through market linkages and building up marketing avenues etc.

Deforestation activists, microclimatic changes and pollution have significantly affected the survival of medicinal plants. Non-availability and poor viability of seeds pose constraints for propagation certain medicinal plants for its perpetuity. During the recent years, therefore interest in using the *in vitro* propagation or micro propagation techniques for rapid and large scale propagation of medicinal and aromatic plants has significantly increased (Bajaj *et al.* 1988, Krishnan & Seeni 1994, Subha & Seeni 1994, Pattnaik & Chand 1996, Patnaik & Debata 1996, Shibata *et al.* 1996, Sha Vali Khan *et al.* 1997, Ajith kumar & Seeni 1998, Eeswara *et al.* 1998, Sahoo & Chand 1998). Propagules can be made available through this technique for large-scale round the year propagation of important plant species. The development of simple and rapid method for the production of a colonial basal population is highly desirable.

Plant tissue culture is one of the important areas of plant biotechnology. It involves propagating plants from very small plant parts, tissues or cells in specialized conditions in which the growing environment and nutrition are strictly controlled and plants are developed in test tubes under laboratory condition. Production of high quality, disease free plants is possible through this technique from vegetative parts which is advantageous to propagate rare or difficult to grow species. Plants can be mass-produced very rapidly which have also disease and pest resistance.

CONSERVATION STRATEGY OF MEDICINAL PLANTS

Demand for medicinal plants is increasing in both developing and developed countries and surprisingly, the bulk of the material traded is still from wild harvested sources on forest lands and only a very small number of species are cultivated. The expanding trade in medicinal plants has serious implications on the survival of several plant species. Many medicinal plants are fast disappearing and some are in danger of extinction. There is a great need to conserve medicinal plants because they contain highly bioactive components which can be developed into pharmacologically-active agents. Medicinal plants are gradually facing extinction due to their inappropriate ways of harvesting like removing all the bark or uprooting the whole plant without leaving part to regrow, bush burning and commercialization of plant sources, lack of awareness that plants are sources of the conventional medicine, povery in arid or semi-arid areas and religious factors. For example, some western religions view the use of traditional medicine as a form of evil worship or witchcraft. Because of the numerous potentials of medicinal plants in the combating of drug resistance by microorganisms, strict conservation measures should be put in place to prevent the total extinction of the medicinal plants from the natural flora.

Harvesting of medicinal plants unrestricted from wild pose threat to their sustainability. Other factors contributing to unsustainability include lack of sufficient data on wild plant populations, marketing, and trading; inadequate regulations and legal protection (including intellectual property rights for locals practitioners with local knowledge); and poor access to appropriate technology for sound harvesting and plantation development.

Now a days there are attempts to cultivate some easily grown species and protect important natural habitats in other to reduce the pressure on these vital resources. Indeed, cultivation offers the best hope for conserving many medicinal plants found in the wild while maintaining harvested supplies at today's levels.

If existing supplies of medicinal plants are to keep up with demands, they will need adequate protection through development of appropriate institutions, policies, and legislation.

Local communities need support and encouragements to protect these resources. To complement cultivation of adaptable species, harvesting from the wild most be guided by accurate inventories and knowledge about the species concerned. Above all, over-exploitation of rare and endangered species must be avoided.

The conservation group has been coordinating since 1993, the country's first medicinal plant conservation programme, which has been implemented by the state forest departments of Tamil Nadu, Kerala and Karnataka, Andhra Pradesh and Maharashtra. This *in situ* conservation initiative has resulted in the setting up of a network of 55 Medicinal Plant Conservation Areas (MPCA) across different forest types and altitude zones in these five states of peninsular India which serves as the gene bank of medicinal plant resources of the region. The network of MPCAs captures the inter and intra specific medicinal plant diversity of peninsular India. The criteria for the selection of the 55 Medicinal Plant Conservation Areas are: (*a*) representation of forest types of the region; (*b*) areas traditionally well known for medicinal plant wealth; (*c*) areas with known high level of endemism; (*d*) areas located across the altitude range; (*e*) sites that are accessible for long-term study. The MPCAs capture around 2000 medicinal plant species, which represent 50% of the medicinal plant diversity of the five states, and significantly includes over 75% of the RED Listed Species of these states. For all the MPCA sites, detailed floristic studies on medicinal plant diversity including the threatened, traded and endemic plants have been undertaken.

CONSERVATION THROUGH EDUCATION

Conservation of medicinal plants through Education involves in creating public awareness on the need for conserving wild populations of the medicinal plant diversity. The target groups include students, tourists, pilgrims and the general public. Demonstration Gardens highlighting important medicinal plants, nature trails to provide a feel of the forests harbouring the medicinal plant and interpretation centres based on thematic presentations on medicinal plants have been established in several MPCAs. The raining of local resource persons to act as guides in medicinal plant identification in nature is undertaken.

MEDICINAL PLANT CONSERVATION PROGRAMME AND POLICIES

The world conservation strategy (IUCN, UNEP & WWF, 1980) defines conservations as "the management of human use of the biodiversity so that it may yield the greatest sustainable benefit to present generation while maintaining its potential to meet the needs and aspirations of future generations". The above definition invokes two complementary components "conservation" and "sustainability". The primary goals of biodiversity conservation as envisaged in the World Conservation Strategy can be summarised as follows :

1. Maintenance of essential ecological processes and life support systems on which human survival and economic activities depend,
2. Preservation of species and genetic diversity, and
3. Sustainable use of species and ecosystems which support millions of rural communities as well as major industries. Medicinal plants are potential renewable natural resources.

Therefore, the conservation and sustainable utilisation of medicinal plants must necessarily involve a long term, integrated, scientifically oriented action programme. This should involve the pertinent aspects of protection, preservation, maintenance, exploitation, conservation and sustainable utilization. A holistic and systematic approach envisaging interaction between social, economic and ecological systems will be a more desirable one. The most widely accepted scientific technologies of biodiversity conservation are the *in-situ* and *ex-situ* methods.

Using IUCN (1994) methods, Botanical Survey of India– the nodal organization responsible for monitoring and preparation of the list of plants to be included in the negative list of export-has so far listed 53 species for restriction in trade. It is roughly estimated that about 10% of higher plants are under- different threat categories. Botanical Survey of India has already published 4 volumes of Red Data Book of Indian plants (RDB) accounting relevant information of more than 800 species. Convention of International Trade in Endangered Species of Wild flora and fauna (CITES), is the international treaty to regulate the international trade of wild species. The legal and policy framework include various Acts such as the Forest Act 1927; the Forest Conservation Act 1980; the Indian Wildlife Protection Act 1972 etc. These are in addition to various international treaties like CITES, Ramsar-CMS, etc. Directly related to conservation of Biological Diversity, which has come into force on 29th December, 1993, which India ratified and joined on 18th February, 1994. It has been decided that for *in-situ* conservation, involvement of indigenous people and local ethnic communities is of utmost importance.

In-situ Conservation

In has been well established that the best and cost-effective way of protecting the existing biological and genetic diversity is the '*in-situ*' or on the site conservation wherein a wild species or stock of a biological community is protected and preserved in its natural habitat.

In-situ conservation of medicinal plants is especially important as their natural habitats have been getting destroyed, modified, shrunk or degraded due to various biotic and environmental factors, and the plant species residing in these habitats, including medicinal plants, face threats to their survival. If the estimated rate of global threat of extinction *i.e.* 27,000 species (flora and fauna) per year (Wilson, 1995) continues, then a large proportion of our plant species would go extinct in the next three generations. Extinction is an irreplaceable loss. The extinction of medicinal plants means not only the loss of valuable plants that can save lives, but also of local cultures associated with their use.

For *in-situ* conservation, a biosphere reserve offers the best site of natural conservation of threatened flora. The concept of preserving biodiversity resulted in the Biosphere Reserve in 1974 as UNESCO MAB (Man and the Biosphere) project no. 8

for the conservation of the natural areas and of the genetic material ecosystems throughout the world were being altered on a massive scale. Therefore, the setting aside of representative sites inclusive of major ecosystem types became absolutely necessary.

The *in-situ* conservation of medicinal plants relates to the conservation of wild population of medicinal plant populations in their natural habitats. Conservation of plants in their natural habitats is important as it is the most cost-effective way of maintaining their gene pools while retaining their full natural evolutionary potential.

With the large number of India's medicinal plant species known to be distributed across diverse ecosystems, there is urgent need to initiate conservation, in all bio-geographic regions of the country. For *in-situ* conservation the Network of 55 forest gene banks have established in peninsular India (Karnataka, Kerala, Tamil Nadu, Andhra Pradesh & Maharashtra) and Plans for extending *in-situ* conservation to Sikkim, Meghalaya, Arunachal Pradesh, Himachal Pradesh, Chhattisgarh, Uttaranchal, Jammu & Kashmir, Orissa, West Bengal (Sundarbans), Rajasthan and Madhya Pradesh is under way.

Ex-situ Conservation or Domestication

Conservation of medicinal plants can be accomplished by the *ex-situ i.e.* outside natural habitat by cultivating and maintaining plants in botanic gardens parks, other suitable sites, and through long term preservation of plant propagules in gene banks (seed bank, pollen bank, DNA libraries, etc.) and in plant tissue culture repositories and by cryopreservation). Botanical gardens can play a key role in *ex-situ* conservation of plants, especially those facing imminent threat of extinction. However, the impracticability of advocating theories of plant reserves for the protection of the flora under climatic conditions of the region is quite obvious, especially because here the plants are represented by species scattered over hundreds of kilometers in the desert. An alternative to this is to start desert gardens, where conditions can be created that are more favorable for the conservation of those, which are in critical stage.

Several gardens in the world are specialised in cultivation and study of medicinal plants, while some contain a special medicinal plant garden or harbor special collection of medicinal plants. India has a network of about 140 botanical gardens which include 33 botanical gardens attached to 33 universities botany departments. But hardly 30 botanical gardens have any active programme on conservation.

Though there are several botanical gardens in our country, the natural genetic wealth, including wild relatives of cultivated plants, and rare and threatened plants are not given priority over ornamental plants and other exotic flora in these gardens. Therefore, for *ex-situ* preservation, special purpose gardens should be established. Practical conservation can always be effective through restrictions in collection and preventing them from being damaged by accelerated human use. Botanic garden should be created, in which all plants can be cultivated, propagated, and kept under conditions similar to those in natural environment. Bulking up such plants in the garden and re-introducing them is essential to restore the critically low population. There are a network of 18 regional community herbal gardens established in the three states of Karnataka, Tamilnadu and Kerala and 894 Medicinal Plant species captured in the community herbal garden network in India. Tropical Botanical Gardens and Research Institute (TGBRI), located in a degraded forest region of Western Ghat mountains in Kerala has an excellent example in *ex-situ* conservation of plant diversity in India. The field gene bank programme launched by TBGRI from 1992-1999 is now well acclaimed as a very effective method of conservation of medicinal and aromatic plant genetic resources. This field gene bank of medicinal and aromatic plants at TBGRI, Thiruvananthapuram is essentially a blend of the *ex-situ* and *in-situ* situations.

MEDICINAL PLANT CONSERVATION EFFORT IN ORISSA

Many commercially important medicinal plants are distributed across different phytogeography including six biodiversity granaries: Similipal, Bhitarkanika-Mahanadi delta,

Gandhamardan, Chilika, Mahendragiri and Deomali. Of the 2727 medicinal plants, 21 species were found to be endemic which are found in these granaries. These medicinal plants constitute the main resource base for primary health care system. The conservation assessment and management prioritisation (CAMP) work shop during October 2007 identified 41 medicinal plant species as red listed. Of these 2 species have been assessed to be critically endangered, 11 as endangered while 26 are vulnerable. Presently 43 important medicinal plants are in common practice and 24 medicinal plants have been economically evaluated for cultivation (OFDC data). Orissa State Vanaspati Van Society : Under Orissa State Vanaspati Van project, 3000 hectares of *in-situ* conservation of medicinal plants has been maintained during 2007-08. OSVVS is functioning since 2003-04 for cultivation and preservation of medicinal seedlings and other activities of the forest at both sides of Gandhamardhan hils *i.e.* Nrusinghanath and Harishankar. This project is for 5 years *i.e.* 2003-04 to 2007-08 with a financial outlay of Rs. 500 lakhs. Till November, 2007 an amount of Rs. 205 lakhs have been released and 175 lakhs has been spent. Under this programme 200 ha of *in-situ* preservation 3,000 ha *in-situ* conservation, 40 ha of *ex-situ* demonstration plot and capacity building in 25 VSS, have been achieved. Similipal Biosphere Reserve (SBR) in Mayurbhanj district of Orissa is the most luxuriant forest and rich in plant wealth comprising of 1076 species of flowering plants among which more than 500 species ate medicinal plants. An orchidarium has been established at Gurguria Range in Karanjia Forest Division and kept 64 orchids in it. Similarly, a medicinal plant nursery has been developed with a stock of 120 plants species at Ramatirtha Crocodile Breeding Center, Jashipur.

1

SIMILIPAL BIOSPHERE RESERVE : THE STUDY AREA

Similipal, "the queen of forests of Orissa", shines on the north eastern tip of the state in the center of Mayurbhanj district (Map : 1). The Similipal hill owe their name to Simili *(Bombax ceiba)* trees which are common in some areas (Saxena and Brahmam, 1989). The famous Oriya Poet Radhanath Roy has referred Similipal as 'Salmali Saila' meaning moss covered titles, indicating that the area is moist due to high precipitation. The virgin forest of Similipal harbors a wide range of flora and fauna for which it is laurated as 'Lungs of eastern India' and also as 'Botanical Garden of India' (Singha, 1998).

The Similipal Biosphere Reserve (SBR) came into existence with affect from June 22, 1994 (Rai, 2000). It is one of the first eight Biosphere Reserve of the country and only one in the State. Therefore it is not only one of the unique forests of Orissa but also of the whole country.

Bio-geographic Region

The Similipal Biosphere Reserve falls within Mahanadian east-coastal biogeographic region of oriental realm and Chhotanagpur biotic province of Deccan peninsular zone. It is the representative ecosystem under Mahanandian region in the eastern end of Central Plateau and the Eastern Ghats of tropical eastern India. However, Similipal shares biotic features of all four biotic provinces for which Orissa is the junction. The provinces are Eastern plateau, Chhotanagpur under the biogeographic zone Deccan peninsula, the lower Gangetic-plain and coastline of 480 km long under the East coast. Infact, geological studies, fossil histories and recent studies indicates that the Similipal is a biological link between the northern and Southern India (Singh, 1998). The entire Similipal massif is separated from the Bengal Bay by a narrow strip of coastal plain. The monsoon and moisture laden bay wind have definite influence on the vegetation pattern. Nature has epitomized all her living resources in this massif.

Location

The Biosphere reserve is located in the central part of Mayurbhanj district of Orissa and close to the interstate boundary with West Bengal in north-east direction and Jharkhand in north-west direction. The reserve is a compact mass of natural forest spreading over an area of 5569 sq. km. lying between 21°–10′ to 22°–12′ North latitude and 85°–58′ to 86°–42′ East longitude. The Similipal Biosphere Reserve has been divided into three zones, *e.g.* (1) Core Zone (2) Buffer Zone and (3) Transition Zone. The core zone comprises 845 sq. km, which is strictly prohibited region where no exploitation activities are entertained. This region is strictly reserved for wildlife habitat development. But the buffer zone, which is around 2,129 sq. km, is partially prohibited. This zone is allowed for some activities like research, education and tourism. On the other hand the transition zone, which lies in the peripheral region covering 2,595 sq. km, is allowed for research, settlement of tribal people, tourism and other environment friendly activities.

Physiography

The physiography of the Similipal Biosphere Reserve is undulating, varying from small hillocks to high mountain peaks. The hills rising very precipitously from the plains of Baripada and Udala extends as far as Jashipur in North and Bisoi in the East and Thakurmunda in the West covering a total area of 2,750 sq. km with their innumerable crests and valleys and perennial streams. Sir William Hunter describes Similipal Hills during 1872 as —

"The hitherto almost unexplored mountains of Mayurbhanj heaped upon each other in noble masses of rock from 3,300ft to 4000ft high. The peaks are densely wooded to the summit, and except the regular passes, are inaccessible to the beasts of burden".

The landscape of Similipal comprises of numerous rolling hills covered with thick forest vegetation. The highest mountain is the peak of Khairiburu which is 1168 m above the sea level. Whereas Meghasini is 1165 m high and Jenabil is 869 m high. The elevation in the central region at Dhudruchampa is 1009 m that of it in the North at Chahala is 774.5 m high only.

River Systems

Similipal is the richest watershed in Orissa giving rise to the perennial rivers like the Budhabalanga, Baitarani and Subarnarekha.The rivers Khairi, Bhandan, West Deo, Salandi, Gobarjhara, Sonai and Tel flow ultimately into Baitarani, where as Sonai, East Deo, Sanjo and Palpala into Budhabalanga which takes its rise from a near a village of the same name in Similipal and Khadkei with its tributaries flows into Subarnarekha. Sona which takes its rise in the Similipal hill drains the forest area at Kaptipada. These rivers are lifeline for the people of Mayurbhanj, Keonjhar, Balasore and Bhadrak districts. There is deep dissection of the plateau surface by these drainage systems giving rise to narrow, deep valleys and water falls. Important water falls are Barheipani Fall (400m) and Joranda Fall (150m) on the Budhabalanga course. The frost valley is also seen sometimes in central and south Similipal.

Climate

In considering climate of the area, the proximity of sea, elevation, direction of the prevailing winds and the configuration of the ground are to be born in mind. Precipitation in Similipal area is more than in the surrounding region as the monsoon winds from the Bay of Bengal when interrupted by the hills, bring about rain. The topography and direction of the prevailing winds results in a general decrease of rainfall from South West to North East but with a good many exceptions.

The climate of the Similipal is warm and humid. Three distinct seasons are felt during the year. Rainy season starts from middle of June till October with rainfall of about 1250 mm in the monsonic leeward valleys, over 2000 mm is the annual receiptal of 2500 mm is experienced in some pockets and more in higher elevations inside Similipal. Winter creeps in gradually from mid October and becomes severe in December lowering temperature to 2°C in many parts of the hill like Upper-barhakamuda, Jenabil and Nawana. The spring is pleasant. The southern and Western aspects are cooler and North Eastern aspects are warmer in Similipal. In hot season from March to June the average maximum temperature rises to 33.5°C and average minimum temperature is 9.8° C during December. The relative humidity is normally high exceeds 70% and prevails throughout the year but it goes up to 90% during rainy season. The difference between relative humidity measured during early morning, mid-day and evening hours is quite tenuous. Spring breeze is quite common all through the reserve. The number of rainy days is ranging from 1800-290 mm precipitation in 135-158 days annually.

In Similipal June to September are the wettest months. These four months account for 79% of the annual mean rainfall. Periodic earth tremors, thunder storms in the rains and dust storms in late May and early June are further characteristic features of Similipal. South Similipal near Devasthali, Upper Barhakamda and towards Bhanjabasa experiences frosts, the signs of which can be seen in sal areas. In a westerly direction severe cold wind blows, popularly called "Kaliani Hawa" in winter (Prusty, 1997).

Geology, Rock and Soil

The Similipal biosphere has the shape of lenticular elongated hill range which forms a special geologic formation that the plateau underlined by an assemblage of volcano-sedimentary rocks consisting of three alternating sequence of quartzite formation and spilitic lavas. Three quartzite formations alternate with three lava flows. They have concentric outcrop patterns, well seen on satellite images. These formations dip towards center forming a basin structure.

The volcano sedimentary assemblage is believed to have been deposited in an oval basin, formed on the pre existing surface underlain by older iron-ore bearing rock assemblage and granite intrusives. During deposition of sediments in the basin, there were repeated submarine volcanic activities giving rise to thick lava flows. Thus we find alternating sequence of sediments and lava flows. Towards the closing phase of sedimentation an important sill, known as 'Amjhori Sill', was intruded into the sequence which now occupy a prominent land at the center of the plateau. The age of the rock is believed to be around 2200 million years and hence belong to the early Proterozoic era.

The sedimentation and volcanic activity in the Similipal basin followed by marginal fractures were intruded by the glabro-arnothosites, pyroxene granite and granophyre suits of igneous rocks. On the west and south of Similipal hills lie the peneplained surface on the Singhbhum granite (Baitarani peneplain) at a level difference of 300 to 400 m. A still lower level peneplain exists on the east now covered by slope debris, laterite and alluvium. The extensive weathering of the volcano-sedimentary suit of rocks under the humid tropical climate has produced thick soil cover which favours the growth of luxuriant vegetation cover. Most of the area in Similipal has rich spread of red loam. Extensive pockets of laterite soil are formed on the plateau. Heavy clay is observed in the flat basins.

The soils of Similipal are acidic in nature, the pH varying from 4.8–6.8 in most of the areas The main soil types are : (*a*) from haematitic rocks, rich red loam soil is derived having intense biotic activity and dense tall trees (*b*) laterites produce deep soil, reddish in colour having the capability to support good tree growth, where ever the depth of the soil is less, it supports poor tree growth but encourage good grass growth for use by animals (*c*) shale on weathering produces substantial deposits of clay and clayey loam soils which are good for plant growth (*d*) outcrops of sub-metamorphic sand stone and quartzite, haematites on disintegration produce reddish sandy soil and in deep layers, it supports good growth of trees and shallow soil produces grass growth.

Tribal Population

The area of Similipal Biosphere Reserve covers the entire Similipal National Park and 10 km boundary in its periphery. Out of 65 villages, 7 villages are located in the core area and 58 villages in the buffer zone. Three villages in the core zone are uninhabited. There are 61 villages within the sanctuary and about 1200 villages all around within a distance of 10km from the periphery. As per the 2001 census figure of 61 villages a total of 12449 population including 72 SC, 11571 ST, 806 Others categories.

In Mayurbhanj district tribes occupy a big chunk of the population constituting 52% of it. Fifty three communities both aboriginal and migrated are found in the district glorifying the rich heritage of tribal culture. The social fabric, cultural behaviour, matrimonial traditions through do not tally with one another yet there is maximum similarity among them. The singing and dancing cultural of tribal life is always correlated into natural forests. The birth and breathing of last in tribal life can not be separated from forest. To him forest is mother, beloved and companion.

So far concerned with tribal population the major tribes Santal, Kolha, Bathudi, Kharias, Mankidias, Gond and Ho are living in the Similipal forest. Besides these other minor tribes like Bhuyan, Paudi Bhuyan are also living in this area. Amongst few tribes living deep inside the Similipal forests prominent are "Kharia" and "Mankidia". They depend solely on their surrounding forest for most of their requirements from food to medicines. The Similipal forest has been the chief source of major and minor forest produce that provides subsistence of the above tribes and forest dwellers residing in the sanctuary area. Besides timber and bamboo, non-timber forest produce also plays a major role in the day-to-day life of tribals. Important items amongst them listed in the table-1 are available from the Similipal forest. Broadly non timber forest products (NTFPs) commonly known as minor forest produce (MFP), mean all biological products of forests other than timber and fuel wood. It includes flora and fauna forming rich biodiversity in the ecological complex and biologically diverse forest ecosystem in Similipal. Non timber forest products are available inside Similipal forest can be classified under various heads (1) fiber and flosses; (2) grass, bamboo and canes; (3) edible minor forest produce; (4) essential oil including those from grasses; (5) medicinal plants; (6) tannins and dyes; (7) gums and resins; (8) leaves, fruits and seeds. Most of the minor forest product like honey, wax, resin, arrowroot etc. are collected by Kharias, Bhagatas, Bhumija and Saouras are not many and do not have any influence on Similipal. The Santals who constitute more than half the population of tribals of the district are the most advanced among tribes. They are hard working, cleanly dressed agriculturists with high sensitivity to environmental aesthetics. The Bhumijas, Bhuyans, Ho and Gond are major groups settled as agriculturists and are advanced. The Pauri Bhuiyans live near the forests and collect food from forest. The Mahalis are basket makers and the Sounties are mostly landless labourers like on wage earning. Mankidias lead nomadic life, collect siali fibre (*Bahunia vahlii)*, make ropes, keep monkey as pet, hence called Mankidias. The Saharas collect fibre wood, herbal plants, roots, fruits, leaves, gums, resin and flowers and sell those in the local market to earn living (Mishra 1973-74, Bose, 1973-74).

Wildlife

The Similipal due to such diverse topography and soil conditions coupled with climatic variation and rich diversity of autotrophs is sure to support a fascinating faunal composition (Pattnaik,1997). The identified species of fauna include 12 species of amphibians, 29 species of reptiles, 264 species of birds and 42 species of mammals. The primary heterotrophs among the mammals are represented by Elephant (*Elephant maximus*), Sambar (*Cervus unicol*), Cheetal (*Axis axis*), Barking deer (*Muntiacus muntjac*), Gaur (*Bos gaurus*), Wildboar (*Susscrofa cristatus*), Mouse deer (*Tragulus memina*), Fourhorned antelope (*Tetraceros quadricornis*), Common langur (*Presbytis entellus*), Rhesus monkey (*Macaca mulatta*), Porcupine (*Hystrix indica*), Giant squirrel (*Ratufa indica*), Flying squirrel (*Petanrista petanrista*) and Indian pangolin (*Manis crassicaudata*) etc.

Among the secondary heterotrophs are tiger (*Panthera tigris*), leopard (*Panthera paradus*), jackel (*Canis aureus*), wilddog, Indian wolf, ratel, jungle cat, civet cat and common mongoose. The scaving anima's are hyena, jungle cat and ratel are found in the Similipal forest. The well known tigress "Khairi" was caught in cub stage from the banks of the river Khairi in Similipal.

Due to its topographical and climatic variation, besides the avifauna common to Peninsular India some Himalayan birds are peafowl, painted spur fowl, black patridge, grey patridge, doves, crested serpent eagle, shahin falcon, flycatcher, hawk, malabar pied hornbill and grey hornbill, owl, hill myna, parakeet, golden oriole, sun birds, common snipe, crow pheasant and red jungle fowl etc. Besides them, water birds like white ibis, spoon bill, herons, egrets, red wattled lapwing, plover, terns, sand piper and king fishers are seen in artificial and natural water bodies in and around Similipal.

Mugger, python, cobra, king cobra, land tortoise and monitor lizard are among the common reptiles found in the forest. Besides them large varieties of fishes, aquatic fauna and insects are found in these forests. A special type of scaled fish Mahasheer locally called 'Khajura' found only in the rivers namely Deo, Khairi and Bhandan of Similipal hill reserve. It is tasty but can not be kept long as after catch it gets decomposed soon. Honey bee is a very important insect of economic importance to the tribes particularly the 'Khadia'.

Vegetation

The Similipal harbours rich flora of 1076 species of vascular plants including 93 species of orchids, 52 species of rare/endangered plants and more than 300 species of medicinal plants. Besides, the hill range forms a biological link and exhibits similarity of floristic and faunal composition between northern and southern India creating a transitional bridge for migration of species from Himalayas to southern peninsula.

The forest of Similipal is among the most luxuriant and valuable forests of the state. The sal (*Shorea robusta*) is the principal species occurring in the Similipal and also economically the most important. But the type of sal varies with the edaphic conditions and its associates will vary with the type. The rolling table land of Similipal has several open grassy areas and large meadows in frosty valleys fringed by annually frost affected cover of bushy sal. Diversity is thus apparent in natural cover. Natural bamboo growth is conspicuously absent in general.

According to the classification made by Champion and Seth (1968), the Similipal holds broadly the following types of forests :

(*a*) Northern Tropical Moist Deciduous Forests;

(*b*) Northern Tropical Semi-evergreen Forests;

(*c*) Deciduous Hill Forests;

(*d*) Level Sal Forests and

(*e*) Grassland and Savannah.

Northern Tropical Moist Deciduous Forests

The top storey in this type consists of predominantly deciduous species but the second storey has some evergreens. These forests are most extensive and occur all over Simlipal often in continuation with the semi evergreen type. By far the predominant species of this type is sal, which forms 59-90 per cent of the crop. The height of sal depends on the site characteristics like gradient, soil depth, temperature, and aspect and soil moisture. Common associates of sal in this type are: *Terminalia alata., T. bellirica, Pterocarpus marsupium, Xylia xylocarpa, Haldinia cordifolia, Emblica officinalis, Lagerstromia parviflora, Bombax ceiba, Grewia* sp., *Syzygium cumini, Litsea* sp., *Dillenia pentagyna, Careya arborea, Kydia calysina, Bridellia retusa, Mitragyna parviflora, Trema orientalis, Ziziphus* sp., *Cassia fistula, Helicteres isora, Croton roxburghii, Buchanania lanzan, Wendlandia* sp., and others. The shrub layer consists of mainly *Ardisia solanacea, Barleria strigosa, Flemingia* spp., *Leea* spp., *Indigofera cassioidesetc*. Climbers are heavy, consisting *of Bauhinia vahlii, Dioscorea* sp., *Smilax* sp., *Millettia extensa, Cissus* sp., *Ampelocissus* sp., etc. Herbaceous flora consists of *Curcuma* sp., *Zingiber* sp., species of Rubiaceae, Asteraceae and Acanthaceae, ferns and orchids. Natural regeneration of sal is generally adequate.

Northern Tropical Semi-evergreen Forests

This type is characterized by a large number of dominant species, heavy climbers and abundant epiphytes. A few of the species of the top canopy of most of the understorey are evergreen and occur intimately mixed with each other. The type is confined to the upper reaches of the damp valleys of perennial streams and rivers, especially in the southern and eastern part of the area. The important constituent species are *Michelia champaca, Mesua ferrea, Mangifera indica, Phoebe lanceolata, Saraca asoca, Diospyros malabarica, Syzygium cumini, Macaranga peltata, Anthocephalus chinensis, Polyalthia cerasoides, Dillenia pentagyna, Turpinia nepalensis, Persea villosa, Neocinnamomum caudatum, Garcinia* sp., *Prunus ceylanica, Vitex* sp., *Elaeocarpus tectorius, Carallia brachiata, Ardisia solanacea, Rubus ellipticus, Cyathea gigantean, Micromelum minutum, Gnetum ula,* etc. and occasionally a few Sal trees. The epiphytic, flora is rich comprising several species of ferns, mosses, lycopods and orchids. Grasses are poor due to heavy shade.

Dry Deciduous Hill Forests

Wherever conditions are hot and dry sal is of poorer quality give rise to this type of forests. Both upper and lower canopies in these forests are composed of deciduous species. This type occurs on steep exposed slopes of mainly South and East Similipal. Sal forms about 26 per cent of the forest vegetation or sometimes more in favourable conditions. Associated with sal are *Anogeissus latifolia, Terminalia alata, Terminalia chebula, Diospyrus melanoxylon, Haldinia cordifolia, Cassia fistula, Mallutus philippensis, Lagerstroemia parviflora, Semecarpus anacardium, Buchanania lanzan, Lannea coromandelica, Garuga pinnata, Protium serratum, Sterculia urens, Sterculia villosa, Chochlospermum religiosum etc.* The shrubs include *Cleistanthus collinus, Nyctanthes arbortristis, Gardenia latifolia, Randia* sp., *Ziziphus* sp. *Helecteres isora, Flacourtia ramontchi etc.* The climbers are not many and consist of *Acacia* sp., *Bauhinia vahlii, Ventilago denticulate, Combretum decandrum*, etc. Epiphytes and ferns are not conspicuous.

High Level Sal Forests

This type of forests extends over an area of about 250 km^2 above 850m elevations on the plateaus. Almost pure stands of sal of very poor quality looking gnarled are found in these areas. The main associates of sal are *Dillenia pentagyna, Syzygium ceresoides* and *Pterocarpus marsupium, Imperata cylindrica* and *Themeda gigantean* with large patches of *Phoenix sylvestris.*

Grassland and Savannah

The area of grasslands in Similipal is between 70-80 km^2 spread allover in small and large patches. It is found on hill tops over 900m high and in the higher frosty valleys. On hill tops the grasslands is perhaps climax type. But in the valleys it used top secondary seral around 1980s, the origin being clearance, either biotic or natural. The grassland stage was arrested by annual fires on the frosty valleys. But sal and other frost tender species appear to have grown above annually bitten field level whippy growth. Attempts have been made to convert these areas to fodder lands by manipulation.

Among the tree species *Syzygium cerasoideum, Symplocos racemosa, Dillenia pentagyna* are common in these areas. Among the grasses, *Imperata cylindrica, Themeda gigantia* and *Saccharum spontaneum* are common. *Phragmites karka* is found on the nala banks. *Phoenix sylvestris* is met with quite frequency. This area has been proved to be the best for animal due to more suitable fodder and provision of well-dispersed edge for cover and shelter.

As stated earlier, it is seen that the grasslands are being gradually encroached upon with sal forests. Management actions are being initiated with suitable habitat manipulation so that grasslands, which are so essential for small herbivores, insects and other invertebrates, continue to contribute to the biodiversity of Similipal.

Abrus precatorius L.

Family

Fabaceae

Vernacular Names

Oriya : Kaincha, Kaicho, Kaincho, Lalgunj, Runjo; **Hindi** : Ratti; **Sans** : Gunja; **Sant** : Gujjbai, Arakeej.

The Plant

A deciduous, climber with tough branches; leaves abruptly pinnae with many pairs of leaflets, the rachis ending in a spine. Flowers pink, clustered on tubercles arranged along the rachis of one-sided pedunculate raceme. Fruits pods, turgid with a sharp deflexed beak. Seeds usually scarlet with a black spot or sometimes pure white. Fl. July-September.

Distribution

Occasional.

Parts Used

Seeds, leaves, root.

Medicinal Properties and Uses

Seeds are purgative, emetic, tonic, antiphlogistic, aphrodisiac and used in nervous disorders, abortifacient, paste as local application in stiffness of shoulder joints, sciatica and paralysis. Leaves are sweetish in taste and are useful in biliousness and in leucoderma and other skin diseases. Leaves decoction used for cough, cold, colic pain. Root is emetic, diuretic, tonic, used in preparations prescribed for gonorrhoea, jaundice and haemoglobinuric bile.

Ethnomedicinal Uses

White seeds kept in unboiled cow milk for the period of

over night and the seed is given to woman in the morning at the end of menstruation cycle for preventing conception. Root pounded with water is sprinkled on head and unripe seed juice is rubbed on scalp new baldness.

Abutilon indicum (L.) Sweet

Family

Malvaceae.

Vernacular Names

Oriya : Pedipedica; **Hindi** : Kanghi; **Sans.** : Atibala; **Sant** : Miru baha.

The Plant

A perennial, softly tomentose, up to 3 m in height. Stems round, frequently tinged with purple. Leaves ovate to orbicular-cordate, 1.9-2.5 cm long. Flowers solitary on jointed peduncles, orange-yellow or yellow; capsules hispid, larger than the calyx, awns erect. Seeds 3-5, reniform, tubercled or minutely stellate-hairy, black or dark brown. Flowers and fruits almost throughout the year.

Distribution

Frequent.

Parts Used

Seeds, leaves, bark, root.

Medicinal Properties and Uses

Seeds are used in piles. Laxative, expectorant. Leaves demulcent, locally applied to boils and ulcers. Decoction is used in tooth ache. Infusion leaves demulcent and diuretic and prescribed in fever, chest affection and urethritis. Bark astringent and diuretic.

Ethnomedicinal Uses

The root is tried on the neck and waist and root paste is orally administered in delivery troubles. Paste of one leaf and seven numbers of *Piper longum* is taken orally for jaundice.

Acacia leucophloea (Roxb.) Willd.

Family

Mimosaceae.

Vernacular Names

Oriya : Kanta siriso; **Hindi :** Safed babul.

The Plant

A moderate sized tree with spreading branches. Leaves bipinnate, main rachis pubescent with a cup-shaped gland between each pair of pinnae. Flowers in large terminal tomentose panicles, heads numerous, globose. Fruits sessile, thin, flat, slightly curved pods, covered with pale brown tomentum.

Distribution

Found in dry deciduous forests.

Parts Used

Bark.

Medicinal Properties and Uses

The bark is astringent, bitter, thermogenic, styptic, alexeteric, anthelmintic, demulcent, constipating, expectorant and antipyretic. It is useful in bronchitis, cough, inflammation, skin diseases, leucoderma, leprosy, vomiting, wounds, ulcers, diarrhoea, dysentery, internal and external haemorrhages, dental cares, oral ulcers and intermittent fevers.

Ethnomedicinal Uses

20 gm bark boil with ½ lit. water allow to reduce up to

½ cup. Filter and add some sugar candy. Take twice a day for five days for anti abortion.

Achyranthes aspera L.

Family

Amaranthaceae

Vernacular Names

Hindi : Circita; **Oriya :** Apamaranga; **Sans :** Apamarga; **Sant :** Buridataran.

The Plant

An erect, straggling or sub scandent herb. Leaves ovate, elliptic, acute, generally appressed hairy beneath, base narrowed, spikes long. Flowers polished green, deflexed, bracteole spinescent. Fl. & Fr. October-February.

Distribution

Throughout India, along roadside and waste places as well as on hills upto 900m.

Parts Used

Whole plant.

Medicinal Properties and Uses

Decoction of herb diuretic, used in renal dropsies. Young leaves are severed as spinach. The whole plant and especially roots are prescribed in the rheumatism, lumbago, osteodynia, dysuria, post-partum haematometra and dysmenorrhoea. The seeds are nutrious when cooked with milk and are a potential source of food. The roots are astringent, their paste is applied to clear opacity of cornea and to wounds as an haemostatic. It is reported to be useful in cancer. A decoction of roots is used for stomach troubles and an aqueous extract for stones in the bladder.

Ethnomedicinal Uses

Twigs are used for brushing teeth. When plants are tied on the body of the cattle it helps in expelling maggot from the wounds. Paste of fruits is applied to the bite of mad dog. Root is boiled in water and decoction is given orally with honey to pregnant mothers. This helps in quick delivery of child. The powdered root of the plant is very useful in cholera.

Achyranthes bidentata Blume

Family

Amaranthaceae.

White, numerous, deflected against the rachis. Utricle oblong-cylindrical, one seeded. Fl. & Fr. November

Distribution

Occasional

Parts Used

Tuberous roots.

Medicinal Properties and Uses

The roots possess anti-inflammatory, hypotensive and uterotonic properties. The drug is indicated for rheumatism, lumbago, hypertension, dysuria and sore throat. It is also used as an oxytocic in dystocia, placenta retention and post-partum haematometra.

Ethnomedicinal Uses

Paste of the leaves is applied externally on the sores and itches and internally taken in stomach pain. Root paste is applied as antidote against snakebite and scorpion stings.

Acorus calamus L.

Family

Araceae.

Vernacular Names

Hindi : Bach, Ghorabach, Safed bach; **Oriya :** Bacha; **Sans :** Bhuta-nashini.

The Plant

A perennial, glabrous, aromatic herb; rhizome creeping, light brown-pinkish outside and white and spongy inside. Leaves sessile, deeply channeled and linear-lanceolate. Flowers small, pale green, in 5-10cm long cylindric spikes called spadix; fruit yellowish in color.

Distribution

The plant is found almost through out India upto an altitude of about 200m growing chiefly in marshy or moist situations.

Parts Used

Rhizome

Medicinal Properties and Uses

The rhizome is bitter, acrid, thermogenic, aromatic, diuretic, purgative, anti-inflammatory, expectorant, aphrodisiac, emetic, antispasmodic, anodyne, antipyretic, sedative and tonic. The under ground rhizome and its oil are used in gastric, repository, diarrhoea, pregnancy, cough, nervine tonic, aphrodisiac. Powder is used in gastric and bronchial troubles of infants. Garland of tuber is tied around neck or belly to get relief from jaundice. Paste is also used in skin diseases and to kill magoots and lices. They yield a yellow aromatic volatile oil which possesses insecticidal properties and is useful against bed bugs, moths lice etc. The root has antibacterial and antifungal properties.

Ethnomedicinal Uses

Rhizome powder 1gm and seed powder 0.5gm of *Piper nigrum* mixed together and the mixture is given to cure colic. An essential oil is extracted from the rhizomes which is utilized in perfumery.

Acronychia pedunculata (L.) Miq.

Family

Rutaceae

The Plant

Small tree, much branched. Leaves opposite, oblong or obovate, entire, coriaceous, glabrous. Inflorescence in axillary or terminal corymb. Flowers white, fragrant. Drupe globose, pale-yellow when ripe.

Distribution

Occasional, Rare.

Parts Used

Root, bark.

Medicinal Properties and Uses

Root and bark used in external application for sores and ulcers. Root is utilized in the therapy of rheumatism, lumbago, and paid in the limbs. Bark tonic used in scabies.

Adenostemma lavenia (L.) Kuntz

Family

Asteraceae

The Plant

Herb, often decumbent. Leaves ovate, coarsely crenate or serrate, acute. Heads white. Fl. & Fr. October-December.

Distribution

Occasional in moist and shady places.

Parts Used

Whole plant

Medicinal Properties and Uses

Plant is used in dysentery and colic.

Adiantum philippense L.

Family

Adiantaceae.

Vernacular Names

Sant : Dodhari, Dodhali; **Hindi :** Kalijhant.

The Plant

Tufted fern with slender fronds, with black, polished, glabrous, wiry stipes. Pinnae alternate, petioled, semiorbicular, simple. Rounded forked, spongia on the recurved lobules or some times on margins. Fertile Sept.-December.

Distribution

Common in forests and shady places.

Parts Used

Rhizome, fronds.

Medicinal Properties and Uses

Used in blood diseases and epileptic fits. Fern also used in case of rabbies. Rhizomes prescribed for strangury and in fever due to elephantiasis. Fronds are burnt in oil and applied to itch.

Ethnomedicinal Uses

2g of fresh leaf paste is taken orally on empty stomach twice a day for 10 days for immediate relief from indigestion.

Adhatoda zeylanica Medic.

Family

Acanthaceae.

Vernacular Names

Hindi : Adusa, Vasika; **Oriya :** Basanga; **Sans :** Vasaka.

The Plant

A tall, much branched, dense, evergreen shrub, with large, lanceolate leaves. Flowers in dense, short spikes. Stalks of the spikes shorter than leaves. Leaf-like structures called bracts present on the spikes. Corolla of the flowers are white with few purplish markings. Fl. & Fr. June-February.

Distribution

This plant occurs through out the plains and submontane regions of India; it is common near habitations.

Parts Used

Roots, leaves, flowers.

Medicinal Properties and Uses

Basanga is a reputed remedy for all sorts of cough and cold, bronchitis and other respiratory disorders due to its expectorant action. Plant is bitter, astringent, diuretic, antispasmodic, expectorant and alterative. It cures vomiting thirst, dermatosis, jaundice, fever and haematomesis. It is particularly useful in fevers associated with bilious and respiratory troubles and also in piles. Roots are expectorant and mild bronchial antiseptic given in intermittent fever pulmonary and catarrhal affection. Leaves and roots are hypoglycemic. Juice of leaves relieves cough by its soothing action on nerves and by liquefying sputum. Fresh leaf juice is beneficial in haemoptysis and menorrhagia. Flowers and roots with ginger are given in rheumatism, constipation, asthma, chronic bronchitis and other chest infections.

Ethnomedicinal Uses

Decoction of the leaves is given with honey twice for 7 days in asthma and cough. Juice of leaves is applied all over the feet and soles in morning and at bed time to cure burn feet.

Aegle marmelos (L.) Correa

Family

Rutaceae.

Vernacular Names

Oriya : Bela; **Hindi :** Bel; **Sans. :** Bilva, Bilwa, Shriphal **Ko. :** Lohagasi.

The Plant

A medium sized deciduous tree bearing strong axillary thorns. Leaves with 3 or 5 leaflets. Flowers greenish white, sweet scented, about 2.5 cm across in small bunches. Fruit 8-20cm diameter, glabrous, green, finally greyish, rind woody, pulp orange coloured, sweet and aromatic. Fl. March-April, Fr. Ripening after one year.

Distribution

Occasional in forest. It is also planted.

Parts Used

Roots, leaves, fruits.

Medicinal Properties and Uses

Fruit is valuable chiefly for its mucilage and pectin. It is very useful in chronic diarrhoea and dysentery, particularly for patients having diarrhoea alternating with spells of constipation. The unripe or half ripe fruits improve appetite and digestion.

The roots are sweet, astringent, bitter, digestive and stomachic. The ripe fruits used for diarrhoea and dysentery. It acts as a laxative and diuretic, in strong doses a cardiac depressant. The leaves are astringent, laxative, febrifuge and expectorant, and are useful in ophthalmia, deafness, inflammations, catarrh, diabetes and asthmatic complaints. The ripe fruits are astringent, sweet, aromatic, cooling and tonic, and are good for the heart and brain and in dyspepsia.

Ethnomedicinal Uses

The expressed juice of green leaves (25ml) is given in empty stomach for stomach disorder. 5 to 7 number of leaves are taken every day in morning in empty stomach in diabetes. Unripe fruit is taken for dysentery and ripe fruit is taken to cure constipation.

Ageratum conyzoides L.

Family

Asteraceae.

Vernacular Names

Oriya : Poksunga; **Sant. :** Heren-ba.

The Plant

Erect hispidly hairy herb. Stem green or purple. Leaves opposite, broadly ovate, coarsely crenate, hairy on both sides. The inflorescence is a terminal corymb of many small heads. Flowers violet or white. Achene minute, black, 5-echinate. Fl. & Fr. all the year round.

Distribution

Fairly common weed.

Parts Used

Whole plant.

Medicinal Properties and Uses

The whole plant possesses anti-inflammatory and anti allergic properties. The juice from the fresh plant and the extract of the dried plant are used for the cure of allergic rhinitis and sinusitis in aqueous solution for nasal instillation. The juice of the fresh plant is also useful in post-partum uterine haemorrhage. A hair wash consisting at a decoction of the fresh plant makes the hair fragrant, soft and dandruff–free, prevents tetanus.

Ethnomedicinal Uses

Boiled leaf paste is applied on skin before bed for the treatment of Khasar (a type of skin disease).

Alangium salvifolium (L.f.) Wang.

Family

Alangiaceae.

Vernacular Names

Hindi : Angol, Dhera, Dhela; **Oriya :** Dhala ankol, Ankula, **Ko :** Ankol. **Sant. :** Dhelakanta.

The Plant

Small bushy tree, often thorny, bark light coloured. Leaves oblong, oblong lanceolate or elliptic, Flowers white or cream fragrant in axillary fascicles from the axils of fallen leaves. Fruits subglobose or ellipsoid, black, succulent with bony endocarp. Fl. March-April, Fr. June-July.

Distribution

In the forests of South India.

Parts Used

Roots, fruits.

Medicinal Properties and Uses

The roots are astringent, emollient, anthelmintic, thermogenic, diuretic and purgative. Root bark is an antidote for several poisons. The roots are useful for external application in rheumatism and leprosy. The fruits are sweet, cooling and purgative and are useful in treating burning sensation and haemorrhages.

Ethnomedicinal Uses

Leaf juice (2ml) with common salt (1gm) is applied drop by drop twicc for five days on eyelids as a cure of eye diseases like redness of eyes. Dried leaf powder along with Gur (molasses) is give for a month or two for piles.

Alsophila gigantea Wall. ex. Hook.

Family

Hymenophyllaceae.

Vernacular Names

Ko. : Sankukuri.

The Plant

Tree fern, stipes bearing scales, rachis almost purple. Fronds bipinnate. Pinnae long glabrous beneath, margin serrate. Sori exindusiate 5-6 pairs arranged in the form of inverted V. Fertile: Oct.-March.

Distribution

Rare in shady valleys along streams.

Parts Used

Rhizome.

Medicinal Properties and Uses

Fresh rhizome 10g mixed 21 black pepper seeds (*Piper nigrum* L.) are powdered and taken orally with milk twice a day for one week in empty stomach against white discharges.

Alstonia scholaris (L.) R.Br.

Family

Apocynaceae.

Vernacular Names

Oriya : Chhatian, Khiromula, Saptaparna; **Hindi :** Chattiyan, Saittan ka jat; **Sans :** Saptaparni; **Sant :** Chatnia; Ko Kanumung.

The Plant

A large evergreen tree reaching up to about 25m high, having bitter milky juice, bark rough, dark grey, branches whorled. Leaves leathery, 10-20cm long, 4-7 in a whorl. Flowers small, greenish white, spice-scented in many flowered clusters. Fruits very long, 30-60 cm, narrow and slender, hanging in pairs and forming dense clusters. Fl. Nov.–Jan., Fr. May-September.

Distribution

Evergreen, frequent, valleys and hill slopes.

Parts Used

Bark, leaves, milky exudates.

Medicinal Properties and Uses

The bark is bitter, astringent, acrid, thermogenic, digestive, laxative, anthelmintic, febrifuge, antipyretic, cardiotonic and tonic. It is useful in fevers, malarial fever, abdominal disorders, diarrhoea, dysentery, dyspepsia, leprosy, skin diseases, chronic and foul ulcers, asthma, bronchitis and debility. The tender leaves, in the form of poultice, are good for ulcers with foul discharges. The milky exudates is bitter and is good for ulcers, vitiated conditions of *vata* and otalgia.

Ethnomedicinal Uses

About 50 gms latex and 10 gms sugar are mixed together and made into 15 doses. It is given thrice daily for four days in spermatorrhoea. Leaf paste is prepared and is used for washing human hair. This cures wasp of human head. About 50 gm latex of this plant and 10 gm sugar are mixed together and made into 15 doses. It is given thrice daily for four days in spermatorrhoea.

Alternanthera sessilis (L.) R.Br. ex DC.

Family

Amaranthaceae.

Vernacular Names

Hindi : Gudrisag; **Oriya :** Madaranga; **Sans :** Matsyaksi, Patturah, Giojihra.

The Plant

A much branched prostrate herb, branches often purplish, frequently rooting at the lower nodes. Leaves simple, opposite, lanceolate, obtuse or subacute, sometimes obscurely denticulate, glabrous, shortly petiolate, Flowers small, white in axillary clusters. Fruits compressed obcordate utricles, seeds suborbicular. Fl. & Fr. June-Dec.

Distribution

Common weed in moist places.

Parts Used

Whole plant.

Medicinal Properties and Uses

The plant is bitter, sweet, astringent, acrid, cooling, constipating, depurative, digestive and is useful in vitiated conditions of *kapha* and *pitta,* burning sensation, diarrhoea, leprosy, skin diseases, dyspepsia and fever.

Ammannia baccifera L.

Family

Lythraceae.

Vernacular Names

Hindi : Dadmari, **Sans :** Kurandika.

The Plant

An erect glabrous reddish herb. Leaves: lower opposite, upper sometimes altrnate, oblong or narrow-elliptic, rounded. Flowers reddish in dense axillary cluster. Fruits depressed globose capsules covered by calyx tube upto the middle. Fl. February.

Distribution

Occasional.

Parts Used

Whole plant.

Medicinal Properties and Uses

The plant is bitter, acrid, cooling, appetizer, stomachic, diuretic and aphrodisiac. It is useful in vitiated conditions of kapha and pitta, burning sensation, anorexia, dyspepsia, flatulence, seminal weakness, rheumatism and herpetic eruptions. Acrid leaves are bruished and used for ringworms and other parasitic skin affections. Plant is used for antityphoid and antitubercular properties.

Ethnomedicinal Uses

Leaves are made into paste and applied on skin infections.

Ampelocissus latifolia (Roxb.) Planch.

Family

Vitaceae.

Vernacular Names

Hindi : Panibel; **Oriya :** Paniamoha, Kanjinoi; **Ko :** Oterori. **Sans :** Icewar.

The Plant

Large climber, glabrous. Leaves simple orbicular, 3-7 angled or lobed, sharply irregularly crenate or dentate, palminerved. Flowers brown red. Berry black, succulent. Fl. June-July, Fr. Aug.-October.

Distribution

Frequent in open forests.

Parts Used

Leaves.

Medicinal Properties and Uses

Juice of tender leaves used in dental troubles and as a detergent for indolent ulcers. Decoction of roots is given in dysentery.

Ethnomedicinal Uses

Paste of the root is applied on eczema.

Anacardium occidentale L.

Family

Anacardiaceae.

Vernacular Names

Hindi : Duk, Kaju; **Oriya** : Kaju, Lanka amba; **Sans** : Kajutaka.

The Plant

A small tree, often banched from near the base. Leaves simple, alternate, obovate, and sometimes broadly elliptic. Coriaceous, glabrous. Flowers pinkish. Drupe reniform, greyish brown, seated on fleshy, yellowish or reddish hypocarp. Seed reniform. Fl -March-April, Fr. April-May.

Distribution

Very commonly planted.

Parts Used

Roots, bark, leaves, fruits.

Medicinal Properties and Uses

The roots are considered purgative. The bark has alterative properties and is used along with the inflorescence for the treatment of snakebite. The bark and leaves are useful in odontalgia and ulitis. The gum from the bark is recommended in leprosy, ringworm and obstinate ulcers. Fruits are acrid, sweet, aphrodisiac and are useful in vitiated conditions of *vata* and *kapha*, skin diseases, dysentery and anorexia. They are used for preventing hair loss and to increase the growth of hair.

Ethnomedicinal Use

The hypocarp mixed with salt is taken to cure sore throat and cough.

Anaphalis adnata DC.

Family

Asteraceae

The Plant

Erect woolly–tomentose herb. Leaves sessile, oblong, acute, thick white–tomentose. Heads sessile in dense rounded terminal corymbs. Florets yellow. Fl. Fr. Jan.–March.

Distribution

Occasional.

Parts Used

Whole plant.

Medicinal Properties and Uses

Flower heads and the hairs are employed to stop bleeding.

Andrographis paniculata Nees

Family

Acanthaceae.

Vernacular Names

Hindi-Kalmegh, Kiryat; **Oriya**-Bhuinimbo, Chirata; **Sans** : Kirata, Bhunimba.

The Plant

An erect, branched annual herb, 0.3 to 0.9m in height with quadrangular branches. Leaves are simple, lanceolate, acute at both ends. Flowers small, solitary in panicles with rose colour corolla, which is hairy extensively. Fl. & Fr. Sept.-May.

Distribution

Frequent in mixed forests.

Parts Used

Whole plant, root.

Medicinal Properties and Uses

Plant is astringent, anodyne, tonic and alexipharmic, antipyretic, hepatoprotective, digestive, anti-inflammatory, cancerolytic, cardioprotective. It is used in dysentery, cholera, diabetes, consumption, influenza, bronchitis, itches and piles. Often substituted for chirayita. Decoction is used for sluggishness of liver and in jaundice. Leaves and roots are used as a febrifuge, cholagogue and anthelmintic.

Ethnomedicinal Uses

Infusion of the leafy twigs is given in empty stomach in the morning for prevention from malaria and also for stomach troubles. 10gm leaf juice is taken everyday for blood purification. Grind 33gm of leaf with 21 gm. black salt and made tablets of wt. 1 gm each and one tablet is given every day to cure cirrhosis of lever.

Angiopteris evecta (Forst.) Hoffm.

Family

Angiopteridaceae

Vernacular Names

Ko : Marang gindung

The Plant

Huge fern with a very stout soft stem. Fronds long, bipinnate, stipes green with scattered, whitish, streaks and cover with small brown hairs. Sori at the ends of the vein, somewhat laterally compressed by one another and opening by a vertical chink. Spores circular. Fertile March-August.

Distribution

In moist valleys along streams.

Parts Used

Leaves

Ethnomedicinal Uses

50g of fresh leaf paste mixed with 1g of common salt and is externally applied for early maturation of boils. The leaf paste mixed with cow ghee i.e. (5:1) ratio is locally applied for burns.

Annona reticulata L.

Family

Annonaceae

Vernacular Names

Oriya : Ramphala; **Hindi :** Luvani, Anta, Nagnewa; **Sans:** Mandargam, Gom; **Ko :** Handiphuta.

The Plant

A small deciduous or semi-deciduous tree. Leaves acuminate. Flowers pale-green, cordate or subglobose. Fruits subglobose yellowish-red when ripe, edible with peculiar aroma. Fl. June, Fr. Dec.-January.

Distribution

Cultivation in India; occasionally found wild.

Parts Used

Bark, fruit, seeds and leaves.

Medicinal Properties and Uses

Root bark contains an alkaloid liriodenine and oxouspinsunine, anonine and a neq alkaloid reticulin. The root is drastic purgative. Seed, leaf, stem and root are insecticidal. Leaves are insecticide and externally useful as suppurant and are used against inflammatory tumors. Bark is a powerful astringent and used as tonic and antidysenteric. Fruit is anthelmintic and antidysenteric. Fruit pulp is sweet and edible.

Ethnomedicinal Uses

Mixture of seed powder with black pepper (*Piper nigrum*) (about 3gm) is prescribed for spoiling of pregnancy up to 3-4 months duration.

Annona squamosa L.

Family

Annonaceae

Vernacular Names

Hindi : Sitaphal; **Oriya :** Atta; **Sant** : Newa, Mondal; **Ko :** Marsinga.

The Plant

A large evergreen staggling shrub or small tree. Leaves simple, alternate, bifarious, oblong-lanceolate. Flowers yellowish green, solitary. Fruit globose, yellowish-green when ripe, edible with aroma. Seeds brownish black, smooth. Fl. March-May, Fr. July-September.

Distribution

Throughout India, cultivated.

Parts Used

Roots, leaves, fruits, seeds.

Medicinal Properties and Uses

The roots are powerful purgative, and are useful in mental depression and spinal disorders. The leaves are suppurative and insecticidal, and are useful in destroying lice, proctopsis in children and as a poultice to produce suppuration. The fruits are sweet, haematinic, cooling, sedative, stimulant, expectorant, maturant and tonic. They are useful in anaemia.

Ethnomedicinal Uses

Dried root powder (5gm) is taken once in morning for five days by women for abortion of 3 to 4 months of pregnancy. The paste of leaves used as an external application from head to toe in scabies and dandruff. The immature fruit rubbed against stone is applied in ulcers and sores. Seed powder with water is applied in scalp and ringed after 10 minutes for treating lice.

Anogeissus latifolia (Roxb.) Wall. ex Bedd.

Family

Combretaceae

Vernacular Names

Oriya : Dhau, Dhaura; **Hindi :** Dhava, Dhaura, Bakali; **Sans :** Dhava.

The Plant

A large or medium sized tree with greenish or greenish white bark. Leaves alternate to opposite broadly elliptic, rarely orbicular, rounded, obtuse, midrib prominent, pink. Flowers sessile in small dense heads. Fruits small many in a globular head, yellowish brown, winged, beaked with the persistent calyx enclosing a single seed.

Distribution

Common in drier places on drier ridges.

Parts Used

Roots, bark, leaves, fruits, gums.

Medicinal Properties and Uses

The roots are astringent, acrid, thermogenic and stomachic. They are useful in vitiated conditions of *kapha* and *vata*, and abdominal disorders. The bark is astringent, acrid, cooling vulnerary, anti-inflammatory, urinary astringent and constipating. It is useful in vitiated conditions of *kapha* and *vata*, wounds and ulcers, inflammations, diabetes, haemorhages, diarrhoea, dysentery, skin diseases, leprosy and general debility. The leaf juice is good for otopyorrhea. The fruits are acrid, astringent, sweet, cooling and constipating. They are useful in vitiated conditions of *kapha* and *pitta*, diarrhoea and dysentery.

Ethnomedicinal Uses

Bark powder is administered twice or thrice daily in dose of about 5 gms for treatment of diarrhoea.

Anthocephalus chinensis (Lam.) Rich. ex. Walp

Family

Rubiaceae

Vernacular Names

Oriya : Kadamba; **Hindi :** Kadamb; **Sans ;** Kadamba.

The Plant

A medium to large sized deciduous tree with clean cylindrical stem horizontal branches and rounded crown. Bark dark grey with longitudinal fissures peeling off in thin scales. Leaves elliptic-oblong or ovate, 30 cm long and 15 cm broad pubescent beneath. Flowers yellow or orange in globose heads. Fruits globose pseudocarpus, yellow when ripe. Fr. February.

Distribution

Occasional in forests, usually along streams.

Parts Used

Bark, leaves, fruits.

Medicinal Properties and Uses

The bark is bitter, astringent, acrid, cooling, anodyne, anti-inflammatory, digestive, carminative, diuretic, expectorant, constipating and tonic. It is useful in vitiated conditions of *pitta*, inflammations, haemoptysis, gastropathy, fever, cough, diarrhoea, vomiting, burning sensation, dipsia, wounds, ulcers and debility. A decoction of the leaves is good for ulcers, wounds and metrorrhea. The fruits are useful in gastric irritability and fever.

Ethnomedicinal Uses

Stem bark paste (3gm) with common salt (1gm) is used as cure for eye inflammation and Juice of leaf (2ml) with common salt (1gm) is taken in empty stomach as a cure for stomach pain. A clove inserted into the bark of a live tree and kept for overnight. Thus swollen clove is taken internally for high sedation.

Ardisia solanacea Roxb.

Family

Myrsinaceae

Vernacular Names

Oriya : Batguri, Bantala, Tinkoli; **Hindi :** Bisi; **Ko :** Gara Boi.

The Plant

Small tree or large shrub. Leaves clustered towards the

ends of the branches, obovate–oblong, entire. Flowers pink. Berry black when ripe, depressed globose. Fl. March–June. Fr. Oct.–January.

Distribution

Common in forests close to streams.

Parts Used

Root

Medicinal Properties and Uses

Leaves are eaten in salads. Roots are used in fever, diarrhoea and rheumatism.

Argemone mexicana L.

Family

Papaveraceae

Vernacular Names

Hindi : Bharband; **Oriya :** Kantakusuma, Sarpuni; **Sans :** Swarna ksiri; **Sant :** Sundi satkeu; **Ko :** Siyalkanta.

The Plant

A strong branched, prickly herb, 2-3 ft. high with yellow latex and pinnatifid green and white leaves. Flowers large and bright yellow. Fruits prickly capsules, oblong-ovoid, opening by 4-6 valves; seeds numerous. Fl. Feb.-June

Distribution

On road sides and waste places.

Parts Used

Whole plant.

Medicinal Properties and Uses

The plant is bitter, acrid, cooling, vulnerary, diuretic, purgative, anti-inflammatory, expectorant, aphrodisiac, emetic, depurative, anodyne, anthelmintic, antipyretic, ophthalmic, stomachic and sedative.

The roots are useful in guinea-worm infestation, skin diseases, leprosy, colic, and malaria fever. The leaves are useful in cough, wounds, ulcers and skin diseases. Seeds yield a nauseous, bitter, non-edible oil, used in cutaneous troubles. It is cathartic. Yellow juice of plant is used in scabies and in ophthalmia. Oil is also used in soap making. Yellow juice of the plant is used in scabies and ophthalmia.

Ethnomedicinal Uses

Seed paste (3gm) mixed with seed oil of *Madhuca longifolia* (1ml) is applied fifteen days continuously on skin for the cure of eczema. The yellow juice is applied to stop bleeding from cuts and wounds. The root juice mixed with pepper is given to children for the disease supposed to be caused by cats. A teaspoonful of latex once a day is given for few days during jaundice.

Argyreia nervosa (Burm.f.) Boj.

Family

Convolvulaceae

Vernacular Names

Oriya : Mundanoi; **Hindi:** Samandar-ka-pat; **Sans** : Samudrapalaka, Vriddadaru

The Plant

Stout climber with woody stems, new shoots densely white tomentose. Leaves broadly ovate, apex rounded, densely white sericeo tomentose beneath. Flowers purple or pink. Fl. July-Sept. Fr. Nov.-April.

Distribution

Frequent in Forests

Parts Used

Roots, seeds.

Medicinal Properties and Uses

The roots are acrid, bitter, astringent, sweet, emollient, thermogenic, roborant, appetizer, digestive, carminative, cardiotonic, anti-inflammatory, expectorant, diuretic, brain tonic, nervine tonic and tonic. They are useful in vitiated conditions of kapha and vata, emaciation, wounds, ulcers, anorexia, dyspepsia, flatulence, colic, constipation, cardiac debility, inflammations, cough, bronchitis, seminal weakness, nervous weakness, cerebral disorders, obesity, anaemia, diabetes and general debility. Seeds show significant hypotensive and spasmolytic activity.

Ethnomedicinal Uses

The leaves used as poultice applied in chronic ulcers.

Argyreia speciosa Sweet

Family

Convolvulaceae

Vernacular Names

Hindi : Samandar-ka-pat; **Oriya :** Mundanoi.

The Plant

Stout climber with woody stems, new shoots densely white tomentose. Leaves broadly ovate, apex rounded, densely white sericeo tomentose beneath. Flowers purple or pink. Fl. July-Sept., Fr. Nov.-April.

Distribution

Frequent in forests.

Parts Used

Roots, leaves, seeds.

Medicinal Properties and Uses

The roots are acrid, bitter, astringent, sweet, emollient, thermogenic, appetizer, digestive, carminative, cardiotonic, anti-inflammatory, expectorant, diuretic, brain tonic, nervine tonic and tonic. They are useful in vitiated conditions of kapha and vata, emaciation, wounds, ulcers, anorexia, dyspepsia, flatulence, colic, constipation, cardiac debility, inflammations, cough, bronchitis, seminal weakness, nervous weakness, cerebral disorders, obesity, anaemia, diabetes and general debility. Seeds show significant hypotensive and spasmolytic activity. Leaves applied externally in cases of itch, eczema and other skin troubles.

Ethnomedicinal Uses

Decoction of root mixed with sugar candy is taken by old people and it is believed that they would become young. For mad dog bite and wound, root powder is snuffed and root paste is applied locally.

Aristolochia indica L.

Family

Aristolochiaceae

Vernacular Names

Oriya : Iswar-mula; **Hindi :** Isharmul; **Sans :** Ishwarimul

The Plant

A twining shrub. Stems woody below, slender and soft

above. Main rootstock woody. Leaves variable in size and shape from linear, to obovate. Flowers small, greenish-white in small branches arising from the axils of the leaves. Flowers purple. Fruit about 5 cm long, longer than broad, opening from below upwards into six valves.

Distribution

Found in hilly region and in plains.

Parts Used

Leaves, root.

Medicinal Properties and Uses

Roots and rhizomes esteemed as a gastric stimulant and bitter tonic. Chief active principle of the drug being aristolochic acid which is used for stimulating phagocytosis in infectious diseases in formulation with antibiotics. Juice of leaves used for cough and seeds for inflammations and biliousness. The dried stem and roots of the plant is useful to promote digestion and regulates menstruation.

Ethnomedicinal Uses

Root powder is snuffed, root juice is taken orally and root paste is applied locally as an antidote for snakebite.

Asplenium indicum Sledge

Family

Aspleniaceae

Vernacular Names

Ko : Kurunga

The Plant

Rhizome short, erect, stipes grey-green, scaly when young

as is rachies with linear-lanceolate, entire brown scales. Laminar linear, simple, pinna ovate, acute.

Distribution

Epiphytic on tree, commonly found in forests.

Parts Used

Rhizome

Medicinal Properties and Uses

Used for enlarged spleen, jaundice, and malaria and also for incontinence of urine.

Ethnomedicinal Uses

5g fresh rhizome paste mixed with 10 ml milk is administered thrice a day for 7 days for treatment of gonorrhoea.

Asplenium laciniatum D. Don

Family

Aspleniaceae

Vernacular Names

Ko : Mardang

The Plant

Small, tufted fern. Fronds linear oblong. Pinnate with numerous alternate or sub-opposite semi-ovate stalked pinnae, Stipes with liner scales, rachies upwards glabrous. Sori linear.

Distribution

Occasion on mossy bark, epiphytic.

Parts Used

Root

Ethnomedicinal Uses

About 10g of fresh root paste along with 100ml of cow urine is taken orally in empty stomach once in the morning for fifteen days to have relief from leucorrhoea.

Asparagus racemosus Willd.

Family

Liliaceae

Vernacular Names

Hindi : Satabari; **Oriya :** Gaisiro, Satawari, Iswar jata; **Sans:** Shatamuli; **Ko :** Huring Atkir, Khajri; **Sant :** Kedar nari.

The Plant

Slender, scrambling or scandent, suffruticose perennial, branches angular with strong, straight or decurved spines, rootstock with elongated tubers. Cladodes 2-8 nate. Flowers white, sweet scented. Berries scarlet when ripe. Fl. Sept.-Dec. Fr. Nov.-Dec.

Distribution

The plant is found almost through out India at low altitude in shades and in tropic climate in areas up to an elevation of 1400m. Fairly common in forests.

Parts Used

Tuberous roots.

Medicinal Properties and Uses

Lactogogue, aphrodisiac, weight increaser, dysentery, diabetes, TB, memory enhancer, appetizer, intrinsic hemorrhage and diarrhoea. Root powder is taken with milk in general debility and leucorrhoea. Tender leaves cooked with ghee are prescribed in night blindness. Powdered tubers taken with milk cure acidity, urine disorders as well as discharge of blood in urine.

The roots are bitter, sweet emollient, cooling, nervine tonic, constipating, galactagogue, ophthalimic, anodyne, diuretic, carminative, appetizer and tonic. They are useful in nervous disorders, dyspepsia, diarrhoea, dysentery, tumerous, inflammations, vitiated conditions of *vata* and *pitta*, burning sensations, hyperdipsia, hepatopathy, scalding of urine, throat infections, tuberculosis and gonorrhoea. Roots form a constituents of medicinal oil used for nervous and rheumatic complaints.

Ethnomedicinal Uses

Root powder (10 gms) is given twice a day with milk for the treatment of noctural pollution. Root paste in water is administered (10 gms) two times a day in gonorrhoea. Root is taken as tonic and aphrodisiac. Roots are boiled and eaten. It is regarded as an auspicious plant and kept on road to achieve good results of any work.

Atylosia scarabaeoides (L.) Benth.

Family

Fabaceae

Vernacular Names

Oriya : Ban Kultha; **Ko** : Gaisani; **Sa** : Birhoree

The Plant

Herbaceous, perennial pubescent climber. Leaflets elliptic, obovate–oblong, densely pubescent, strongly nerved. Flowers yellow or tinged with reddish-brown. Pods oblong, covered with long soft brownish hairs, with deep transverse or obliquely transverse depressed lines between the seeds. Seeds 4–6, grey brown, oblong rounded. Fl. Aug.-Dec. Fr. Oct.–April.

Distribution

Very common in open forests.

Parts Used

Whole plant.

Medicinal Properties and Uses

The plant cures diarrhoea in cattle.

Ethnomedicinal Uses

Pasty mass of seeds is taken with hot water twice continuously for fifteen days as a cure for tape–worm. The whole plant is boiled in water and bathed to children in skin diseases.

Azadirachta indica A. Juss.

Family

Meliaceae

Vernacular Names

Hindi : Nim, Nimb; **Oriya :** Nima; **Sans :** Nimba; **Sa:** Nimba-daru.

The Plant

It is a very well known tree of India. The tree has pinnate leaves. Flowers small, white, in short axillary bunches. Fruits 1.2-1.8 cm long. Green or yellow, seed one in each fruit. Fl. Feb.-May, Fr. June-July

Distribution

Cultivated all over India near habitations and on road side.

Parts Used

Bark, leaves, flowers, seeds, oil.

Medicinal Properties and Uses

The bark is bitter, astringent, acrid, depurative, demulcent, liver tonic and urinary astringent. It is used in skin trouble. The leaves are bitter, astringent, antiseptic, and appetizer, insecticidal, demulcent and refrigerant. They are useful in vitiated conditions of *pitta,* burning sensation, leprosy, skin diseases, ulcers and malarial and intermittent fever. Leaves are also considered antiseptic, applied to boils in the form of poultice; decoction is given for ulcers and eczema. Flowers are used as tonic and are stomachic. The seeds are bitter, refrigerant, ophthalmic, stomachic and tonic. Berries are purgative and emollient. They are useful in tumours, leprosy, skin diseases, intestinal worms and diabetes. The oil is bitter, anthelmintic, anodyne and depurative. It is useful in vitiated conditions of vata, chronic diseases, scabies, intestinal worms, chronic malaria, fever and leprosy.

Ethnomedicinal Uses

Aqueous extract of leaves (15ml) is taken once a day in empty stomach continuously one month for treatment of diabetes. Leaves extract is given as a blood purifier and for removal of intestinal worms. Leaf paste is applied on skin diseases and in small pox. Young shoots are used as tooth brush. Young leaves and flowers are eaten as vegetable. Oil extracted from seeds is applied on body as a mosquito repellent. Powder of dry leaves is mixed with rice and eaten by the tribal. The expressed juice of leaves (25ml) is taken internally for 5 days in chronic skin troubles.

Bacopa monnieri (L.) Pennell

Family

Scrophulariaceae

Vernacular Names

Hindi : Barami, Jalnim, Safed Chamni; **Oriya :** Brahmi, Panikundi, Jalbrahmi; **Sans :** Saumyalata, Nira-brahmi

The Plant

A prostrate or creeping, juicy, succulent, glabrous annual herb rooting at the nodes with numerous ascending branches; leaves simple, opposite, decussate, sessile, obovate-oblong or spatulate, entire, fleshy; flowers pale blue or whitish, axillary, solitary, on long slender pedicles. Fl. & Fr. April-December.

Distribution

Common in wet places near water courses.

Parts Used

Whole plant

Medicinal Properties and Uses

The plant is astringent, bitter, sweet, cooling, laxative, intellect promoting, carminative, digestive, anti-inflammatory, cardiotonic. It is useful in vitiated conditions of *kapha* and *vata,* biliousness, inflammation, epilepsy, insanity, ulcers, constipation, bronchitis, sterility, fever and general debility. Also used to improve intellect.

Ethnomedicinal Uses

The powdered leaves of about 5 gm with 2-3 black pepper are given in a single dose in bone fracture. The extract juice of leaves is mixed with milk and honey, then given in epilepsy.

Baliospermum montanum (Willd.) Muell-Arg.

Family

Euphorbiaceae

Vernacular Names

Oriya : Dumbojoda, Konaka; **Hindi :** Danti; **Sans :** Danti.

The Plant

A stout, under shrub, herbaceous plant. Leaves simple, sinuate-toothed, sometimes palmately 3-5 lobed; Flowers numerous, axillary racemes with male flowers above and a few females below; Fruits capsule; Seeds ellipsoid, smooth, mottled. Fl. & Fr. Oct.-April.

Distribution

Found in humid valleys.

Parts Used

Roots, leaves, seeds.

Medicinal Properties and Uses

Roots are purgative, anti-inflammatory, digestive, anthelmintic, diuretic, diaphoretic, febrifuge and tonic. They are useful in dropsy, constipation, jaundice, leprosy, skin diseases, anemia and leucoderma. The leaves are good for asthma and bronchitis. Seeds are drastic purgatives and stimulant and are useful in inflammations and flatulence.

Ethnomedicinal Uses

Seed are used in gastric disorders, gouts and rheumatism.

Barleria cristata L.

Family

Acanthaceae

Vernacular Names

Sans : Jhunti; **Oriya** : Banpatoli, Daskarada, Banfetali.

The Plant

Erect or diffuse under shrub, stems subterete strigose. Leaves subsessile, lanceolate, ovate, pubescent or thinly strigose on nerves both sides. Flowers blue (bright rose coloured or sometimes white), solitary or paired in the leaf axils or forming dense capitate, often few flowered spikes on the branchlets. Capsule glabrous, shining, compressed. Fl. & Fr. Sept.–February.

Distribution

Common in grasslands and hill sides.

Parts Used

Leaves, roots

Medicinal Properties and Uses

Leaves and roots are used for cough and inflammations.

Ethnomedicinal Uses

The green leaves are eaten to check stomachache. Root infusion is given twice a day for 5-7 days during acidity.

Barleria strigosa Willd.

Family

Acanthaceae

Vernacular Names

Sans : Nilakusuma; **Oriya :** Sapta phena, Banamali; **Ko :** Gasar

The Plant

Under shrub, branches strigose. Leaves large elliptic or ovate, acuminate. Flowers blue, in dense secund spikes. Capsule 1.8cm long, 4 seeded. Fl. Sept.–Nov., Fr. Feb.–May.

Distribution

Fairly common is moist and shady places in forests.

Parts Used

Leaves, roots.

Medicinal Properties and Uses

Leaves and roots are used for cough and inflammations.

Ethnomedicinal Uses

Root is made into paste, few drops of mustard oil is added to it, the preparation if inhaled for sometime relieves headache. Three table spoons of decoction of whole plants is given daily for six months in tuberculosis.

Barringtonia acutangula (L.) Gaertn.

Family

Barringtoniaceae

Vernacular Names

Hindi : Samudraphal, Hyal; **Oriya :** Hinjal, Hingala; **Sans:** Nichula; **Ko:** Dundi

The Plant

A moderate sized glabrous tree with brown somewhat fibrous bark; leaves simple, alternate, obovate-oblong, the margins minutely denticulate or crenulate, main nerves 10-13 pairs; flowers fragrant, dark scarlet in pendulous many flowered racemes; fruits bluntly quadrangular. Fl. April-June, Fr. September.

Distribution

Frequent on the banks of streams and rivers.

Parts used

Roots, leaves, fruits.

Medicinal Properties and Uses

The roots are bitter, cooling, aperient, antipyretic, stimulant and emetic. They are useful in catarrh, intermittent fevers, splenomegaly and constipation. It is similar to 'cinchona' in action when administered in malarial fever. The leaves are bitter, constipating and tonic and useful in diarrhoea and dysentery.

The fruits are acrid, bitter, anthelmintic and antipyretic. They are useful in vitiated conditions of pitta, colic, intestinal worms, ulcers, leprosy, cough and intermittent fevers.

Ethnomedicinal Uses

The leaves made into a fine paste mixed with butter milk is taken internally to check dysentery. The young leaves are cooked and eaten. Seed paste is applied on stomach to cure tympanitas.

Bauhinia purpurea L.

Family

Caesalpiniaceae

Vernacular Names

Oriya : Borda, Barada, Kuilari, Debkanchan; **Hindi :** Kaliari, Khairwal; **Sans :** Vanaraja; **Ho. :** Simidi, Singa.

The Plant

Moderate sized tree, bark ashy or dark brown, branchlets glabrous. Leaves often oblong, deeply lobed, scarcely overlapping. Flowers purple, large in terminal panicled racemes. Pods long, narrow below, somewhat broadening upward, flat dehiscent when ripe. Fl. Sept.-Feb. Fr. Feb.-March.

Distribution

Frequent in mixed forests.

Parts Used

Root, bark.

Medicinal Properties and Uses

Root carminative. Bark used in diarrhoea. Flowers are laxative and anthelmintic.

Ethnomedicinal Uses

Seeds are roasted and eaten by children. Leaves and flowers are cooked and eaten as vegetable. Flower buds are cooked as vegetables. Seeds are roasted and eaten by children. It is believed that consumption of leaves gives stamina; enable one to walk over long distances.

Bauhinia vahlii Wight & Arn.

Family

Caesalpiniaceae

Vernacular Names

Oriya : Siali, Sialipatra; **Hindi :** Malghan, Maljan, Jallur.

The Plant

An immense climber, shoots and young parts tomentose. Simple circinate tendrils mostly leaf opposed, deeply 2 lobed, deeply cordate leaves. Flowers white or cream, large in tomentose often panicled. Pods woody. Seeds oblong-ellipsoid, compressed, polished. Fl. April-June, Fr. Dec.-March.

Distribution

Common in mixed and Sal forests.

Parts Used

Root, bark, flowers.

Medicinal Properties and Uses

Roots carminative. Bark used in diarrhoea. Flowers are laxative and anthelmintic.

Ethnomedicinal Uses

The roasted seeds are eaten. Stem fibers are used for making ropes and leaves are used for making baskets and plates.

Barks of the stem and lime made into paste and are taken orally, twice a day for 3 days to cure dysentery. The decoction of leaves is taken internally to check chronic diarrhoea.

Bauhinia variegata L.

Family

Caesalpiniaceae

Vernacular Names

Oriya : Kanchano, Kanchu, Boraro Thero; **Hindi :** Kachnar, Mohota; **Ko :** Buj, Jururu, Burunga

The Plant

A moderate sized deciduous tree with vertically cracked grey bark. Leaves of 2 leaflets, connate for about two-thirds up, leaflets ovate, rounded at apex. Flowers white or pink, the uppermost petal darker and variegated. Fruits flat dehiscent pods. Fl. Feb.-March, Fr. April-May.

Distribution

Frequent in forests.

Parts Used

Root, bark.

Medicinal Properties and Uses

The root and bark are astringent, acrid, cooling, constipating, depurative, anthelmintic, vulnerary, anti-inflammatory and styptic. They are useful in diarrhoea, dysentery, skin diseases, leprosy, intestinal worms, tumours, wounds, ulcers, cough, menorrhagia and diabetes. Dried buds are used as laxative in dysentery, piles, diarrhoea and worms and against tumors.

Ethnomedicinal Uses

Root bark decoction (15ml) is taken once a day

continuously one month in empty stomach for reducing bulkiness of the body.

Bidens pilosa L.

Family

Asteraceae

Vernacular Names

Oriya : Magha latenga

The Plant

Erect annual herb, striate, hairy. Leaves opposite, leaflets ovate–lanceolate, serrate, acuminate. Heads ray florets white, disc florets yellow. Fl. & Fr. Sept.-April.

Distribution

Common weed.

Parts Used

Whole plant

Medicinal Properties and Uses

Herbs tonic and stimulant. It is used in leprosy and other skin troubles, fistulae, tumours. Decoction used for prickly heat and as a diuretic and febrifuge. Infusion of leaves, sudorific, juice used for eyes and ear troubles. Flowers used in diarrhoea. Seeds anathematic. Infusion of roots used for colic.

Bischofia javanica Blume

Family

Euphorbiaceae

Vernacular Names

Hindi : Paniala; **Ko :** Hajam.

The Plant

Tree up to 30 m tall. Leaves alternate, trifoliate, leaflets ovate-elliptic with toothed margins. Flowers minute, unisexual, cream to yellowish, borne in may-flowered axillary panicles. Fruits small brown globose berry with thin flesh. Fl. March-April, Fr. Oct.-Dec.

Distribution

Occasional near streams.

Parts Used

Leaves, stem and bark.

Medicinal Properties and Uses

The bark is used to treat stomach ulcer, mouth ulcer, and athelete's foot. Leaves are used in treating stomachache. Infusion of the bark is used in mouth infections. The plant is used to treat tuberculosis.

Bixa orellana L.

Family

Bixaceae

Vernacular Names

Oriya : Kumkum, Sundri, Sakta, Gulbas; **Hindi :** Sinduriya, Latkan; **Sans :** Sinduri

The Plant

A small handsome evergreen tree, leaves large, cordate, acuminate, glabrous. Flowers white or pink in terminal panicles. Fruits reddish brown or green capsules, clothed with soft bristles. Seeds trigonous covered with a red pulp. Fl. July-Oct. Fr. Oct.-May.

Distribution

Widely cultivated throughout India.

Parts used

Roots, bark, seeds

Medicinal Properties and Uses

The roots, bark and seeds are antiperiodic, antipyretic and astringent. They are useful in intermittent fevers and gonorrhoea. The pulp surrounding the seed is a mosquito repellant, and is useful to treat dysentery. A non-toxic dye 'Annatto dye' obtained from the pulp is used for colouring edible materials.

Blechnum orientale L.

Family

Blechnaceae

Vernacular Names

Oriya : Raktamahajal, Brahma rakshasani; **Hindi** : Hatthajori

The Plant

Large fern with an erect stout caudex clothed with fibrillose dark brown scales. Fonds simply pinnate; pinnae sessile, entire, linear, with caudate tips, uppermost with decurrent bases. The lower pinnae reduced to small rounded auricles on the stipes. Sori forming a continuous line from the base nearly to apex of pinna.

Distribution

Common in forests near streams both in open and moderate shade.

Parts Used

Rhizomes

Medicinal Properties and Uses

Rhizomes are used in urinary disorders and as an anthelmintic. Their poultice applied to boils.

Ethnomedicinal Uses

The leaf juice, 2-3 drops is put as ear drops in case of severe pain.

Blumea lacera (Burm. f.) DC.

Family

Asteraceae

Vernacular Names

Oriya : Pokasunga; **San :** Kukundarah; **Hindi :** Kukaraundha, Jangli muli

The Plant

Variable aromatic herb. Leaves simple, alternate. Flowers yellow, numerous in heads, both terminal and axillary, Corolla looks glabrus. Fruits subtetragonous achenes. Fl. & Fr. Feb.-June.

Distribution

Frequent weed.

Parts Used

Whole plant.

Medicinal Properties and Uses

The plant is bitter, astringent, acrid, anti-inflamatory, digestive, livertonic, antipyretic, diuretic and stimulant. It is useful in vitiated conditions of *pitta* and *kapha*, wounds, abdominal disorders, intestinal worms, cough, bronchitis, fever and cholera.

Boerhavia diffusa L.

Family

Nyctaginaceae

Vernacular Names

Oriya : Kharkharia, Parni; **Hindi** : Punarnava, Survari; **Sans** : Raktakanda, Raktapunarnava; **Ko** : Kenchua.

The Plant

A much branched herb, generally spreading on the ground or partly ascending. Leaves two on each mode, one smaller than the other, base of the leaves cordate. Lower surface of leaves whitish, upper green. Flowers very small, reddish, in short clusters on long axillary stalks. Fruit with five ridges, glandular. Fl. & Fr. throughout the year.

Distribution

A widely occurring weed.

Parts Used

Whole plant.

Medicinal Properties and Uses

The drug contains the alkaloid, Punarnavine. The main use of the drug is as a diuretic. It is also laxative. In moderate doses, it is recommended for asthma. Large doses can bring about vomiting.

Ethnomedicinal Uses

Tender shoots are eaten as potherb. The plant juice is antidote to rat poisoning.

Buchanania lanzan Spren g.

Family

Anacardiaceae

Vernacular Names

Oriya : Chara; **Hindi :** Chironji, Piyal; **Sans :** Priyala; **Ko :** Tarub.

The Plant

Small tree, bark rough, dark grey or black. Leaves alternate, simple, petioled, ovate–oblong, entire, rounded pubescent beneath. Flowers small, greenish, white, in terminal and axillary panicles which are shorter than the leaves. Fl. Jan.-Mar., Fr. April-May.

Distribution

Common in forests.

Parts Used

Bark, roots, leaves, fruits, oil.

Medicinal Properties and Uses

Infusion of bark is given to cure mouth sores. Paste of tender leaves is given to cure the chronic constipation. Oil is used for glandular swellings of the neck. Tree yields a gum is used in diarrhoea and intestinal pain. The roots are acrid, astringent, cooling and constipating and are useful in vitiated conditions of *pitta* and *kapha,* leprosy, skin diseases and diarrhoea. The fruits are sweet, sour, cooling, depurative, anti-inflammatory, nervine, tonic and are useful in vitiated conditions of *pitta* and *vata,* leprosy, skin diseases, nervous debility, hyperdipsia, cardiac debility, abdominal disorders and seminal weakness.

Ethnomedicinal Uses

Fruits are edible. Infusion of the bark is given to cure mouth sores. Paste of tender leaves and flower buds is given as a laxative for the treatment of chronic consumption. Wood is used for making *"Khot khora"* (bed legs) for long lasting and less weight. Infusion of the bark is administered (10ml) to cure mouth-sores. Paste of the tender leaves and flower buds is given as a laxative for the treatment of chronic constipation. The ripe fruits are eaten as tonic for strength. The root and bark made into paste is applied to chronic wounds.

Butea monosperma (Lam.) Taub.

Family

Fabaceae

Vernacular Names

Oriya : Palas; **Hindi :** Dhak, Palas; **Sans :** Palasha.

The Plant

Small or medium sized tree, trunk crooked, bark rough, dark brown. Leaves rarely 1 foliolate, linear – lanceolate, deciduous leaflets rigidly coriaceous. Flowers bright orange-red or rarely yellow. Pods stalked. Seeds oval, compressed, and brown. Fl. Feb.-April, Fr. May-July. Leafless during flowering.

Distribution

Fairly common throughout India.

Parts Used

Bark, leaves, flowers, seeds.

Medicinal Properties and Uses

The bark is acrid, bitter, astringent, thermogenic, digestive, constipating and tonic. It is useful in vitiated conditions of *pitta* and *kapha,* dyspepsia, diarrhoea, dysentery, intestinal worms, bone fractures, ulcers, tumours, hydrocele and diabetes. The leaves are astringent, anti-inflammatory, tonic, diuretic and aphrodisiac and are useful to cure boils, pimples, tumours and haemorrhages. The flowers are astringent, sweet, cooling, constipating, aphrodisiac, haemostatic, diuretic and tonic. They are useful in vitiated conditions of *pitta* and *kapha,* diarrhoea, haemorrhoides, menorrhagia, strangury, fever, leprosy, skin diseases, swellings and are very efficacious in birth control. The seeds are purgative, ophthalmic, anthelmintic and tonic. They are useful in herps, skin diseases, ringworm, epilepsy, round worm, flatulence, constipation and diabetes.

Ethnomedicinal Uses

Roots are used in tuberculosis. Pastes of seeds are applied on skin diseases. Latex mixed with honey cures piles, bite and stomach trouble. 3 gm bark paste is mixed with ghee and taken for 3 days during menstruation period for anti-abortion.

Butea superba Roxb.

Family

Fabaceae

Vernacular Names

Oriya : Nai Palaso; **Sans :** Latapalasha; **Hindi :** Palasa lata **Ko :** Morud.

The Plant

Large woody climber with smooth brownish bark, exuding a reddish gum from the wounds. Leaflets green and thinly hairy. Flowers bright orange red, borne in great profusion along the leafless branches. Pods longer stalked. Fr. March-Apr., Fr. June-July. Leafless Feb.-May.

Distribution

Occasional in forest.

Parts Used

Gum

Medicinal Properties and Uses

Gum is used as tonics and poultices. Decoction of shoots is considered emollient and sedative, used in piles. Seeds sedative and anthelmintic.

Ethnomedicinal Uses

Root powder is mixed with ghee or honey and given for some days to cure impotency.

Callicarpa macrophylla Vahl.

Family

Verbenaceae

Vernacular Names

Hindi : Priyamgu, Daya; **Sans :** Priyangu, Phallini; **Ko :** Bunduan

The Plant

Stout shrub, branches densely stellate tomentose. Leaves elliptic, broadly oblong or oval lanceolate, crenate-serrate. Flowers pink, in dense, dichotomous cymes. Drupe white, glabrous. Fl. Aug.–Oct., Fr. Nov.–January.

Distribution

Occasional in forests.

Parts Used

Flowers, fruits, roots, leaves.

Medicinal Properties and Uses

The flowers and fruits are bitter, sweet, astringent, acrid, cooling, digestive, depurative and febrifuge. They are useful in rheumatoid, arthritis, burning sensation, ulcers, dyspepsia, flatulence, colic, diarrhoea and dysentery, skin diseases, diabetes, fever and general weakness. The leaves are useful in gout and arthralgia. Roots yield aromatic oil which is used in stomach disorders.

Callicarpa tomentosa (L.) Murr.

Family

Verbenaceae

Vernacular Names

Oriya : Bodopatri; **Sans :** Priyangu

The Plant

Small or moderate sized tree. 4-angled, densely tomentose, bark light or brown. Leaves large–elliptic ovate, lanceolate, entirely or slightly toothed. Flowers small, purple in dichotomous corymbose. Drupe purple, finally black. Fl. April–May. Fr. August.

Distribution

Frequent

Parts Used

Bark, leaves

Medicinal Properties and Uses

Decoction of the bark used for skin troubles, hepatic, obstructions and fever. Leaves boiled in milk and used as a wash for apathies of the mouth.

Calotropis gigantea R.Br.

Family

Asclepiadaceae

Vernacular Names

Oriya : Aroko, Urak; **Hindi :** Madar; **Sans :** Swetarka; **Ko :** Patladhudha; **Sant :** Parkha.

The Plant

A large hard much-branched milky shrub, very pale in colour, the branches, leaves and inflorescence covered with loose soft white wool. Leaves opposite, subsessile or shortly petioled, obovate, obtuse, rounded. Flowers beautiful lilac, rosy or purple tinted in umbellate lateral cymes. Fruits fleshy follicles, green, seeds with abundant with coma.

Distribution

Frequent in open waste ground.

Parts Used

Whole plant.

Medicinal Properties and Uses

The dried whole plant is good tonic, expectorant, depurative and anthelmintic. The dried root bark is a substitute for ipecacuanha. The root bark is febrifuge, anthelmintic, depurative, expectorant and laxative and is useful in cutaneous diseases, intestinal worms, cough, ascites and anasarca. The powdered root promotes gastric secretions and is useful in asthma, bronchitis and dyspepsia. The leaves are useful in treatment of paralysis, arthralgia, swellings and intermittent fevers.

The flowers are bitter, digestive, astringent, stomachic, anthelmintic and tonic. They are useful in asthma, catarrh, anorexia, inflammations and tumours. In large doses it is purgative and emetic.

Ethnomedicinal Uses

Decoction of root (3 ml) with paste of Piper longum (1gm) is given to women in empty stomach continuously ten days for the treatment of leucorrhoea. Dry and root powder is mixed with leaf juice and made tablets. One tablet is taken one week with hot water to cure colic.

Calycopteris floribunda Lam.

Family

Combretaceae

Vernacular Names

Oriya : Dubopatli, Kokundia, Sil; **Hindi :** Kokkarai.

The Plant

A scandent woody shrub with slender brown streaked diffuse branches occasionally twining around supports and storing water abundantly. Leaves simple, opposite, elliptic or ovate, acute or acuminate, surfaces tomentose. Flowers yellowish green. Fruits 5-ribed, one seeded, crowned with strongly 3-nerved persistent calyx lobes. Fl. Mar.-April, Fr. May.

Distribution

Frequent in forests.

Parts Used

Leaves, fruits

Medicinal Properties and Uses

The leaves are bitter, astringent, laxative, anthelmintic, depurative, diaphoretic and febrifuge. They are useful in intestinal worms, colic, leprosy, malarial fever, dysentery, ulcers and vomiting. The fruits are useful in jaundice, ulcers, pruritus and skin diseases.

Camellia sinensis (L.) Kuntz

Family

Theaceae

Vernacular Names

Oriya : Cha, Chagaccho, Tea plant; **Hindi :** Chai; **Sans :** Syamaparni.

The Plant

An evergreen shrub or tree. Leaves simple, alternate, elliptic-ovate or lanceolate with serrate margins, usually glabrous, leathery. Flowers white, fragrant. Fruits depressed capsules. Fl. Feb.-March, Fr. May-June.

Distribution

Planted

Parts Used

Leaves

Medicinal Properties and Uses

The leaves are astringer [illegible] itter, thermogenic, appetizer, digestive, carminative, diure[illegible] n[illegible] nervine tonic. They are useful in hyperdipsia, hemicrania o[illegible]halmia, inflammations, abdomina[illegible] disorders and fatigue.

Canscora decussata ([illegible]b.) Schult.

Family

Gentianaceae

Vernacular Names

Oriya : Paincki mircha; **Hindi :** Sankhapuli; **Ko :** Kalmeg

The Plant

An erect dichotomously branched annual upto 60cm in height with 4-winged stems and decussate branches. Leaves sessile, lanceolate, ovate or oblong. Flowers white or pinkish. Capsule oblong. Seeds very small, brown, reticulate. Fl. & Fr. Sept.-December.

Distribution

Common in moist and shady places.

Parts Used

Whole plant

Medicinal Properties and uses

The plant is bitter, acrid, astringent, thermogenic, laxative, vulnerary, emollient, alexeteric, anthelmintic, appetizer, intellect promoting, aphrodisiac, depurative, rejuvenating and tonic. It is useful in vitiated conditions of kapha, inflammation, ascites, abdominal disorders, intestinal worms, insanity, epilepsy, nervous debility, forgetfulness, leucoderma, leprosy, skin diseases, tuberculosis, ulcers and general debility.

Ethnomedicinal Uses

Dried stems (not leaves or flowers) are kept in water overnight, tea coloured filtrate is orally taken in stomachache an as blood purifier.

Canscora diffusa (Vahl) R. Br.

Family

Asteraceae

Vernacular Names

Oriya : Burrurria

The Plant

Repeated dichotomously branched herb, stems 4-angled. Leaves sessile or sub sessile, ovate, oblong or narrowly lanceolate. Flowers small pink. Fl. & Fr. most part of the year.

Distribution

Fairly common in moist places, river banks.

Parts Used

Whole plant.

Medicinal Properties and Uses

Fresh juice is prescribed in insanity, epilepsy and nervous debility.

Ethnomedicinal Uses

Plant is used in headache and malarial fever.

Canthium dicoccum (Gaertn.) Teijsm. & Binnend.

Family

Rubiaceae

Vernacular Names

Oriya : Kumar chinki, Dolsingh, Karuna; **Ko :** Jordaru.

The Plant

Low branched tree or large shrub with spreading or dropping branchlets flattened at the upper extremities. Bark smooth but with vertical cracks, dark grey. Leaves ovate or lanceolate, acuminate, shining above, pale beneath. Flowers greenish or white. Fruits black, globose or sub globose. Fl. Feb.-Apr., Fr. April-May.

Distribution

Common in mixed forests.

Parts Used

Bark

Medicinal Properties and Uses

Bark employed as a febrifuge and applied externally to fracture. The bark is used for killing fishes due to presence of tannin.

Ethnomedicinal Uses

Infusion of powdered bark is given in doses of 30 ml to children suffering from stomach-ache and worms.

Carica papaya L.

Family

Caricaceae

Vernacular Names

Oriya : Amrutabhanda, Bhanda, Papaya; **Hindi :** Papaya, Papeeta; **Ko :** Jhoda.

The Plant

A small, soft wooded, fast growing, short lived laticiferous tree. Leaves deeply lobed, palm like with characteristically long, hollow petiole. Flowers white or yellowish white, rarely bisexual, males in long drooping panicles; females in short clusters. Fruits one-chambered, succulent, indehiscent, spherical or cylindrical. Seeds many, yellowish brown, ash coloured or black. Fl. & Fr. Most parts of the year.

Distribution

Cultivated in garden throughout India.

Parts Used

Fruits, latex

Medicinal Properties and Uses

The fruits are bitter, acrid, thermogenic, anodyne, stomachic, appetizer, digestive, carminative, anthelmintic, anti-inflammatory and diuretic. They are useful in vitiated conditions of vata, cough, bronchitis, stomachalgia, dyspepsia, anorexia, intestinal worms, haemorrhoides, inflammations, ringworm, skin diseases, urinary calculus and injures of the urinary tract. The latex is anthelmintic, anodyne, laxative, digestive, galactagogue, depurative, febrifuge and tonic. It is useful in round worm infestation, stomachalgia, dyspepsia, constipation, menorrhoea, skin diseases, leprosy, fever and general debility.

Ethnomedicinal Uses

Latex is taken for some days as livertonic.

Cassia fistula L.

Family

Caesalpiniaceae

Vernacular Names

Oriya : Sonari, Bara chakunda; **Hindi :** Baahawaa, Amaltas **Sans :** Suvarnaka, Aragwadha.

The Plant

Small or medium–sized tree, bark smooth, pale or whitish leaflets 4–8 pairs, ovate, lanceolate, accuminate, glabrous. Flowers light yellow in long pendulous racemes. Pods short stipitate. Seeds many. Fl. Apr.-June, Fr. found on the tree during most part of the year. Deciduous: March.

Distribution

Common in forests.

Parts Used

Root, leaves, fruits.

Medicinal Properties and Uses

Leaves made into paste is orally taken to purify blood. Leaves are used in skin diseases. Dried fruits used as a purgative, laxative for habitual constipation. Root is used in common cold.

Ethnomedicinal Uses

5 gm gum is mixed with warm milk and given to cure constipation. Bark paste is applied locally for healing and raw juice of fresh bark is taken orally for dysentery.

Cassia occidentalis L.

Family

Caesalpiniaceae

Vernacular Names

Oriya : Kasinda, Kala Chakunda; **Hindi :** Raantaakalla, Kasondi; **Ko :** Kaiu, Chakodara.

The Plant

Erect, glabrous herb or under shrub, whole plant foetid. Leaves 15-30 cm long, leaflets 4-5 pairs, ovate–lanceolate. Flowers yellow in axillary and terminal racemes. Pods short stipitate, flattened. Seeds ovoid.

Distribution

Common weed

Parts Used

Leaves, root, seed.

Medicinal Properties and Uses

The leaves and seeds are used in cough, ulcers, and leprosy and also in skin diseases. Roots are bitter, acrid, diuretic, anti-inflammatory, digestive, stomachic and tonic. They are useful in inflammation, diabetes, elephantiasis, ringworm, colic flatulence and epilepsy. Root is considered expectorant. It is used in snakebite. A paste made out of roots is specific for ringworm, eczema and other skin ailments. Bark in infusion or the powdered seeds with honey are given in diabetes.

Ethnomedicinal Uses

The leaves, roots and seeds are used in cough and whooping cough and also in skin diseases. Roots are used in gastric disorders. Leaves and seeds are made into paste and applied on skin infections.

Cassia tora L.

Family

Caesalpiniaceae

Vernacular Names

Oriya : Chakunda; **Hindi :** Taakalla, Panevar, Chakunda, Cakvat; **Sans :** Chakramarda.

The Plant

A herbaceous foetid annual weed. Leaves pinnately compound, leaflets three pairs, obovate-oblong, oblique. Flowers yellow. Fruits subtetragonous obliquely septate pods. Fl. Sept.-Nov., Fr. Nov.-December

Distribution

Common in forests as weed.

Parts Used

Leaves, seeds.

Medicinal Properties and Uses

The leaves and seeds are acrid, thermogenic, laxative, depurative, antiperiodic, anthelmintic, liver tonic, expectorant, and are useful in ringworm, leprosy, skin diseases, hepatopathy, flatulence, colic, dyspepsia, intermittent fever, constipation, cough, bronchitis, cardiac disorder and haemorrhoids. Leaves pounded are applied on cuts, act like tincture iodine, applied against eczema. Seeds are used externally and internally for all sorts of eye diseases and are recommended for arthritis and hemicrania.

Ethnomedicinal Uses

Seed paste is used in the treatment of ringworm and itch. The crushed seeds about 5gms are taken with water in cough.

Catharanthus roseus (L.) G. Don

Family

Apocynaceae

Vernacular Names

Oriya : Sadabihari, Ainsakati; **Hindi** : Sadabahar

The Plant

Perennial herb or sub shrubs. High stems pinkish – red, much branched. Leaves opposite, obovate, oblong, rounded at apex, glabrous, polished. Flowers white or pink. In the axil of the leaves. Follicle cylindrical, narrow, slightly arched-recurved in pairs. Seeds numerous, tiny, blackish-brown. Fl. & Fr. All the year round.

Distribution

Commonly cultivated in garden.

Parts Used

Roots, leaves.

Medicinal Properties and Uses

The leaves are useful in treating oliguria, haematuria, diabetics mellitus and menstrual disorders. The roots and leaves in the form of decoction or extract are active on hypertension. The purified alkaloids extracted from the leaves are effective in treating leukemia and those from the roots are used to induce cerebra vascular dilation and for hypertension.

Ethnomedicinal Uses

Root paste is applied twice a day continuously seven days for healing of septic wounds and fresh leaf juice (few drops) mixed with a cup of water and is taken in empty stomach for the treatment of blood dysentery.

Catunaregam spinosa (Thunb.) Tirveng

Family

Rubiaceae

Vernacular Names

Oriya : Kalai kanta, Potua; **Ko :** Potua; **Hindi :** Mainphal, Karhar

The Plant

Small tree or large shrub usually armed with straight axillary spines, bark grey, fissured. Leaves mostly clustered, obovate, obtuse or shortly acuminate. Flowers white, turning yellow, solitary. Berry yellow, when ripe, globose or ovoid. Fl. March-June, Fr. Nov.-January.

Distribution

Common in open or dense forests.

Parts Used

Bark, fruit, root.

Medicinal Properties and Uses

The bark is astringent, emetic, abortifacient, anodyne, constipating and antiseptic. It is useful in ostalgia during fever, diarrhoea, dysentery, cuts and vitiated conditions of *vata*. The fruits are bitter, astringent, acrid, sweet, thermogenic, anti-inflammatory, carminative and are useful in vitiated conditions of *pitta* and *kapha*, pains and sprains, inflammations, gout, leprosy, and asthma. Roots possess insecticides and insect repelling properties.

Ethnomedicinal Uses

Seed paste with resin of Sal (*Shorea robusta*), fermented rice water or curd is applied over infected skin till disappearance of disease.

Celastrus paniculatus Willd.

Family

Celastraceae

Vernacular Names

Oriya : Pengu, Katta pangu, Laibeheda; **Hindi :** Malkamni, Malkungi; **Sans :** Jyotismati; **Ko :** Kujri

The Plant

An unarmed large perennial deciduous climbing or scrambling shrub. Leaves simple, alternate, ovate or obovate, crenulate, glabrous, lateral nerves arching. Flowers greenish white in terminal drooping panicles. Fruits capsules, depressed-globose, 3-lobed, bright yellow when ripe. Fl. Apr.-June, Fr. Oct.-January.

Distribution

Common in forests.

Parts Used

Bark, leaves, seeds, oil

Medicinal Properties and Uses

Various parts of plant are used in sore throat, anaemia, colic, syphills, carbuncle. Leaves are emmenagogue. Leaves and roots used as poultice to cure headache. Bark is abortifacient. Decoction of bark used in bronchitis. Seeds are bitter, emetic, alterative, laxative, stimulant, nervine and aphrodisiac. Decoction of seeds is given in rheumatism, leprosy, gout, various fevers, paralysis. The seed oil is bitter, thermogenic and intellect promoting and is useful in abdominal disorders, beri-beri and sores.

Ethnomedicinal Uses

Oil from seeds is used as mosquito repellent, leeches and other biting insects. Stem bark and seed oil is taken in acute stomach pain. The bark of the root is prescribed to take orally to increase urine flow and to induce vomiting.

Celosia argentea L.

Family

Amaranthaceae

Vernacular Names

Hindi : Safed murgha; **Oriya** : Lobanga, Sirali, Manjur, Chulia.

The Plant

Erect glabrous herb or sub shrub. Leaves lanceolate oblong. Spikes very often excessively developed, cocks comb-like, variously branched, red or yellow. Fl. & Fr. Aug.-January.

Distribution

Common weed in cultivated land and waysides.

Parts Used

Flowers, seed.

Medicinal Properties and Uses

Flowers are astringent. They are used in diarrhoea. Seeds are demulcent and are prescribed in painful micturition, cough and dysentery.

Centella asiatica (L.) Urb.

Family

Apiaceae

Vernacular Names

Oriya : Thalkudi; **Sans :** Mandukaparni; **Hindi :** Brihmi, Brahma manduki, Brahmi; **Ko :** Thalkudi

The Plant

The plant trails on the ground and its creeping stems bear roots on their nodes. Leaves small, 2-4 cm diameter, sometime, more rounded or broad kidney shaped, their margins toothed. Flowers minute, pinkish red, 3-6 in a cluster. Fruits small, like a grain of barley, 7-9 ridged. Fl. & Fr. most part of the year.

Distribution

Common in wet places.

Parts Used

Leaves, stem.

Medicinal Properties and Uses

The leaves or entire plant parts are boiled in water and this decoction is given in treatment of leprosy. The plant is also considered useful in certain kinds of tuberculosis and as an alternative and tonic for brain.

Ethnomedicinal Uses

The bruished leaves mixed with turmeric is applied externally in skin allergies. A decoction is prepared with the leaf of *Ocimum tenuiflorum* and seeds of *Piper nigrum* and given thrice daily for 7 days to cure fever.

Centipeda minima (L.) A. Braun & Asch.

Family

Asteraceae

Vernacular Names

Oriya : Nakchika; **Hindi :** Nak-chikni, Pochitti.

The Plant

Small prostrate herb with many branched stems spreading from the root. Leaves oblanceolate or ovate oblong, coarsely toothed or lobed. Heads very small, sessile, globose. Achenes minute. Fl. & Fr. March-January.

Distribution

Occasional in open moist places.

Parts Used

Leaves, seeds.

Medicinal Properties and Uses

Powdered leaves and minute seeds used in the preparation of snuff. Infusion of the herb used in ophthalmia. Seeds considered vermifuge.

Chlorophytum arundinaceum Baker

Family

Liliaceae

Vernacular Names

Hindi : Sufed musli; **Oriya :** Saphed musali, Bhinka, Jhinka, Musli; **Sans :** Musali; **Ko :** Jaringa.

The Plant

Herb, root fiber at the ends with thick, cylindrical tubers. Leaves petiolate, oblong, lanceolate or oblanceolate, acuminate, many nerved. Flowers white, star like. Seeds 1-6 per cell. Suborbicular, black, minutely tessellate or punctate. Fl. March-July. Fr. Sept.-December.

Distribution

Common in forests.

Parts Used

Root

Medicinal Properties and Uses

Root is used as health tonic. Aqueous extract of root is taken orally to cure cough. Decoction is given to cure the arthritis.

Ethnomedicinal Uses

Roots are taken as food in fever. The tubers of about 20g is boiled with milk and is taken twice a day for a month incase of impotency and weakness.

Christella parasitica (L.) Lev.

Family

Thelypteridaceae

Vernacular Names

Ko : Paranga

The Plant

Rhizome long, creeping. Stipes long, laminar long, pinnae acuminate, somewhat narrowed to their bases which are slightly auricled on acroscopic side. Pinnae lobed. Sori on adjacent veins oftern contiguous. Fertile most part of the year.

Distribution

Frequent in hill forests.

Parts Used

Root

Ethnomedicinal Uses

5g fresh root along with 1g fresh root of *Asparagus racemosus* Willd. and 5g of sugar boiled in 250 ml of water. The decoction orally administered for 10 days to cure spermatorrhea

---

Chrysanthemum indicum DC.

Family

Asteraceae

Vernacular Names

Oriya : Sonna rasi; **Hindi :** Guldaaudi

The Plant

Annual or perennial herb. Stems sulcate, glabrous. Leaves alternate, deeply lobed and irregularly toothed. Inflorescence axillary or terminal corymb of many heads. Flowers yellow. Fl. & Fr. June-December.

Distribution

Occasional in open grassy places.

Parts Used

Flowers

Medicinal Properties and Uses

The flowers possess antibacterial and antihypertensive properties. They are utilized in medication for photopsia, vertigo, fever, headache, ophthalmia, hypertension and phelgmon. Their long-term use is rejuvenating. They are also a constituent of composite prescriptions. Washing with the decoction and poultices of pounded flowers are effective in furunculosis and impetigo.

Cissus quadrangularis L.

Family

Vitaceae

Vernacular Names

Oriya : Hadjoda, Hadabhanga; **Hindi :** Harjora

The Plant

Rambling shrub, often climbing over bushes and trees to some length. Stems fleshy, 4-angled, jointed, 4-winged or margined, leafless or bearing leaves at the nodes during rainy and cold season. Leaves short petioled. Flowers greenish-white in short penduncle, small. Seeds ellipsoid. Fl. & Fr. Apr.-January.

Distribution

Common on rocks and planted in gardens.

Parts Used

Roots, stem, leaves.

Medicinal Properties and Uses

Plant is light, sweet, hot, alterative, carminative,

anthelmintic, aphrodisiac and stomachic. It is useful in dyspepsia, indigestion, piles, worms and asthma. It has ability to rejoin broken bones. Juice of plant is beneficial in scurvey. Infusion of plant is purgative. A paste of the stem is plastered over the fracture and swellings. Powdered dry shoots are used in digestive troubles. It is also applied in cases of otorrhoea and epistaxis and used as alterative. The stem beaten into a paste is given in asthma and powdered root is a specific in the treatment of fractured bones. Fresh shoots are pounded and applied for burns and wounds.

Ethnomedicinal Uses

Paste of the stem and banana flower is applied to the head of the women for ten days or so for preventing conception.

Citrus aurantium L.

Family

Rutaceae

Vernacular Names

Oriya : Kamala; **Hindi :** Khatta, Santre.

The Plant

A medium sized thorny tree or a shrub with greenish white, glabrous, young shoots. Leaves foliolate. Flowers white, large, very fragrant. Fruit round, orange coloured, bright yellow when ripe.

Distribution

Cultivated and sometime self-sown.

Parts Used

Leaves, fruits.

Medicinal Properties and Uses

The fruits are sour, bitter, astringent, thermogenic, laxative, appetizer, stomachic and digestive. Plant is used against enlarged spleen, stomach-ache and menorrhagia. Leaves used as tea in headache and stomach pain.

Ethnomedicinal Uses

Leaf juice of *tulsi* and and *lembu* are given twice a day for 1-2 days in dysentery. Leaf juice of *tulsi* and seeds are given twice a day in stomach-ache.

Citrus medica L.

Family

Rutaceae

Vernacular Names

Oriya : Jambira, Janglilembbu; **Hindi :** Baranimbo, Bijaura

The Plant

An evergreen armed shrubs with straggling thorny branches and smooth yellowish brown bark. Leaves oblong or elliptic with acute or rounded apex, coriaceous, glabrous and dull dark green above. Flowers white. Fruits large berries, oblong or globose, yellow when ripe. Fl. Jan.-June, Fr. Nov.-December.

Distribution

Wild along streams in the moisture valleys.

Parts Used

Fruit, leaves, seeds.

Medicinal Properties and Uses

The roots are laxative, anthelmintic and diuretic and are useful in constipation, colic, flatulence, strangury, renal and vesical calculi, tumours, vomiting and dental caries. The leaves are anodyne. The ripe fruit is stimulant and tonic. Fruit is expellant of poisons. Yellow pulp is aromatic and stomachic. Fruit juice is astringent, digestive and refrigerating. The seeds are stimulant, anti-inflammatory, and are useful in inflammations, skin diseases, amenorrhoea and haemorrhoids.

Clausena excavata Burm. f.

Family

Rutaceae

Vernacular Names

Oriya : Agnijal; **Ko** : Ote armu, Dukipotum.

The Plant

Undershrub, shoots herbaceous, tomentose. Leaves 9-many foliolate, rachis tomentose, leaflets alternate, hairy especially on the nerves. Flowers greenish white. Berry ellipsoid or ovoid. Fl. April-May, Fr. June-July.

Distribution

Frequent in forests.

Parts Used

Root, leaves, flowers.

Medicinal Properties and Uses

Plant is diuretic and is useful for digestion. Infusion of the roots, flowers and leaves is used for colic.

Cleome viscosa L.

Family

Capparidaceae

Vernacular Names

Oriya : Anasoriso; **Hindi** : Hulhul, Hurhur; **Sans** : Adityabhakta, Arkakanta; **Ko** : Chamani

The Plant

An annual sticky herb with strong penetrating odour. Leaves 3-5 foliolate, gradually becoming shorter upwards. Flowers yellow in lax raceme. Fruit capsule, compressed, hairy throughout. Fl. & Fr. May-October.

Distribution

Occasional

Parts Used

Leaves

Medicinal Properties and Uses

Leaves are applied to arthritic joints. Plant is diuretic. The juice is reputed to relieve headaches and migraine if sniffed, but as this might destroy the mucous.

Ethnomedicinal Uses

The powdered root is put on the lips to restore consciousness, when a person faints.

Clerodendrum indicum (L.) Kuntze

Family

Verbenaceae

Vernacular Names

Oriya : Nagri, Jathia, Pudanargi; **Hindi** : Bharangi, Barangi; **Sans** : Bhargi

The Plant

Shrub or herb with strict, annual, hollow, glabrous stem. Leaves rarely opposite, lanceolate, coarsely toothed. Flowers white or cream. Drupe blue. Fl. June-Aug., Fr. Aug.-December.

Distribution

Occasional in grassland.

Parts Used

Root

Medicinal Properties and Uses

Root used in asthma, cough and scrofulous affections. Leaves vermifuge.

Ethnomedicinal Uses

Young shoots are given to cattle in diarrhoea, worms and flatulence. Leaf paste is applied over forehead in headache. Dried root powder is smoked once a day continuously one month for the treatment of asthma and fresh leaf paste with long peppers (*Piper longum*) is used in the ratio of 2: twice a day in the early morning and before sleep continuously twenty days as cure for swelling of legs.

Clerodendrum serratum (L.) Moon

Family

Verbenaceae

Vernacular Names

Hindi : Barangi; **Oriya :** Samarkand, Buda rasana; **Sans :** Bharangi; **Kol :** Saramlutum.

The Plant

Shrub or undershrub with herbaceous stems from a

perennial root stock, branches 4 angled above. Leaves opposite or ternate, shortly petiolate, oblong obovate, coarsely serrate. Flowers blue (pale pink or white) in large terminal cymose panicles. Drupe broadly obovoid. Fl. June–Oct. Fr. Nov.–December.

Distribution

Common in forests and grasslands..

Parts Used

Root, leaves, seed.

Medicinal Properties and Uses

Roots are used in rheumatism and dyspepsia. Seeds aperient and are used in dropsy. Leaves are used as febrifuge and also employed in external applications for cephalagia and ophthalmia. Seeds aperients and are used in dropsy. Leaf paste is applied in cuts and wounds. The roots are employed against snake–bite.

Ethnomedicinal Uses

Root paste (5gms) is given twice daily in diarrhoea.

Clerodendrum viscosum Vent. Jard. Malm.

Family

Verbenaceae

Vernacular Names

Hindi : Bhant; **Sans :** Baribarha; **Oriya :** Kunti, Madhvi; **Ko :** Chamgar, Kula-marsal.

The Plant

Shrub or under shrub, branches hairy. Leaves ovate or

broadly ovate, entire or dentate, acuminate, base cordate or rounded. Flowers white with pink center or pink spotted, in large terminal corymbose panicles. Drupe bluish–black, usually of a single globose drupel, at first enclosed by the calyx which opens widely on maturity. Fl. Jan.–March, Fr. April–July.

Distribution

Common in shady waste places, along streams,

Parts Used

Leaves.

Medicinal Properties and Uses

Leaves are used as bitter tonic, vermifuge, laxative and cholagogue. Fresh leaf juice is introduced into the rectum for removal of ascarids. Leaves and roots are used in external applications for tumours. Leaves warmed with ghee are applied to the head in catarrhal colds.

Ethnomedicinal Uses

Leaf paste rubbed over scalps, stops falling hairs, relieves headache and promotes hair growth. Plant paste is applied on cuts and wounds. Roots are given in gastric disorder as well as in pains and body aches.

Clitoria ternatea L.

Family

Fabaceae

Vernacular Names

Oriya : Aparajita; **Hindi** : Aparajita; **Sans** : Aparajita.

The Plant

A good looking perennial twining herb with terete stem and branches. Leaves imparipinnate, leaflets mostly 5, elliptic.

Flowers blue rarely white, solitary or axillary penduncles. Pods linear flat. Seeds 6-10, smooth, yellowish brown. Fl. July-Oct., Fr. Nov.-December.

Distribution

Throughout India in hedges and thickers, also cultivated in garden.

Parts Used

Root, leaves, seeds

Medicinal Properties and Uses

Roots are bitter, refrigerant, ophthalmic, laxative, intellect promoting, diuretic, anthelmintic, depurative and tonic and are useful in ophthalmopathy, tubercular glands, amentia, burning sensation, helminthiasis, asthma, leprosy, bronchitis, pulmonary tuberculosis and ulcers. The leaves are useful in otalgia, hepatopathy and eruptions. The seeds are cathartic and are useful in visceralgia.

Ethnomedicinal Uses

Root paste is used as antivenus.

Coccinia grandis (L.) Voigt

Family

Cucurbitaceae

Vernacular Names

Oriya : Bano kundri, Kundri; **Hindi :** Kundru; **Sans :** Bimbi

The Plant

A perennial much branched handsome tendril climber, root some times tuberous. Leaves ovate or orbicular entire. Male flowers clustered, white. Fruit oblong, red when ripe. Seed oblong, compressed, yellowish green. Fl. & Fr. most part of the year.

Distribution

Found growing wild and common in hedges.

Parts Used

Roots, leaves, fruits.

Medicinal Properties and Uses

The roots are cooling and aphrodisiac and are useful in vomiting, burning sensation and uterine discharges. The leaves are bitter, sweet, astringent and cooling and are useful in vitiated conditions of *kapha* and *pitta*. The fruits are cooling, sweet, astringent, depurative, antipyretic, galactagogue and expectorant, and are useful in burning sensation, leprosy, skin diseases, intermittent fever, asthma, cough, bronchitis and jaundice. The fruits and leaves of the bitter variety are bitter, acrid, thermogenic, emetic, purgative, vulnerary, anti-inflammatory, liver tonic and are useful in wounds ulcers, inflammations, helminthiasis, dyspepsia, hepatopathy, jaundice, skin diseases, leprosy, fever, asthma, cough, diabetes and anaemia.

Ethnomedicinal Uses

Leaves are mashed in water and bandaged over filarial swellings.

Cochlospermum religiosum (L.) Alston

Family

Cochlospermaceae

Vernacular Names

Oriya : Kontopalas, Kopasia, Pithalu; **Hindi :** Kumbi, Galgal; **Sans :** Girisalmalika; **Ko :** Opubaha, Hupu.

The Plant

A small deciduous tree with smooth, ash coloured, fibrous, deeply furrowed bark containing a gum. Leaves palmetely 5-lobed, tomentose beneath. Flowers large, golden yellow in terminal panicles appearing after the leaf fall. Fruits large, pear shaped. Fl. Feb.-Mar. Fr. Apr.-June.

Distribution

Frequent in dry deciduous forests.

Parts Used

Leaves, flowers, gum

Medicinal Properties and Uses

Dried leaves and flowers are used as stimulant, and the young leaves are used as a cooling wash for the hair. The gum is sweet, thermogenic, anodyne and sedative, and is useful in cough, diarrhoea, dysentery and trachoma.

Ethnomedicinal Uses

The gum mixed with raw sugar as taken internally for dysentery.

Combretum roxburghii Spreng.

Family

Combretaceae

Vernacular Names

Oriya : Atundi, Korakokundia; **Ko :** Phalandu

The Plant

Large sarmentose or scandent rusty pubescent shrub. Leaves oblong or obovate – oblong, shortly suddenly acuminate, coriaceous, glabrous. Spikes rusty villous, large axillary and terminal panicles with conspicuous large white bracts. Flowers 5 merous. Fruits oblong or elliptic. Fl. Nov.-Feb., Fr. March-June. Leaves on the panicle turning white or yellowish-white during November.

Distribution

Fairly common especially in valleys and also in scrub forests.

Parts Used

Root, bark.

Medicinal Properties and Uses

The root or bark paste is orally administered twice a day, first in empty stomach next after meal in loose motion. Leaf paste is used on sore and infusion of the leaf is used as blood purifier.

Ethnomedicinal Uses

The root or bark paste is orally administered twice a day, first empty stomach, next after meal in loose motion, leaf paste is used on sore and infusion of the leaf is used as blood purifier.

Commelina benghalensis L.

Family

Commelinaceae

Vernacular Names

Hindi : Kanchira; **Sans :** Kanchata; **Oriya :** Kaniseera, Khet papra, Ranasiri

The Plant

Diffuse, branched, sub succulent herb, stem often creeping and rooting below, glabrous, often pilose below the nodes.

Leaves ovate, often inequilaterally, obtuse, acute or rounded at the tip. Spathe 1-3 together, conduplicate with the margins connate. Flowers small blue. Capsule membranous, pyriform. Seeds rugose, closely pitted. Fl. & Fr. July-November.

Distribution

Common weed in wet places.

Parts Used

Whole plant.

Medicinal Properties and Uses

Mucilaginous and starchy rhizomes are cooked and eaten. Herb considered demulcent, emollient, laxative and refrigerant. It is used in leprosy.

Ethnomedicinal Uses

The green leaves are eaten as vegetables.

Costus speciosus (Koenig) Sm.

Family

Zingiberaceae

Vernacular Names

Hindi : Keu; **Sanskrit** : Kushta; **Oriya** : Gaigobra, Kena, Keukand, Kokola; **Ko** : Kero.

The Plant

Herb. Leaves elliptic-oblong, acute, acuminate, glabrous above, pubescent and paler beneath. Flowers white, very large, in densely terminal spikes, bracts red. Fl. & Fr. July–Dec.

Distribution

Common throughout the area, especially in shady places.

Parts Used

Stems, rhizomes.

Medicinal Properties and Uses

The rhizomes possess anti–inflammatory activity. It is indicated in the treatment of fever, urodynia, rheumatism, lumbago and neuralgia. The juice of pounded fresh tops of young branches is instilled in the ear of otitis. The plant can be used as raw material for diosgenin extraction.

Etnomedicinal Uses

The rhizome is rich in starch and cooked for eating.

Croton roxburghii Balak.

Family

Euphorbiaceae

Vernacular Names

Hindi : Chucka; **Oriya** : Putidi,Masud, Devchandan, Masundi; **Kol** : Gote.

The Plant

Trees, branchlets lepidote, bark smooth. Leaves large, ovate, elliptic, crenate–dentate, serrate or coarsely toothed, coriaceous. Flowers dioecious or monoecious, in long racemes. Flowers yellowish green. Fl. Jan.–Feb. Fr. March–April.

Distribution

Frequent in forests.

Parts Used

Root, bark

Medicinal Properties and Uses

The root is mashed in water and taken in sore throat. The

bark and roots are given as a purgative and also as an alternative in dysentery. The root is used as antidote against snakebite and scorpion sting. It is also used for antifertility purposes.

Ethnomedicinal Uses

Paste of root-bark is heated and applied to boils for either subsiding or hastening suppuration.

Crinum defixum Ker-Gawl.

Family

Amaryllidaceae

Vernacular Names

Oriya : Kondai; **Sans** : Vishamandala.

The Plant

Stout herb, leafy stem not dying down annually. Leaves erect in water or spreading on the soil, margins smooth. Flowers white. Fruit globose. Fl. June-November.

Distribution

Occasional along streams.

Parts Used

Bulbs

Medicinal Properties and Uses

Bulbs diaphoretic and emollient, used for burns, whitlow and carbuncles.

Curculigo orchioides Gaertn.

Family

Amaryllidaceae

Vernacular Names

Oriya : Talmuli, Kua kanda; **Hindi** : Kali musli, Musli; **Sans** : Mushali

The Plant

A herbaceous tuberous geophilous perennial with a short or elongate root stock bearing several fleshy lateral roots. Leaves simple, crowded on the short stem, sessile or short petioled with sheathing leaf bases. Flowers bright yellow. Seeds black, oblong, deeply grooved in wavy lines. Fl. May.-August.

Distribution

Fairly common

Parts Used

Root – stock

Medicinal Properties and Uses

The root stocks are sweet, cooling, bitter, emollient, diuretic, aphrodisiac, depurative, appetizer, carminative, antipyretic and tonic and are useful in vitiated conditions of *pitta* and *vatta,* lecorrhoea, pruritus, skin diseases, asthma, diarrhoea, cuts and wounds, dyspepsia, colic and gonorrhoea.

Ethnomedicinal Uses

The root paste is applied on wounds of finger tips to allay pus formation. It is also given in diarrhoea. Tuber paste with curd is taken orally for three days to regularize menstruation.

Curcuma amada Roxb.

Family

Zingiberaceae

Vernacular Names

Oriya : Ban haldi, Amada; **Hindi** : Ama-haldi; **Sans** : Amrardrakam

The Plant

A rhizomatous aromatic herb. Leaves long, petiolate, oblong-lanceolate, tapering at both ends, glabrous, green on both sides, flowers white or pale yellow in spikes in the centre of the tuft of leaves. Fl. Aug.-November.

Distribution

Fairly common in forests.

Parts Used

Rhizomes

Medicinal Properties and Uses

The rhizomes are bitter, sweet, sour, aromatic, cooling, appetizer, carminative, digestive, stomachic, demulcent, laxative, diuretic and antipyretic. They are useful in anorexia, dyspepsia, flatulence, colic, bruises, wounds, chronic ulcers, skin diseases, fever, constipation, cough, bronchitis, sprains, gout and inflammations.

Ethnomedicinal Uses

Rhizome is rubbed in stone with water and few drops of this is administered into the nostril for two to four hours for a day in case of snakebite. Plant paste (3gm) with paste of 7 long peppers (*Piper longum*) (1gm) is used twice for seven days after food for the treatment of piles and decoction of rhizome (3ml) with common salt (2gm) is taken twice for five days against cold and cough.

Curcuma aromatica Salisb.

Family

Zingiberaceae

Vernacular Names

Oriya : Banhaladi, Palua; **Hindi :** Ban-haridra, Jangli-haldi; **Sans:** Aranyaharidra, Vanaharidra; **Ko :** Paro

The Plant

A perennial tuberous herb with annulate aromatic yellow rhizome which is internally orange-red in colour. Leaves elliptic or lanceolate-oblong, caudate-acuminate. Flowers pink, lip yellow. Fl: April-May.

Distribution

Common in forests.

Parts Used

Rhizomes

Medicinal Properties and Uses

Rhizomes are bitter, carminative, appetizer and tonic and are used in combination with astringents and aromatics for bruises, sprains, bronchitis, cough, leucoderma and skin eruptions.

Cyathocline purpurea (Buch.–Ham.ex. D.Don) Kuntze

Family

Asteraceae

Vernacular Names

Ko : Garu puru.

The Plant

Erect or sometimes decumbent, aromatic herb stems hairy. Leaves sessile, lobes toothed, more or less. Pubescent, basal leaves larger. Heads bright rose purple. Fl. & Fr. Nov.–June.

Distribution

Frequent in moist places

Parts Used

Leaves

Medicinal Properties and Uses

The plant is used as tonic and anthelmintic. Decoction of whole plant is used against cold.

Cymbopogon martinii (Roxb.) Wats.

Family

Poaceae

Vernacular Names

Oriya : Dhanantri; **Hindi :** Gandhabel, Rusa ghas; **Sans :** Dhyamakha, Rohisah; **Ko :** Taser, Sailtati

The Plant

A perennial, sweet-scented grass. Leaves linear-lanceolate, subcordate, finely caudate. Flowers in spikelets, in panicles, turning reddish brown when mature. Fl. & Fr. Oct.-Dec.

Distribution

Frequent

Parts Used

Whole plant

Medicinal Properties and Uses

The plant is acrid, bitter, thermogenic, appetizer, carminative, digestive, cardiotonic, depurative, diuretic and febrifuge and is useful in vitiated conditions of *kapha* and *vata,* bronchitis, cough, catarrh, dyspepsia, colic, cardiac, debility, leprosy, skin diseases and fever.

Ethnomedicinal Uses

Half a cup of whole plant juice is given every morning in empty stomach for few days to cure reproductive disorders. A spoonful roots dried in shade and pounded to fine powders is given twice day to cure hysteria.

Cynodon dactylon (L.) Pers.

Family

Poaceae

Vernacular Names

Oriya : Dhuba; **Hindi** : Dub, Durba; **Sans** : Niladurva, Durva; **Ko** : Dhuba

The Plant

A prostrate, extensively creeping glabrous, highly branched perennial grass, rooting at every nods. Leaves narrow, linear, soft and smooth. Inflorescence terminal spikes. Fruits, oblong, laterally compressed. Fl & Fr. most of the year.

Distribution

Fairly common.

Parts Used

Whole plant.

Medicinal Properties and Uses

The plant is astringent, sweet, cooling, depurative, diuretic and tonic and is useful in vitiated conditions of *pitta* and *kapha*, haematuria, haemorrhages, wounds, skin diseases, vomiting, abortion and general debility. Rhizome used in genito-urinary troubles.

Ethnomedicinal Uses

Plant decoction is diuretic, useful in dropsy and anasarca.

Leaves are crushed and the juice (2-3 drops) is poured in the nose to check nose bleeding. This is repeated 3-4 times at half an hour intervals. Leaf juice is taken daily with honey to improve general debility.

Cyperus rotundus L.

Family

Cyperaceae

Vernacular Names

Hindi : Mutha; **Sans :** Musta; **Oriya :** Mutha, Motha; **Ko:** Rotesila

The Plant

Perennial, rhizome, emitting long, slender, wiry stolons ending in tubers, tubers fragrant. Leaves several, mostly radical. Inflorescence simple or compound, spikes green. Fl. & Fr. July-December.

Distribution

Common weed.

Parts Used

Rhizomes

Medicinal Properties and Uses

The rhizomes give successful results in the treatment of irregular menstruation, dysmenorrhoea, gastralgia, dyspepsia, diarrhoea and vomiting.

Ethnomedicinal Uses

The tubers mixed with various other substances are given internally to heal ulcers. Plant paste is applied on breast for some days to increase milk of mother.

Dalbergia lanceolaria L.f.

Family

Fabaceae

Vernacular Names

Oriya : Puradubi, Chakundia, Sujanipati; **Hindi:** Takoli, bithua; **Ko :** Koiad, Kaichalam

The Plant

Medium sized tree, bark white or grey. Leaves lenear, oblong with thin scattered, short hair beneath or both surfaces. Flowers pink, purple or nearly white or sometimes blue. Fl. April-May, Fr. Sep.-January.

Distribution

Frequent in forests.

Parts Used

Bark, seed.

Medicinal Properties and Uses

Decoction of bark used in dyspepsia. Seed oil for rheumatism.

Dalbergia latifolia Roxb.

Family

Fabaceae

Vernacular Names

Oriya : Sissoo; **Hindi :** Shisham, Sissu; **Sans :** Shinsapa; **Ko :** Kiri

The Plant

A deciduous tree with a crooked trunk, light crown and pubescent or tomentose young parts. Leaves imparipinnate; leaflets 5-7, very unequal sized on the same rachis, suborbicular. Flowers white, in numerous lax panicles. Fl. Aug.-Sept., Fr. Jan.-February.

Distribution

Common in moist deciduous forest

Parts Used

Root, bark, leaves, heartwood

Medicinal Properties and Uses

The roots are astringent and constipating and useful in diarrhoea and dysentery. The leaves are bitter, ophthalmic, styptic, diuretic and stimulant and are useful in gonorrhoea, menorrhagia, colic, vomiting and burning sensation. The bark and heartwood are acrid, bitter, thermogenic, depurative, antipyretic and appetizer and are useful in leprosy, skin diseases, ulcers, scabies and gout.

Ethnomedicinal Uses

Oil extracts from firing the heart wood pieces cures skin diseases.

Datura metel L.

Family

Solanaceae

Vernacular Names

Oriya : Datura, Dudura; **Hindi** : Sadahdhatura; **Sans** : Dhatura

The Plant

Small herbaceous plant. Branches pubescent when young, marked with leaf scars. Leaves alternate, unequal at the base, minutely pubescent on both surfaces, margins wavy. Flowers large purple or white. Fruit inclined or nodding, globose. Seeds numerous, blackish-brown. Fl. & Fr. most part of the year.

Distribution

Common in waste places.

Parts Used

Leaves, flowers.

Medicinal Properties and Uses

The leaves possess antispasmodic, sedative and anodyne properties. They are used for treating cough, asthma and rheumatism. Chilblains, gastric ulcers, haemorrhoids, sea sickness and air sickness. The dried leaves and flowers are cut into small chips and used in antiasthmatic cigarettes. A poultice of the pounded fresh leaves has an anodyne effect. Warning should be given of their high toxicity.

Ethnomedicinal Uses

Oil is mixed with the leaf juice and heated it then applied on hydrocil.

Dendrophthoe falcata (L.f.) Etting.

Family

Loranthaceae

Vernacular Names

Oriya : Datura, Dudura; **Hindi :** Sadahdhatura; **Sans :** Dhatura

The Plant

A stem parasite with smooth, grey bark. Leaves usually opposite, thick, variable in shape from ovate to linear-oblong, mid rib prominent. Flowers orange-red or scarlet in short spreading, stout, axillary, racemes, calyx present, often as a rim. Fruit oblong or ellipsoid, glabrous. Fl. & Fr. Nov.-April.

Distribution

Common on wide variety of hosts.

Parts Used

Whole plant

Medicinal Properties and Uses

The plant is cooling, bitter, astringent, aphrodisiac, narcotic and diuretic and is useful in pulmonary tuberculosis, asthma, menstrual disorders, swellings, wounds, ulcers and vesical calculi.

Desmodium gangeticum (L.) DC.

Family

Fabaceae

Vernacular Names

Oriya : Salparni, Salpheni; **Hindi :** Salpan, Salvan

The Plant

An erect, diffusely branched undershrub with short woody stem and numerous prostrate branches provided with soft grey hairs. Leaves unifoliate, ovate, membranous and mottled with grey patches. Flowers white, purple or lilac in elongate lax, terminal or axillary racemes. Fruits moniliform, jointed glabrescent pods. Seeds compressed reniform. Fl. & Fr. May-January.

Distribution

Fairly common in forest, wasteland and cultivated land.

Parts Used

Roots

Medicinal Properties and Uses

The roots are bitter, sweet, thermogenic, nervine tonic, aphridisiac, carminative, constipating, diuretic, febrifuge, cardio-tonic, anti-inflammatory and tonic and are useful in vitiated conditions of *vata*, anorexia, dyspepsia, dysentery, stragury, fever, gout, inflammations, cough, asthma, bronchitis, cardiopathy and debility.

Ethnomedicinal Uses

Decoction of root (15ml) is taken in empty stomach once for seven days for the treatment of Malaria.

Desmodium oojeinensis (Roxb.) Ohashi

Family

Fabaceae

Vernacular Names

Oriya : Bandhan, Banjan; **Hindi** : Sandan, Panan; **Ko** : Ruta, Panjan.

The Plant

Tree, usually small and crooked, bark dark brown, deeply cracked. Leaves pinnately 3 foliolate, cordate. Flowers white or pink, small, mostly 3 nate, in the axils of bracts in dense facicled racemes. Stamens 9+1. Pod linear, joints flat, large. Seeds 1 –5, compressed, reniform. Fl. Feb,-March, Fr. Mar.-April

Distribution

Frequent in mixed forests.

Parts Used

Root, leaves, seeds

Medicinal Properties and Uses

Roots and cumin seeds marshed in water and orally taken in orchitis. Leaves possess antibacterial and anti-inflammatory properties. They are indicated in the treatment of dysentery and diarrhoea.

Ethnomedicinal Uses

Plant is pounded, mixed with water and given in stomach pain and fever.

Desmodium triflorum (L.) DC.

Family

Fabaceae

Vernacular Names

Oriya : Kuradiagachha, Katkana; **Hindi :** Kudaliya, Jangli methi; **Sans :** Tripadi

The Plant

A small perennial much branched prostrate trailing herb with slender stems rooting at the nodes. Leaves trifoliate, leaflets membranous, obovate, cuneate or emarginated or rarely rounded. Flowers pink or white. Fruits pods. Fl. & Fr. most of the year.

Distribution

Very common in open near water cources, road sides, grasslands.

Parts Used

Whole plant

Medicinal Properties and Uses

The plant is acrid, sweet, cooling, expectorant and is useful in vitiated conditions of *pitta,* cough, bronchitis, wounds, abscess, sores, dysentery, flatulence and burning sensation.

Ethnomedicinal Uses

The root is used as abortifacient and in menstrual disorder.

Dioscorea pentaphylla L.

Family

Dioscoreaceae

Vernacular Names

Oriya : Pittalo kanda, Karwa, Karaba alu; **Hindi :** Bhusa, Kanta alu; **Sans :** Kantak alu; **Ko :** Merantua sanga, Itulad-sanga.

The Plant

Stem twining to the left, prickly towards the base, glabrous, tubers oblong. Leaves very variable in different varieties, 3-5 foliolate, simple, ovate, acuminate. Flowers shortly pedicelled or sessile above the bract. Fl.& Fr. Oct.-December.

Distribution

Fairly common in forests.

Parts Used

Tubers

Medicinal Properties and Uses

Tubers considered tonic, also used for swellings.

Ethnomedicinal Uses

Dry rhizome ground with water is applied on cuts, boils and pimples.

Diospyros malabarica (Desr.) Kostel.

Family

Ebenaceae

Vernacular Names

Oriya : Mankara Kendu, Kola Kendu; **Hindi :** Kala tendu, Gab; **K :** Gara tiril

The Plant

Tree with low spreading branches, bark black. Leaves acute, glabrous, shining above. Flowers white fragrant. Fruit globose. Seeds large. Fl. Mar.-April, Fr. ripens following March, April.

Distribution

Common in valleys along streams.

Parts Used

Bark, leaves, flowers, fruits.

Medicinal Properties and Uses

The bark is astringent, acrid, cooling. Constipating and febrifuge and is useful in vitiated conditions of *pitta*, diarrhoea, dysentery, leprosy, skin diseases, dyspepsia, diabetes, fever and vaginal disorders. The leaves are diuretic and aphrodisiac and are useful in anaemia and scabies. The fruits are bitter, cooling, digestive, carminative and useful in aphthae and vitiated conditions of *pitta* and *vata*.

Ethnomedicinal Uses

Fruits pulp is applied on cracks of feet.

Diospyros melanoxylon Roxb.

Family

Ebenaceae

Vernacular Names

Oriya : Kendu; **Hindi :** Bhum; **Sans :** Dirghapatrika; **Ko:** Tiril, Terel

The Plant

Small and bushy or large tree with grey or rusty tomentose branchlets, bark black, rough. Leaves mostly sub opposite, broadly ovate, old leaves corriaceous. Male flowers in pendun-cled. Female flowers solitary. Fruit globose, yellow when ripe. Fl. Apr.–May, Fr. ripens following May.

Distribution

Common in mixed forests.

Parts Used

Bark, leaves, flowers.

Medicinal Properties and Uses

Leaves diuretic, laxative, carminative and styptic; dried flowers used in urinary and skin troubles. Decoction of the bark used in diarrhoea and dyspepsia.

Ethnomedicinal Uses

Mixture of decoction of young leaves (3ml) with unboiled egg (2gm) and rice bran oil (2ml) is prescribed for the treatment of night blindness.

Drosera indica L.

Family

Droseraceae

The Plant

A slender erect tuberous herb. Leaves are of two types; the basal leaves are clustered just above the soil surface, deflexed up to 2.5cm long; the upper leaves alternate, narrow, linear with many sticky glandular tentacles above and hairless below. Flowers pink to rose. Fl. & Fr. Aug.-Oct.

Distribution

Occasional on moist soil among grasses and sedges.

Parts Used

Whole plant.

Medicinal Properties and Uses

The plant is considered to be a rejuvenating herb and more widely used in Alchemy. Also used to cure corns.

Diplazium esculentum (Retz.) Sw.

Family

Athyriaceae

Vernacular Names

Ko : Dukhuri

The Plant

Large fern with erect stout and a terminal tuft of fonds. Fonds bipinnate slightly scented, stipes pale, slightly scaly and grooved. Sterile fonds almost dimorphic. Sori linear, long. Fertile: March

Distribution

Frequent near streams.

Parts Used

Roots

Ethnomedicinal Uses

About 20g of fresh root is boiled in 1 liter of water till to be one fourth of its volume. 3 ml of this decoction along with 2 ml of honey is taken orally in empty stomach twice a day for 15 days to cure spermatorrhea.

Drynaria quercifolia (L.) J. Sm. Hook.

Family

Drynariaceae

Vernacular Names

Oriya : Gorurpanki; **Sans :** Ashvakatri; **Ko :** Dunguri

The Plant

Rhome creeping, short with lanceolate subulate, cordate. Sterile fronds glossy, pinnatifid or lobbed soon turning brown. Fertile fronds long. Sori on the anastomosis, small.

Distribution

Common on branches of the tree.

Parts Used

Fronds, rhizomes.

Medicinal Properties and Uses

Fronds used for poulticing swellings. Rhizomes astringent, aqueous extract possesses antibacterial properties.

Ethnomedicinal Uses

Young shoots are shade dried, powdered and mixed with root powder of *Saraca asoca* (Roxb.) de Wilde, in 1:1 ratio and administered with one glass of milk after dinner for 15 days for one week to generate strength & sexual vigor.

Eclipta prostrata (L.) L. Mant.

Family

Asteraceae

Vernacular Names

Oriya : Kasarda, Bhrungaraj; **Hindi** : Bhangra; **Sanskrit:** Bhrngaraj, Pittapriya, Ajagara

The Plant

An erect or prostrate annual succulent herb, frequently rooting at the lower nodes. Leaves shortly petioled, oblong or elliptic, toothed. Heads sub globose. Fl. & Fr. Aug.-April.

Distribution

Occasional in moist places along streams and borders of rice field.

Parts Used

Leaves and roots

Medicinal Properties and Uses

It is good for the hair and skin, expels intestinal worms, cures cough and asthma and strengthens body. It is specific in night blindness, eye diseases, headache and diseases pertaining to hair and its growth. Herb is used as tonic and deobstruent in hepatic and spleen enlargements, emetic, used in skin diseases. Leaves used in scropion sting. Root is applied externally as antiseptic to ulcers and wounds in cattle.

Ethnomedicinal Uses

The roots used as antidote to snakebite and scropion stings. Infusion of leaves given in malarial fever.

Elephantopus scaber L.

Family

Asteraceae

Vernacular Names

Oriya : Mayur chandrika, Mayur chulia, Chhota rasna; **Hindi :** Pituret; **Sans :** Gojihva; **Ko :** Chaulichapi

The Plant

Erect rigid herb, stem slender, dichotomously branched, radical leaves or clustered and erect, obovate or oblanceolate. Clusters of partial heads with conspicuous cordate leafy bracts. Fl. & Fr. Aug.-December.

Distribution

Common in forests.

Parts Used

Root, leaves, flowers.

Medicinal Properties and Uses

The plant is bitter, acrid, astringent, antipyretic constipating, diuretic and tonic. A decoction of the roots and leaves is given dysuria, intermittent fevers, diarrhoea and bronchitis. The root decoction is specific for haemorrhoic and a paste made out of leaves is very specific for skin diseases. The flowers are astringent, bitter, sweet, and expectorant and are recommended for vitiated conditions of *pitta*, bronchitis, cough and swellings.

Ethnomedicinal Uses

Root paste is applied to the forehead to relieve headache. Root paste (10gm) is taken twice a day after food for a week for the treatment of pain during discharge of urine. Root paste is mixed in raw milk is taken orally as laxative. Root paste with rice washed water is taken in empty stomach for 3-5 days for irregular menstruation.

Embelia tsjeriam-cottam (Roem. & Schult.) DC.

Family

Myrsinaceae

Vernacular Names

Oriya : Baibirango, Nununia; **Hindi :** Baibirang, Gaiya; **Ko :** Gointamata

The Plant

A shrub or small tree, young branches covered with brownish hairs, mature branches glabrous, branches specked with white glands. Leaves upto 12 cm long, narrowed at both ends dotted all over with glands, margins simpler or toothed, leaves sometimes reddish on lower surface, hairy on nerves. Flowers minute, pale green in short axillary, densely hairy clusters. Fruit small, globose, pointed, red when ripe. Fl. May-July, Fr. Oct.-January.

Distribution

Frequent in open forests.

Parts Used

Fruit

Medicinal Properties and Uses

The main use of this drug is in treatment of tapeworms. Given in suitable doses, the drug kills tapeworms. The drug also showed some antibacterial and antitubercular activity.

Enydra fluctuans Lour.

Family

Asteraceae

Vernacular Names

Oriya : Hidmicha; **Hindi :** Harakuch

The Plant

Prostrate herb, rooting at the nods. Stems succulent with short ascending flowering hairy branches. Leaves narrowly oblong, serrate. Heads yellow, terminal and axillary. Fl. & Fr. Dec.-February.

Distribution

Occasional in wet places along river beds and pond.

Parts Used

Leaves

Medicinal Properties and Uses

Leaves eaten as a vegetable. Leaves are used to cure headache, eye diseases, hook worms and bile products. It is also considered laxative, antibilious and demulcent and used in cutaneous and nervous affections.

Ethnomedicinal Uses

Leaves and twigs are used as vegetable. Pure mustard oil mixed with leaf juice and given to cure headache. Leaf juice mixed with honey is given three times a day in cough.

Equisetum ramossissimum Desf.

Family

Equisetaceae

Vernacular Names

Ko : Ghoda languid

The Plant

Scrambling plant, branches sparse, branchlet slender 2-3 in a whorl in each node. Strobilus long, sessile, epiculate, peltate sporophylls orbicular or oblong, sporangia oblong, yellow. Fertile: Aug.-October.

Distribution

In open and shaddy places closed to stream.

Parts Used

Whole plant.

Ethnomedicinal Uses

Whole plant paste is externally applied to cure scabies, itches and allied skin infections.

Erioglossum rubiginosum (Roxb.)Bl.

Family

Sapindaceae

Vernacular Names

Oriya : Menhga koli, Sona mahanga, Nunga; **Hindi :** Ritha

The Plant

Small tree, branchlets rusty-tomentose. Leaves impari-pinnate, leaflets opposite, entire, acuminate. Flowers whitish, tomentose. Fruit of 1-3, fleshy, young fruits villous, red turning black on ripening. Fl. April-May, Fr. May-June.

Distribution

Common in damp forests.

Parts Used

Seed

Medicinal Properties and Uses

Decoction of seeds used for whooping cough.

Erycibe paniculata Roxb.

Family

Convolvulaceae

Vernacular Names

Oriya : Chain katho, Jorai kuli, Durkuri, Jodakoli; **Ko** : Kari; **Sans** : Kari

The Plant

Climbing shrubs, young branchlets rusty pubescent or tomentose. Leaves obovate, elliptic-oblong. Flowers white or yellowish-white. Fruit black. Seeds ellipsoid. Fl. May-June. Fr. Following March-May.

Distribution

Common in forests

Parts Used

Bark

Medicinal Properties and Uses

Bark used in cholera.

Ethnomedicinal Uses

Bark (5cm long and 1 cm broad piece) is chewed twice daily for two days to cure fever. The bark juice is given in cholera. Barks pasted and used against intermittent fever.

Eryngium foetidum L.

Family

Apiaceae

Vernacular Names

Oriya : Jangli dhania, Bilati dhania

The Plant

Erect, perennial, dichotomously branched, aromatic herb. Leaves sessile, oblanceolate, spinosely serrate, obtuse, base crenate. Flowers sessile in the axils of narrow membranous margined bracts.

Distribution

In Damp places close to stream in cool valleys.

Parts Used

Whole plant, root.

Medicinal Properties and Uses

The plant has strong smell of coriander and is used occasionally as a condiment. Root stomachi.

Ethnomedicinal Uses

Leaf paste is eaten as 'chatini' and mixed with curry for its sweet flavour.

Euphorbia hirta L.

Family

Euphorbiaceae

Vernacular Names

Oriya : Cheldudhi, Chitakuli,Chitakuti, Harihari; **Hindi:** Dudhi; **Sans :** Dugdhika; **Ko :** Pusi toa.

The Plant

Erect, ascending or prostrate hairy herb. Leaves opposite, ovate oblong, broadly oblong, often unequalised, serrulate. Involucre campanulate, hairy or strigose. Male florets ebracteolate. Female florets laterally pendulous. Seeds oblong, reddish. Fl. throughout the year.

Distribution

Fairly common weed.

Parts Used

Leaves, latex, root.

Medicinal Properties and Uses

A specific treatment for bronchial asthma. Pill bearing spurge relaxes the bronchial tubes and eases breathing. Latex is used in eye trouble and plant paste is applied to keep the eye cool. The root is given to allay vomiting. The plant is given to nursing mothers as a galactogue. Leaves are used as antidote to snakebite and scropion sting.

Ethnomedicinal Uses

The paste of whole plant mixed with mango leaves is taken internally for malarial fever. The latex is applied to the eye lids in conjunctivitis. Whole plant juice is given for three days to enhance lactation.

Euphorbia nivulia Buch.-Ham.

Family

Euphorbiaceae

Vernacular Names

Oriya : Siju, Kath siju; **Hindi :** Kata thohar; **Sans:** Patrasnuhi, Vajri; **Ko :** Etke

The Plant

Large glabrous, erect, fleshy shrub or small tree. Leaves alternate towards the ends of the branches, fleshy. Involucre yellow. Fl. March-April.

Distribution

Common in scrub forests and rocky places.

Parts Used

Whole plant.

Medicinal Properties and Uses

The entire plant possesses antibacterial and galactagogic properties. It is used in treating bacillary dysentery, boils, hypogalactia and infantile lientery. A combination in equal parts with *Portulaca oleracea* is also used for dysentery. The plant is also used as an insecticide. Juice purgative and diuretic. Root bark is used in dropsy.

Ethnomedicinal Uses

Latex is used in eye trouble and plant paste is applied to keep the eye cool. The root is given to allay vomiting. The plant is given to nurshing mother as a galactagogue.

Exacum bicolor Roxb.

Family

Gentianaceae

Vernacular Names

Hindi : Bara charayata

The Plant

Erect herb, stem 4 angled, often slightly winged. Leaves

sessile, lanceolate, ovate or oblong-lanceolate. Flowers tetramerous, pink, blue or white blue. Fl. & Fr. Sept.–November.

Distribution

Frequent in grassland.

Parts Used

Whole plant

Medicinal Properties and Uses

Tonic and stomachic, employed as a substitute for chirayata and gentian.

Flacourtia indica (Burm.f.) Merr.

Family

Flacourtiaceae

Vernacular Names

Oriya : Baincho, Kontaikoli; **Hindi :** Katahi, Bilangoa, Kanjubench; **Sans :** Swadukantaka; **Ko :** Merle

The Plant

A small deciduous thorny shrub. Leaves simple, elliptic, acute or acuminate, coarsely crenate or serrate. Flowers greenish yellow. Fruits globose, dark purple drupe with juice pulp and hard endocarp. Fl. Dec.-March, Fr. March-May.

Distribution

Common both in plains and hills.

Parts used

Root, leaves, fruits.

Medicinal Properties and Uses

The roots are sweet, refrigerant, depurative and diuretic. They are useful in vitiated conditions of *pitta* and *vata*. Aphthae, poisonous bites, skin diseases, pruritus, erysipelas, strangury, nephropathy and psychopathy. The leaves are useful in pruritus and scabies. The fruit is sweet, appetizer, digestive and diuretic and useful in strangury, jaundice, gastropathy and splenomegaly.

Ethnomedicinal Uses

Infusion of crushed fruits is taken (150ml) in the morning for three days in painful urination. Bark paste is applied by rubbing the skin for the treatment of eczema. Root paste is mixed with seeds of *Piper nigrum* taken twice a day to cure cough.

Flacourtia jangomas (Lour.) Raeusch.

Family

Flacourtiaceae

Vernacular Names

Oriya : Baincho; **Hindi :** Paniyala, Paniyamalak.

The Plant

A large deciduous shrub or a small spreading tree upto 9m in height often armed low down with stout sharp decompound spines on the trunk. Leaves simple, oblong or ovate, crenate-serrate, dark green above and shining surface. Flowers small, in glabrous racemes. Fruits ovoid, green, turning brownish purple on ripening. Fl. June, Fr. Oct.-January.

Distribution

Common in cool valleys.

Parts Used

Bark, leaves, fruits

Medicinal Properties and Uses

The bark and leaves are astringent, acrid, sour, refrigerant, stomachic and diaphoretic. Leaves are used in jaundice and for snake bite. Decoction of leaves used as gargle for sore throat, infusion in dysentery. Fruit is astringent and purgative. Seeds are cordial, astringent, febrifuge and a good remedy for gonorrhoea, antiperiodic and antipyretic. Seed pulp is astringent, haemostatic, antidysentery, diuretic, laxative febrifuge and helps digestion. Prescribed in epilepsy and skin diseases. Fresh pulp applied to burns to prevent blisters and scars. Seed fatty acid used in leprosy. Pulp useful in kidney diseases. Pulverised seeds are antisecretary; aqueous extract is antispasmodic and hypotensive.

Ethnomedicinal Uses

Stem bark paste is applied by rubbing the skin for the treatment of Eczema.

Flemingia strobilifera (L.) R.Br.

Family

Fabaceae

Vernacular Names

Hindi : Kussunt

The Plant

Shrub, branches terete or slightly angular. Leaves 1-foliolate, lanceolate, ovate, elliptic. Flowers white or purple. Fl.&Fr. Feb.-April.

Distribution

Frequent in shady ravines in hilly areas.

Parts Used

Root

Medicinal Properties and Uses

Root used in epilepsy and hysteria, also used to induce sleep and relieve pain. Leaves used as vermifuge.

Floscopa scandens Lour.

Family

Commelinaceae

The Plant

Erect herb, stem glabrous or thinly pubescent, rooting below. Leaves sessile, lanceolate, oblong, scaberulous above, base narrowed. Flowers in dense terminal panicles, pink or white. Seeds pale glaucous Fl. & Fr. June-November.

Distribution

Frequent in damp places.

Parts Used

Whole plant.

Medicinal Properties and Uses

Whole plant is used in application for fractured bones. Juice of stem is used for sore eyes.

Gardenia gummifera L. f.

Family

Rubiaceae

Vernacular Names

Oriya : Bhurudu, Kurlu; **Hindi :** Dikamali; **Ko :** Bururi, Bhudrukoli; **Sans :** Nadihingu.

The Plant

A small tree or large shrub, 3-7 m tall. Branchlets twisted, crooked, brittle. Bark thin, smooth, greyish brown. Leaves opposite, inverted, egg-shaped to oblong, heart shaped, apex obtusely acute, margin entire, with a dot like gland known as 'domatia' at the axil of each nerve. Flowers bisexual, solitary, axillary, corolla tube 3-5cm long with 5 spreading lobes at apex which is about 5cm across, white turning yellow, fragrant. Berries ellipsoid to oblong, about 4×3cm. Smooth, not prominently ribbed. Seeds many, minute. Fl. Mar. -May, Fr. June-August.

Distribution

Drier hills or open forests.

Parts Used

Resin.

Medicinal Properties and Uses

Resin from leaf buds is used in curing wounds, indigestion, gas trouble, piles, chronic coughs, neuropathy, anorexia, colic, foul ulcers, intestinal worms, cardiac debility, leprosy, enlargement spleen and obesity. The plant is one of the ingredients of a veterinary herbal antiseptic ointment MELICON V., which is effective in healing wounds, fungal infections and other skin lesions in cattle. The ointment showed prominent antimicrobial effect.

Ethnomedicinal Uses

The wood is used as tanning material in leather making in home. Fruits are eaten. Paste made with the gum and lime is used as strong leak proof paste to check the leakage of earthen pot.

Glochidion lanceolarium (Roxb.) Dalz.

Family

Euphorbiaceae

The Plant

Small glabrous tree or shrub, branchlets green, rather flexuous and angular, bark grey, smooth. Leaves elliptic, glabrous, coriaceous, dark green, shining. Male flowers numerous, axillary clustered, yellow. Female 1-3 or more together, green narrow campanulate. Seeds red, persisting after dehiscence. Fl. Apr.-May, Fr. June-August.

Distribution

Common in forests

Parts Used

Bark, seed.

Medicinal Properties and Uses

Bark is employed for stomach ailments and seed oil is used as an illuminant.

Gloriosa superba L.

Family

Liliaceae

Vernacular Names

Hindi : Languli, Kulhari, Kaliari; **Sanskrit** : Visalya, Langali; **Oriya** : Panchangulia, Durga phulo; **Ko** : Bing-ki-chung

The Plant

Pretty climbing or usually scrambling, glabrous herb. The leaves are ovate, lanceolate, acuminate, the tips spirally twisted to serve as tendrils. Flowers solitary axillary on reflexed pedicels, flowers inverted, sepals long by beautifully waved and crisped lower half yellow, upper half red. Sporadic in open forests. Fl. Sept.-Nov. Fr. Nov.-Dec.

Distribution

Sporadic in open forests.

Parts Used

Seeds, tubers.

Medicinal Properties and Uses

The tuberous roots are useful in curing inflammations, ulcers, scrofula, bleeding piles, white discharge, skin diseases, leprosy, indigestion, helminthiasis, snake bites, baldness, intermittent fever and debility. Root is given internally as an antidote for snake poison. Considered useful in prompting labour and expulsion of the placentae. If consumed in large doses, it is highly poisonous, it causes vomiting, purging, stomachache and burning sensation. Seeds are used for relieving rheumatic pain and as a muscle relaxant. Seeds are used for treating gout, rheumatism, piles, arthritis and body pain. Root is used for preparation of tonic, against snakebite and anthelmenthic.

Ethnomedicinal Uses

Tuber paste (3 gm) with paste of long peppers (*Piper longum*) (1gm) is prescribed once a day for twenty days as a cure for rheumatism. Tuber paste is applied over the abdomen and kept for hours. It is repeated for few days till abortion.

Gmelina arborea Roxb.

Family

Verbenaceae

Vernacular Names

Oriya : Gambhari; **Hindi :** Gambhari, Sewan; **Ko :** Kasmar; **Sans :** Gambhari, Kasmari

The Plant

Large or moderate sized tree, bark light grey. Leaves broadly ovate, entire, acuminate, glabrous above, white or grey stellate tomentose beneath, base cordate, strongly 3–5 nerved. Flowers yellow or yellow–brown in terminal panicles. Drupe obovoid, usually 2–1 celled and seeded. Fl. March–April, when more or less leafless. Fr. May–June.

Distribution

Frequent in forests.

Parts Used

Leaves, root, fruit.

Medicinal Properties and Uses

The roots are acrid, bitter, sweet, atomachic, tonic and anthelmintic. It is useful in fever, dyspepsis, haemarrhoids and burning sensation. Leaves are demulcent and used in gonorrhea, cough and ulcers. Root is an ingredient of 'Dasamula' an Ayurvedic preparation. Fruits enter into cooling decoction and is used in fevers and bilious affections. They are used for promoting the growth of hair and for anaemia, leprosy, ulcers, constipation and leucorrhoea.

Ethnomedicinal Uses

Decoction of root bark is used for washing and healing of septic wounds. Ripe fruits are eaten by goats and seeds collected from the faecal pellets germinate easily. An aliquot of 20-30 ml bark juice is taken daily for fifteen days or till the disappearance of white discharge during irregular menstruation.

Grewia hirsuta Vahl

Family

Tiliaceae

Vernacular Names

Oriya : Kulo, Kukurbendi; **Hindi** : Kakarundah, Kukurbicha; **Ko** : Seta andir

The Plant

Shrub branchlets stellate-tomentose. Leaves lanceolate to ovate, serrate, acute. Flowers white or yellowish. Fl. July-Sept., Fr. Oct.-December.

Distribution

Common in open forests.

Parts Used

Fruits

Medicinal Properties and Uses

Fruits are used in diarrhoea and dysentery. Paste of the root applied to hasten suppression.

Ethnomedicinal Uses

A piece of root is rubbed in stone with water and applied in eyes to cure white spots in children.

Grewia tilifolia Vahl

Family

Tiliaceae

Vernacular Names

Oriya : Dhamuro, Bhangia; **Hindi :** Dhaman; **Sans:** Dhanvangha, Dhanurvrksah; **Ko :** Ahsing, Gonyet

The Plant

A medium sized tree with grey to blackish brown rough fibrous bark peeling off in thin flakes; leaves simple, alternate, ovate with oblique base. Flowers yellow, small on thick axillary peduncles. Fruits globose drupes, black when ripe. Fl. Apr.-June, Fr. Sept.-October, Deciduous: April-May.

Distribution

Frequent in hill forests.

Parts Used

Bark, fruits

Medicinal Properties and Uses

The bark is astringent, sweet, acrid, refrigerant, expectorant, emetic, styptic and tonic. It is useful in burning sensation, hyperdipsia, cough, skin diseases, wounds, ulcers, diarrhoea and general debility. The fruits are sweet, sour, cooling and edible and are useful in vitiated conditions of *vata* and *kapha*.

Ethnomedicinal Uses

The leaf paste is used as antiseptic.

Haldinia cordifolia (Roxb.) Ridsd.

Family

Rubiaceae

Vernacular Names

Oriya : Haldu, Koim, Kurum; **Hindi** : Haldu, Kadami; **Ko:** Kumba, Kurumba

The Plant

A tall deciduous tree with large crown and buttressed at the base. Bark smooth, light coloured, exfoliating in patches. Leaves broadly ovate, shortly abruptly acuminate. Heads yellow, axillary, usually in vertical rows of three. Fruits capsules, splitting into two dehiscent cocci. Seeds many, narrow, small, tailed above. Fl. June-July, Fr. Nov.-March. Deciduous: Feb.-May.

Distribution

Common in deciduous forests.

Parts Used

Bark, roots.

Medicinal Properties and Uses

The roots are astringent and constipating and are useful in diarrhoea and dysentery. The bark is acrid, bitter, astringent, refrigerant, diuretic, demulcent, aphrodisiac and tonic. It is useful in vitiated conditions of *pitta*, wounds and ulcers, strangury, skin diseases, gastropathy, fever and burning sensation.

Ethnomedicinal Uses

Powdered dried fruit buds are used for headache and bodyache. Leaves have antiseptic property.

Hedychium coronarium Koenig

Family

Zingiberaceae

The Plant

A robust rhizomatous tall herbaceous plant. Leaves arranged in two rows, lanceolate to oblong-eliptic, apex gradually tapering into acuminate with a tall like lip. Flowers pure white or tinged with yellow, fragrant. Seeds many, small, black covered with crimson red coloured aril. Fl. Aug.-October.

Distribution

Frequent near streams

Parts Used

Flowers, rhizomes

Medicinal Properties and Uses

Rhizomes are used as carminative and stimulant. Rhizome paste is applied to bruises and sprains.

Helicteres isora L.

Family

Sterculiaceae

Vernacular Names

Oriya : Murmuria, Kurkurbicha; **Hindi :** Morphali; **Sans:** Avarttani; **Ko :** Poto-poda, Sinkari; **Sant :** Petkamra.

The Plant

A large shrub or small tree with grey bark. Leaves simple, alternate, bifarious, obovate, cordate, serrate, scabrous above. Flowers red in axillary clusters. Fruits greenish, brown beaked, cork screw like follicles, seeds numerous, angular, testa, wrinkled. Fl. Apr.-December, Fr. Oct.-January.

Distribution

Widely distributed in forests.

Parts Used

Root, bark, fruits.

Medicinal Properties and Uses

The roots and bark are expectorant, demulcent, constipating and are useful in colic, scabies, gastropathy, diabetes and dysentery. The fruits are astringent, acrid, refrigerent, demulcent, constipating and urinary astringent. They are useful in vitiated conditions of *pitta,* colic, flatulence, diarrhoea, wounds, ulcers and diabetes.

Ethnomedicinal Uses

Fruits and raw turmerie are added in mustard oil and kept for a few days. This oil is applied to the defective limbs of the children. Fibers from the bark are used for making ropes. The seed powder about 20gms is used thrice a day for one week in the treatment of dysentery and stomach pain.

Heliotropium indicum L.

Family

Boraginaceae

Vernacular Names

Oriya : Hati-sundha; **Hindi :** Hattajuri, Siriari; **Sans:** Bhurundi, Hati-sunda

The Plant

A coarse, somewhat succulent foetid herbaceous annual plant. Leaves simple, alternate, ovate, obtuse, narrowed or cordate at base. Flowers pale violet. Fl. & Fr. June.

Distribution

Common weed, found in waste places

Parts Used

Leaves, flowers

Medicinal Properties and Uses

The plant is emolient, vulnerary and diuretic, used as local applications for ulcers, sores, wounds, gum boils and skin affections. Decoction of leaves used in urticaria and fevers, that of roots in cough and fevers. Flowers considered emmenagogue in small doses and abortifacient in large doses.

Hemidesmus indicus (L.) R. Br.

Family

Periplocaceae

Vernacular Names

Oriya : Dudhi, Sugandhi; **Sans :** Anantamula, Swetasariva; **Hindi :** Anontmul; **Ko :** Guadhemda.

The Plant

Slender, glabrous twiner with aromatic root stock. Leaves in distant pairs, linear, oblong, ovate. Flowers green outside and purplish-brown within. Fl. chiefly Aug.-Oct., Fr. Dec.-February.

Distribution

Frequent in forests, wasteland.

Parts Used

Roots, leaves, stem.

Medicinal Properties and Uses

Root is sweet, bitter, cooling, tonic, astringent and demulcent. Cures leprosy, leucoderma, itching, skin diseases, fevers and bronchitis. It is an ingredient of several medicinal preparations. The leaves are useful in vomiting, wounds and leucoderma. The stems are bitter, diaphoretic and laxative and are useful in inflammations.

Ethnomedicinal Uses

Root paste (about 10gms) is taken in empty stomach continuously seven days for the treatment of leucoderma. Root paste with one-fifth amount of piper and taken for colic pain. The root decoction (about 10ml) is used thrice a day for one month as blood purifier and in skin diseases.

Hemionitis arifolia (Burm.f.) Moore

Family

Hemionitidaceae

Vernacular Names

Ko : Chakula

The Plant

Small tufted fern with ovate-cordate fronds. Fertile fronds are long, brown, fibrillose towards the base. Stiffs of sterile frond curious with thin long hair beneath. Sponrangia densely covering under surface but following reticulate veins. Fertile: Aug.-January.

Distribution

Occasional in shady places.

Parts Used

Root

Medicinal Properties and Uses

Juice of the fronds applied to burns.

Ethnomedicinal Uses

About 10g of root powder is taken orally with water in empty stomach twice a day for 10 days for treatment of hypertension.

Heteropogon contortus (L.) Beauv.

Family

Poaceae

Vernacular Names

Oriya : Dauria, Sin kola, Sukla; **Hindi :** Kher, Sura; **Ko:** Saiyu

The Plant

Perennial, culms tufted. Leaves acute, scabrid above and on midrib below. Fl. & Fr. Aug-September.

Distribution

Fairly common in grassland, open ground.

Parts Used

Root

Medicinal Properties and Uses

Roots stimulant, diuretic.

Ethnomedicinal Uses

The root of 'Dauria' and the root of *Achyranthes aspera* is grounded and applied to the tooth-ache problem.

Hiptage benghalensis (L.) Kurz.

Family

Malpighiaceae

Vernacular Names

Oriya : Banomali, Natanageswar; **Sans :** Madhavi; **Hindi:** Madhumalati, Aneta

The Plant

Large woody climbing shrub. Leaves ovate-oblong, elliptic, shortly acuminate. Flowers white, fragrant. Fl. Feb.-March, Fr. Mar.-May.

Distribution

Occasional along streams in forests.

Parts Used

Leaves, bark

Medicinal Properties and Uses

Leaves are useful in chronic rheumatism, skin diseases and asthma. Juice of leaves is used for insecticide application for scabies. Bark is useful in bronchial asthma and rheumatoid arthritis.

Ethnomedicinal Uses

Leaves are cooked with rice and eaten to cure body pain.

Holarrhena pubescens (Buch.-Ham.) Wall.ex G. Don

Family

Apocynaceae

Vernacular Names

Oriya : Kherwa, Pitakorwa, Kurmi, Kuda, Indrajalo, Kurchi; **Hindi:** Kurchi, Karchi, Karra, Kora, Kuar, Kureya, Kura; **Sans:** Kutajah, Kalinga; **Ko :** Kuar, Tuar, Gotel, Gotik

The Plant

Large shrub or small tree, bark thick, smooth. Leaves opposite, oval, subsessile. Flowers white in axillary or terminal corymbiferous cyme. Follicles cylindrical in pairs. Long narrow, incurved. Seeds numerous, brownish, crowned with a tuft of long hairs one end. Fl. May-July, Fr. Oct.-February.

Distribution

Fairly common in the forests in wastelands.

Parts Used

Bark, seeds.

Medicinal Properties and Uses

The bark possesses amoebicidal properties. It is effective against amoebiasis. The sum of the alkaloids and conessine are also used. A bath containing a decoction of bark or leaves cures scabies. An alcoholic maceration of pounded roots is also used topically against scabies. Bark is astringent, anthelmintic, stomachic, antipyretic, tonic and antidysenteric, used in amoebic dysentery and diarrhoea. Contains alkaloids conessine, a gum resin and tannin. Bark of the plant and black pepper are powered together and orally taken against malaria fever.

Ethnomedicinal Uses

Stem bark infusion with honey in the ratio of 3:1 is taken once a day in empty stomach for cure of dysentery. Bark of the plant and black pepper are powered together and orally taken against malarial fever. Oral use of pounded bark with honey is given to cure dysentery. On the occasion of festival the peduncle of flowers are used by tribal women at the time of dancing.

Holoptelia integrifolia (Roxb.) Planch.

Family

Ulmaceae

Vernacular Names

Oriya : Charla, Dauranja, Jirappa; **Hindi :** Kanju, Banchilla, Begana; **Sans :** Chirabilva, Putikaranjah

The Plant

A medium sized to large glabrous deciduous tree with whitish or yellow grey bark. Leaves simple, alternate, elliptic, entire, glabrous with rounded or cordate base. Flowers green, in very numerous fascicles, male and female flowers in same clusters. Fl. Mar.-April, Fr. May-June.

Distribution

Occasional

Parts Used

Bark, leaves.

Medicinal Properties and Uses

The bark and leaves are bitter, astringent, acrid, thermogenic, anti-inflammatory, digestive, carminative, laxative, anthelmintic and urinary astringent. They are useful in vitiated conditions of *kapha* and *pitta*, inflammations, dyspepsia, flatulence, colic, leprosy, diabetes and rheumatism.

Ethnomedicinal Uses

The paste of bark is used in orchitis.

Homonoia riparia Lour.

Family

Euphorbiaceae

Vernacular Names

Oriya : Pani begunia, Godamalla; **Sans :** Pashanabhedaka

The Plant

Large evergreen shrub with numerous erect stems marked with prominent leaf-scars, bark brown. Leaves linear, entire with wavy margins. Male spikes long. Fl. March-April.

Distribution

Common along streams and rivers.

Parts Used

Root

Medicinal Properties and Uses

Root laxative, diuretic, used in piles, stone in bladder and vesical calculi, strangury and urinary discharges.

Hygrophila auriculata (Schum.) Heine

Family

Acanthaceae

Vernacular Names

Oriya : Koelekha; **Hindi :** Talmakhana, Kamtakaliya; **Sans:** Kokilaksha

The Plant

Rubust under shrub, hairy stems and whorled spines at the nodes. Leaves sessile often 6 in a whorl, two outer ones often larger, entire or minutely dentate. Flowers purple, in axillary whorls. Fl. & Fr. Oct.-Feb.

Distribution

Common along water courses.

Parts Used

Root, leaves, seeds.

Medicinal Properties and Uses

Roots are sweet, sour, bitter, diuretic, and anti-inflammatory. They are useful in dropsy, inflammation, ascities, hyperdipsia, jaundice and dysentery. The leaves are sweet; sour, bitter, stomachi and tonic. They are useful in jaundice, dropsy, rheumatism, lumbago, and diseases of the urogenital tract, cough and gastropathy. The seeds are acrid, bitter, diuretic and liver tonic aphrodisiac. They are useful in gonorrhoea, promoting sexual vigour and strength, arresting absorption, burning sensation, gout and general debility.

Ethnomedicinal Uses

Extract of leaf juice is taken twice a day for 15 days for the treatment of cirrhosis of lever. Seed powder is mixed with curd and given thrice a day to cure cholera.

Hypericum japonicum Thunb.

Family

Hypericaceae

The Plant

Herb. Leaves sessile, oblong or elliptic, acute to obtuse. Flowers yellow. Capsule ovoid. Seeds oblong. Fl. & Fr. Jan.-June.

Distribution

Common in moist places

Parts Used

Leaves

Medicinal Properties and Uses

Astringent and vulnerary, used in asthma and dysentery and as a styptic.

Hyptis suaveolens (L.) Poit.

Family

Lamiaceae

Vernacular Names

Oriya : Ganga tulsi, Ban tulsi; **Hindi :** Wilayati tulsi

The Plant

Tall, branched, hairy, aromatic herb. Leaves ovate, crenate-dentate. Flowers blue, small. Nutlets compressed, ovoid-oblong. Fl. & Fr. Sept.-January.

Distribution

Common in open places

Parts Used

Leaves

Medicinal Properties and Uses

The plant is stimulant, carminative and lactagogue. Infusion used in catarrhal conditions, uterus affections and parasitical cutaneous diseases. Leaf juice given in colic.

Ethnomedicinal Uses

Whole plant paste is applied externally four times a day for 3 days to get relief from fever.

Ichnocarpus frutescens (L.) R.Br.

Family

Apocynaceae

Vernacular Names

Oriya : Dudhilata, Madhobi, Swanati; **Hindi :** Kalidudhi, Dudhi; **Sans :** Ulpalasariba; **Ko :** Onol-sing

The Plant

A much branched extensively climbing rusty villous evergreen, laticiferous woody climber. Leaves simple, opposite, elliptic-oblong to broadly lanceolate, acute or acuminate, main nerves 5-7 pairs. Flowers greenish white, fragrant, numerous in axillary or terminal panicles of cymose clusters. Fl. Sept.-Dec., Fr. Jan.-April.

Distribution

Common in forests.

Parts Used

Roots.

Medicinal Properties and Uses

The roots are sweet, refrigerant, febrifuge, aphrodisiac, alternant, diaphoretic, diuretic, depurative, demulcent and tonic. They are useful in vitiated conditions of pitta, burning sensation hyperdipsia, fever, seminal weakness, nephrolithiasis, strangury, skin diseases, leprosy, pruritus, dyspepsia, vomiting, diabetes, cephalalgia and general weakness.

Ethnomedicinal Uses

The leaves are used in stomach pain and stems in problem of toothache and gums. A mashed plant taken with water relieves fever.

Imperata cylindrica (L.) P. Beauv.

Family

Poaceae

Vernacular Names

Hindi : Dabh, Siru, Ulu Oriya: Juna; **Sans :** Darbha; **Ko:** Chero.

The Plant

Perennial herb. Rhizome hard coriaceous, descending deeply into the soil. Leaves narrow and long, prominently nerved. Inflorescence of many spikes, silver white, densely silky. Fl. April-May.

Distribution

Frequent in low lying ground.

Parts Used

Rhizome

Medicinal Properties and Uses

Rhizome, a diuretic and febrifuge, is used in the treatment of urodynia, pollakiuria, haematuria and fever. Roots emollient, hemostastic and antifebrile.

Indigofera glabra L.

Family

Fabaceae

The Plant

Diffuse herb, stems many. Leaves membranous, impari-pinnate, petiole short, stipules lanceolate, acute, hairy, leaflets opposite. Flowers pink or reddish, small, usually in lax racemes. Pods slender, glabrous. Seeds cylindrical, truncate at both ends.

Distribution

Frequent in sandy soils.

Parts Used

Leaves

Medicinal Properties and Uses

Leaves used as a bitter tonic and febrifuge, also used as an emollient in external applications.

Ethnomedicinal Uses

One fresh flower with one black pepper is given daily before sun rise for seven day in filaria.

Iphigenia indica (L.) A. Gray ex Kunth

Family

Liliaceae

Vernacular Names

Ko : Chulia chandbol

The Plant

Erect herb, stem flexuous, leafy, corm globose, covered with brown sheaths. Leaves sessile, linear, and acuminate. Flowers dark purple, axillary or terminal. Capsule oblong. Fl. & Fr. June-November.

Distribution

Occasional in open grassy places.

Parts Used

Corm

Medicinal Properties and Uses

Corm used in colic. Flowers yield a red dye.

Ethnomedicinal Uses

In epilepsy the bulb is put around the neck with the help of a thread to cure convulsion.

Ipomoea nil (L.) Roth

Family

Convolvulaceae

Vernacular Names

Oriya : Khami khondo Krushnavela; **Sans** : Kaladana; **Hindi** : Kaladana, Mirchai

The Plant

Hairy twiner, stems retrorsely hirsute. Leaves ovate, pubescent or thinly hairy. Flowers bluish-purple or pinkish-purple. Capsule subglobose, glabrous. Fl. Sept.-Nov, Fr. Dec.-February.

Distribution

Frequent in open places, in hedges and along streams.

Parts Used

Seeds and leaves.

Medicinal Properties and Uses

Seed is acrid, light, hot, anthelmintic, purgative and blood purifier. It cures inflammations, abdominal diseases, fevers, headache and bronchitis. It is a mild purgative useful to eliminate bile, cough and worms. Juice of leaves is also used for the same purposes.

Ethnomedicinal Uses

For dandruff, dried seeds roasted and powdered are applied in scalp with water. It is kept for 5-10 minutes and rinsed in water. It is repeated thrice in a week.

Ixora pavetta Andr.

Family

Rubiaceae

Vernacular Names

Oriya : Kalakrya, Kila kerua, Patra Koria, Lohajharia; **Hindi** : Lohajanghia; **Ko** : Pete

The Plant

Large shrub or usually a small tree, bark pale grey, nearly smooth. Leaves sub sessile, oblong or elliptic, obtuse or rounded, coriaceous, smooth. Flower white. Fruit shinning black, depressed globose. Fl. March-May, Fr. May–June.

Distribution

Common in forests

Parts Used

Bark

Medicinal Properties and Uses

Decoction of bark is used for general debility and anemia.

Jasminum arborescens Roxb.

Family

Oleaceae

Vernacular Names

Oriya : Bana mali, Kalamukhi; **Hindi** : Bela, Kameli; **Sans:** Nagamali; **Ko** : Hundi

The Plant

A large suberect shrub with hairy climbing branchlets. Leaves simple, opposite, ovate or ovate-oblong, acuminate, grey tomentose on both surface. Flowers white, fragrant in lax trichotomous pubescent panicles. Fruit single. Fl. March-May, Fr. June-October.

Distribution

Common in forests

Parts Used

Leaves

Medicinal Properties and Uses

The leaves are bitter, astringent, sweet, stomachic, emetic and tonic. They are useful in obstruction of the bronchial tubes, menstrual disorders, colic, flatulence, cough and general debility.

Jasminum scandens Vahl.

Family

Oleaceae

Vernacular Names

Oriya : Ban malli

The Plant

Scandent shrub, climbing by means of recurved, hardened petiole bases. Leaves ovate, ovate-lanceolate, acuminate, glabrous, base rounded. Flowers white. Fl. Nov.-Feb., Fr. Mar.-May.

Distribution

Occasional in open forests.

Parts Used

Leaves, flowers.

Medicinal Properties and Uses

Dried leaves are good for indolent ulcers. The flowers are sweet, bitter, acrid, refrigerant, laxative, cardiotonic, alexipharmic depurative and digestive. They are also useful in vitiated conditions of *pitta*, inflammations, rheumatism and cephalagia.

Jatropha gossypifolia L.

Family

Euphorbiaceae

Vernacular Names

Oriya : Johaji, Baigoba; **Hindi** : Verenda, Bherenda.

The Plant

Small dark coloured glandular-hairy shrub. Leaves sub orbicular, palmately 3-5 lobed, lobes obovate, entire margin densely glandular-hairy. Flowers red with yellow center. Capsule 1 cm long. Fl. & Fr. July-October.

Distribution

Common in waste places, village hedges and waysides.

Parts Used

Bark, root, leaves.

Medicinal Properties and Uses

Stems are used as tooth brushes to cure teeth diseases. Roots are employed against leprosy. Decoction of leaves is employed as a purgative and stomachic. Latex is used for ulcers. Leaves are employed as febrifuge in intermittent fevers. Decoction of bark is used as emmenagogue. Seeds are purgative and yield a fixed oil, which is purgative and emetic.

Justicia adhatoda L.

Family

Acanthaceae

Vernacular Names

Oriya : Vasak, Basango, Basak; **Hindi :** Arusha, Adulasa

The Plant

Shrub, 1-2m. height. Leaves large, elliptic, elliptic-lanceolate or ovate lanceolate, acuminate, base cuneate, Flowers white, subsessible large, in axillary and terminal. Capsule clavate oblong. Seeds compressed, rugose. Fl. & Fr. June–Feb.

Distribution

Common.

Parts Used

Leaves

Medicinal Properties and Uses

Fresh or dried leaves constitute the drug vasaka, used in bronchial troubles and congestion. Leaf juice used also in diarrhoea, dysentery and glandular tumours.

Powdered and leaves are used for skin infections. Chief principle is vasicine which has been found to be a promising utero-tonic and abortifacient. It is also used in stopping post-partum haemorrhage.

Ethnomedicinal Uses

5 pieces of root paste with 2-3 pieces of roots of *Abrus precatorius* L. and 3-4 pieces of roots of *Achyranthes aspera* is mixed and the grinded pasty mass taken twice a day after meal for twenty days as cure for the treatment of piles.

Justicia betonica L.

Family

Acanthaceae

Vernacular Names

Ko : Had-pat.

The Plant

Erect under shrub. Leaves ovate, lanceolate. upwards smaller, entire or some what crenate-dentate. Flowers white, rose spotted, in mostly terminal. Capsule clavate. Seeds corrugated or rugose. Fl. & Fr. Oct.-March.

Distribution

Common in ravines and along streams banks.

Parts Used

Whole plant

Medicinal Properties and Uses

The plant is used in applications for boils and swellings, and also used in diarrhoea.

Kaempferia rotunda L.

Family

Zingiberaceae

Vernacular Names

Oriya : Bhuin champa; **Hindi** : Bhui champa; **Sans:** Bhumichampaka, Hallakah

The Plant

Herb with tuberous rootstock. Leaves large, erect, oblong or ovate lanceolate. Inflorescence radical. Flowers fragrant, bluish, crowded in spike. Fl. April-May.

Distribution

Occasional in moist places.

Parts Used

Whole plant, tubers

Medicinal Properties and Uses

The whole plant, when reduced to podwer is used in the form of ointment and has wonderful efficacy in healing fresh wounds, and if taken internally it removes any coagulated blood. The root is useful in swellings. Tuberous rhizomes and young leaves are used as a flavouring agent. Rhizomes are also used in cosmetics and as a dye. Rhizomes are considered stomachic and used in gastric complaints. Juice of tubers is used in dropsical infections. Powdered tubers are applied to mumps with coconut oil and is used as a cicatrizant. The tubers are useful in vitiated conditions of *vata* and *kapha,* gastropathy, dropsy, inflammations, ulcers, tumours and cancerous swellings.

Ethnomedicinal Uses

Bulb paste is applied locally to take out pus from boils and nuts formed in part of spine.

Kalanchoe pinnata (Lam.) Pers.

Family

Crassulaceae

Vernacular Names

Oriya : Amarpoi, Hemsagar; **Hindi :** Zakham-haiyal; **Sans:** Parnabijah; **Ko :** Patragaja

The Plant

Perennial succulent herb. Stems tubular and glabrous, mottled with purple. Leaves opposite, entire or 3 lobed, blade thick and fleshy, margins crenate. Inflorescence in terminal paniculate cyme with long stalk. Flowers pendulous, red or orange-red. Fl. Jan-February, Fr. March.

Distribution

Occasional

Parts Used

Leaves.

Medicinal Properties and Uses

The fresh leaves, which possess antibacterial and demulcent properties are used in the treatment of burns, wounds, ulcer and congestive ophthalmial. They are also haemostatic and depurative. Poultices and ointments are prepared with fresh leaves for external application.

Ethnomedicinal Uses

Leaves used to cure acute diarrhoea.

Lablab purpureus (L.) Sweet

Family

Fabaceae

Vernacular Names

Oriya : Simba; **Hindi** : Bhatvas; **Sans** : Nispavah; **Ko** : Sim, Sirmi

The Plant

A tall, nearly glabrous, twining, perennial herb. Leaves long. Flowers in racemes, white or pink, fruits white pods, green or purple margined. Seeds white, yellow, purple or black. Fl. Oct.-Jan., Fr. cold season.

Distribution

Cultivated

Parts Used

Leaves, seeds

Medicinal Properties and Uses

Leaves are alexipharmic and emmenagogue and are given in colic. Seeds are sweet, astringent, sour laxative, diuretic, galactagogue, stomachic and antispasmdic. They are useful in inflammations, strangury and agalactia and vitiated conditions of *kapha*.

Lagerstroemia parviflora Roxb.

Family

Lythraceae

Vernacular Names

Oriya : Sidha, Chhena, Salora; **Hindi :** Lendia, Bakli, Sidi; **Ko :** Sekre

The Plant

Trees, bark grey or reddish, smooth, young branches often 4-winged. Leaves narrowly elliptic or oblong, ovate lanceolate, acute or acuminate, glabrous above. Flowers white, axillary and terminal downy panicles. Fl. April–May. Fr. Dec.-January.

Distribution

Common in forests.

Parts Used

Bark, leaves, fruits

Medicinal Properties and Uses

Decoction of the bark is given in nursing mother to dilute breast milk. Leaves purgative, diuretic and deobstruent. Decoction of dried fruits as well as of leaves used in diabetes.

Ethnomedicinal Uses

Leaf paste is applied over fresh cut or wound as antiseptic and quick healing of the wound.

Lagerstroemia reginae Roxb.

Family

Lythraceae

Vernacular Names

Oriya : Patoli; **Hindi :** Jarul; **Ko :** Sekra

The Plant

Branched tree, bark light grey or pale brown, smooth, peeling off in irregular flaxes. Leaves elliptic, oblong lanceolate, acuminate. Flowers purple. Fl. Apr.–August. Fr. Sept.–Dec. but remaining on the tree till the following flowering season.

Distribution

Planted.

Parts Used

Leaves, fruits

Medicinal Properties and Uses

Leaves purgative, diuretic and deobstruent. Decoction of dried fruits as well as of leaves used in diabetes.

Ethnomedicinal Uses

Bark boiled with mustard oil is applied to get relief from pain.

Lagerstroemia speciosa (L.) Pers.

Family

Lythraceae

Vernacular Names

Oriya : Patoli; **Hindi :** Mota-bondara, Jarul; **Ko :** Sekra

The Plant

Branched tree, bark light grey or pale brown, smooth, peeling off in irregular flaxes. Leaves elliptic, oblong lanceolate, acuminate. Flowers purple. Fl. Apr.-Aug., Fr. Sept.-December.

Distribution

Planted

Parts Used

Leaves, bark, root, seeds, fruits.

Medicinal Properties and Uses

Root, astringent, stimulant and febrifuge. Bark and leaves, purgative. Aqueous extract of leaves has hypoglycemic activity. Leaves purgative, diuretic and deobstruent. Decoction of bark is used in fever. Fruit is used as local application for aphthae of mouth. Seeds are narcotic. Decoction of dried fruits as well as of leaves used in diabetes.

Ethnomedicinal Uses

Decoction of the bark is given to nurshing mother to dilute breast milk.

Laggera alata (D. Don) Sch.-Bip.ex Oliver

Family

Asteraceae

Vernacular Names

Oriya : Golak ladaka, Gota khadaka.

The Plant

Much branched herb. Leaves sessile with the decurrent bases forming wings, oblong-lanceolate, apex acute or obtuse. Heads purple. Fl. & Fr. March.

Distribution

Occasional in forests and wasteland.

Parts Used

Whole plant.

Medicinal Properties and Uses

Plant used in Malagasy as a disinfected. Leaves yield an essential oil.

Lannea coromandelica (Houtt.) Merr.

Family

Anacardiaceae

Vernacular Names

Oriya : Moi, Raji-mohi, Jhingan; **Hindi** : Jhingan, Mohin; **Sans** : Jhingini, Jingini; **Ko** : Nanam.

The Plant

A medium sized to large tree with greyish bark. Leaves imparipinnately compound, crowded at the end of branches. Flowers small, yellowish or purplish. Fruits reniform, compressed. Fl. Mar.-April, Fr. Apr.-June, Leafless: Nov.-May.

Distribution

Fairly common in the forests through out the area.

Parts Used

Bark, leaves.

Medicinal Properties and Uses

The bark is acrid, astringent, sweet, thermogenic, stomachic and anodyne. It is useful in cuts, wounds, bruises, ulcers, ophthalmia, gout, ulcerative stomatitis, diarrhoea and dysentery.

The leaves are useful in elephantiasis, inflammations, neuralgia, sprains and bruises.

Ethnomedicinal Uses

The bark decoction is used to treat toothache and gum trouble.

Lantana camara L. var. *aculeata* (L.) Mold.

Family

Verbenaceae

Vernacular Names

Oriya : Nagaboiri, Naguari; **Sans :** Caturangi, Vanacchedi; **Ko :** Putus

The Plant

Straggling or subscandent, aromatic shrub. Leaves ovate or ovate oblong, crenate–serrate, glabrescent or shortly villous on the nerves beneath, prickly. Flowers usually white pink or orange yellow or various coloured in gardens scented in short capitate spikes. Drupe black globose, Fl. & Fr. all the year round.

Distribution

Common roadside and forests

Parts Used

Leaves

Medicinal Properties and Uses

Leaves yield an essential oil. The oil is used for itch and may also be useful as an antiseptic for wounds. Plant is credited with vulnerary, diaphoretic, carminative and antispasmodic properties. It is used in fistulae, pustules, and tumours. Decoction is given in tetanus, rheumatism and malaria and for a taxy of abdominal viscera.

Ethnomedicinal Uses

Decoction of plant (15ml) is taken for the treatment of tetanus and there is strict prohibition of taking of sour food during treatment and decoction of leaf is taken twice a day for a week after food for the treatment of malaria fever.

Lawsonia inermis L.

Family

Lythraceae

Vernacular Names

Oriya : Manjuati; **Hindi :** Mehndi; **Sans :** Madayantika

The Plant

A glabrous much branched shrub or small tree, branches often ending in thorns. Leaves elliptic or broadly lanceolate. Flowers white or cream coloured, fragrant. Capsules red when young. Seeds numerous, smooth, pyramidal. Fl. Aug.-Oct. Fr. Nov.-December.

Distribution

Scarcely in dry deciduous forests.

Parts Used

Roots, leaves, flowers, seeds.

Medicinal Properties and Uses

The roots are bitter, refrigerant, depuratve, diuretic, emmenagogue, abortifacient and trichogenous and are useful in burning sensation, dipsia, leprosy, skin disease, amenorrhoea, dysmennorhoea and premature graying of hair. The leaves are bitter, astringent, acrid, refrigerant, diuretic, emetic, expectorant, anodyne, constipating, depurative, liver tonic, haematinic, styptic febrifuge and trichogenous. They are useful in wounds, ulcers, bronchitis, vitiated conditions of *kapha* and *pitta*, burning sensation, cephalalgia, hemicrania, lumbago, rheumatalgia, inflammations, diarrhoea, dysentery, falling of hairs, greyness of hair and jaundice. The flowers are intellect promoting, cardiotonic, refrigerant, soporific, febrifuge and tonic. They are useful in cephalagia, burning sensation, sardiopathy, insomnia and fever.

Ethnomedicinal Uses

The decoction of root is given to pregnant women at bed time to remove constipation. Juice extract of fresh leaves are given in morning and evening for 10 days in case of white discharge menstruation. Paste made from leaves is applied on affected areas in morning and evening 5 to 6 days in fungal infection.

Leea asiatica (L.) Ridsdale

Family

Vitaceae

Vernacular Names

Ko : Hom

The Plant

Erect undershrub; leaves elliptic oblong or ovate, coarsely serrate, long, acuminate. Flowers greenish white. Berry glaucous or steel grey, finally black. Fl. June-Sept., Fr. Nov.-December.

Distribution

Frequent in forest.

Parts Used

Root

Medicinal Properties and Uses

Root tubers are used against guinea worms.

Leea indica (Burm. f.) Merr.

Family

Vitaceae

Vernacular Names

Oriya : Kalad chana, Kukurbiri; **Hindi :** Kurkurjihva; **Sans:** Chatri

The Plant

A large shrub with numerous tough branches, the young ones green. Leaves glabrous, very large, much divided, leaflets oblong. Flowers white in large branched corymbose cymes. Fruits black purple, depressed globular berries. Fl. & Fr. Aug.-December.

Distribution

Common in hill forests.

Parts used

Roots, leaves.

Medicinal Properties and Uses

The roots are astringent, acrid and cooling, anthelmintic and sudorific. They are useful in diarrhoea, dysentery, colic, hyperdipsia, ulcers and skin diseases. The young leaves are digestive and are applied to the head in vertigo.

Leea macrophylla Roxb.

Family

Vitaceae

Vernacular Names

Oriya : Hanshia dabar, Jibni; **Hindi :** Dholasmudra; **Sans:** Dholasmudrika, Hastikarna; **Ko :** Hom, Horom

The Plant

Robust herb or shrub. Leaves unifoliolate, trifoliolate, with very large stipules, serrate, Flowers greenish or white. Fl. Aug.-Sept., Fr. Oct.-February.

Distribution

Occasional in forests.

Parts Used

Root

Medicinal Properties and Uses

Mucilaginous root tubers anodyne, used on wounds and sores.

Ethnomedicinal Uses

The roots mixed with chillies made into a fine paste is given internally for all heart ailments.

Leucas indica (L.) Druce

Family

Lamiaceae

Vernacular Names

Oriya : Goiso; **Hindi :** Guma halkusa, Kumbha; **Ko:** Kapura

The Plant

Erect herb, stems usually much branched. Leaves linear–lanceolate, entire or remotely shallowly crenate-serrate. Flowers white. Fl. & Fr. Aug.-June.

Distribution

Common, waste places, cultivated field.

Parts Used

Leaves

Medicinal Properties and Uses

Plants are aromatic and used for flavouring. Decoction of leaves is used as a sedative, stomachic, and vermifuge. Poultice of fresh leaves is applied to old sores and dermatosis.

Ethnomedicinal Uses

Leaf juice is used for chronic skin eruption and painful swellings.

Leucas mollissima Wall. ex Benth.

Family

Lamiaceae

Vernacular Names

Ko : Gitil arak

The Plant

Slender herb with straggling or often climbling branches with adpressed hairs. Leaves petioled, ovate, and serrate, white tomentose. Whorls many flowered, distant, axillary, bracts, minute, linear. Nutlets obliquely truncate at the apex., Fl. & Fr. Sept.-June.

Distribution

Common in forests and waste ground.

Parts Used

Whole plant

Medicinal Properties and Uses

Leaves are eaten as a pot herb. Plant is diuretic and is used for digestion and antiseptic.

Ethnomedicinal Uses

Leaf is eaten as pot herb to cure asthma.

Limnophila indica (L.) Druce

Family

Scrophulariaceae

Vernacular Names

Oriya : Keralata; **Hindi** : Kuttra; **Sans.** : Ambusa

The Plant

Small marsh herb. Leaves pinnatifid, whorled. Flowers white or pale purple. Capsule subovoid. Fl. & Fr. February-November.

Distribution

Common along wet lands.

Parts Used

Whole plants.

Medicinal Properties and Uses

Plant considered antiseptic and carminative. It is useful in elephantiasis, infusion of leaves given for dyspepsia and dysentery.

Lindernia crustacea (L.) F. Muell.

Family

Scrophulariaceae

The Plant

Glabrous herb. Leaves ovate, entire, serrate or crenate, obtuse, base broad or narrowed. Flowers bluish or blue violet.

Seeds pale yellow, granular. Fl. & Fr. July-December.

Distribution

Fairly common in moist places.

Parts Used

Leaves

Medicinal Properties and Uses

Used for bilious infections and dysentery. Also used in poultices for boils, sores, itch and ring worms.

Ethnomedicinal Uses

15-20 ml decoction of whole plant is taken orally to treat headache.

Linum usitatissimum L.

Family

Linaceae

Vernacular Names

Oriya : Pesu; **Hindi :** Alsi, Tisi; **Ko :** Unchi

The Plant

An erect annual herb. Leaves subsessile. Linear or linear-lanceolate, entire, acute to acuminate. Flowers blue. Seeds compressed, shining brown. Fl. & Fr. Oct.-January.

Distribution

Cultivated

Parts Used

Leaves, bark, flowers, seeds, oil.

Medicinal Properties and Uses

Dried ripe seeds are used as demulcent and in form of poultices useful for rheumatic and gouty swellings and as laxative in cases of haemorrhoides. They are internally used for gonorrhoea and irritation of genito-urinary system. Bark and leaves are used in gonorrhoea. Flowers are nervine and cardiac tonic. Oil mixed with limewater is used as an application to burns.

Litchi chinensis Sonner

Family

Sapindaceae

Vernacular Names

Oriya : Lichu; **Hindi** : Lichi; **Sans** : Lishi

The Plant

Small evergreen tree. Leaves paripinnate, leaflets 2-6 pairs, ovate lanceolate, entire, glabrous, shining. Flowers small, greenish-white or yellowish. Fruit globose reddish when ripe. Seed one with large fleshy aril. Fl. Feb-March. Fr. May-June.

Distribution

Planted.

Parts Used

Seed.

Medicinal Properties and Uses

Seeds used as anodyne in neuralgic disorders and orchitis.

Ethnomedicinal Uses

The seed eaten is said to purify blood.

Litsea glutinosa (Lour.) Robins.

Family

Lauraceae

Vernacular Names

Oriya : Ledha chhali; **Hindi :** Maida, Menda.

The Plant

Small or medium sized tree, bark grey, smooth or dark grey and slightly rough in old trees. Leaves very variable in size and shape, elliptic lanceolate. Flowers white or yellowish, in coymbose or racemose, few flowered umbels. Fruit black, globose. Fl. June-July. Fr. Sept.-November.

Distribution

Common in valleys.

Parts Used

Bark, leaves, flowers, root.

Medicinal Properties and Uses

Mucilaginous bark used in diarrhoea and dysentery, also used for sprains, bruises and rheumatic gouty joints and as an emollient and styptic. Leaves and flowers are employed in poultices for bruise and wounds. Decoction of root is used as an emmenagogue.

Ethnomedicinal Uses

Bark and leaves are pounded and applied on sores and ulcers of the animals, powdered leaf applied on deep bruises.

Litsea monopetala (Roxb.) Pers.

Family

Lauraceae

Vernacular Names

Oriya : Bastura, Baghoari, Mosonea; **Hindi :** Maida, Meda, kalmara; **Ko :** Pojo

The Plant

Small tree, bark dark grey, smooth, branchlets brown pubescent. Leaves alternate, ellipitic, oblanceolate–oblong, obtusely acute. Umbels tomentose, stout pedicelled clustered along the branchlets and axillary, flowers white or yellowish. Fl. Mar.-May. Fr. July-August.

Distribution

Common in valleys.

Parts Used

Bark, seed.

Medicinal Properties and Uses

Bark is astringent and used in diarrhoea. It is also used in external applications for sprains and bruises. Seeds yield fat which is used for candle manufacturing and in ointments for rheumatism.

Ethnomedicinal Uses

The incense stick (Dhoop) is made from bark paste due to having the banded capacity. Bark paste is used to cure boils.

Ludwigia octovalvis (Jacq.) Raven

Family

Onagraceae

Vernacular Names

Oriya : Kapasia; **Hindi :** Banlumga; **Sans :** Bhulavangah.

The Plant

An erect much branched perennial suffrutiocose under shrub upto 1.2m in height with stiff, terete branches. Leaves alternate, neatly sessile, broadly elliptic to lanceolate, acute or more or less wooly, main nerves numerous. Flowers yellow, tetramerous, axillary and solitary. Fruits subquadrangular, truncate, 8 ribbed capsules, breaking up between the ribs clove like in appearance, seeds numerous, minute, ovoid. Fl. & Fr. Oct.-April.

Distribution

Common in wet places along streams.

Parts Used

Whole plant.

Medicinal Properties and Uses

The plant is astringent, carminative, vermifuge, laxative, diuretic, anti-inflammatory, expectorant and febrifuge. It is useful in dyspepsia, verminosis, flatulence, strangury, dropsy, cough, asthma, vitiated conditions of *vata,* neuropathy, diarrhoea, dysentery, leucorrhoea, cervical adenitis and fever.

Lygodium flexuosum (L.) Sw.

Family

Lygodiaceae

Vernacular Names

Oriya : Kalamahajal; **Sant :** Nanjomrehet; **Ko :** Karlitulia.

The Plant

Climbing fern. Primary pinnae bearing a pair of 1-2 pinnate divaricate secondary pinnae in well grown fronds. Fertile pinnules rather narrower, pectinately lobed with spongial spikes which are long. Fertile: Aug.-February.

Distribution

Common in forests.

Parts Used

Root

Medicinal Properties and Uses

Used as an expectorant. Fresh roots used in external applications for rheumatism, sprains, scabies, eczema and wounds. It is useful particularly for carbuncles.

Ethnomedicinal Uses

Powdered root 2g mixed with 1g *Piper nigrum* L. and 100ml of water are orally administered twice a day for 3 days to check blood dysentery.

Lygodium microphyllum R. Br.

Family

Lygodiaceae

Vernacular Names

Oriya : Kalamahajal.

The Plant

Ferns with twining fronds. Main pinnae ending in a tuft of golden hairs. Lateral pinnae with delicate zigzag rachies. The pinnae more slender, pinnules broadly ovate to lanceolate. Margin minutely crenulate. Fertile pinnules orbicular or ovate, long, stalks very slender. Fertile: Nov.-December.

Distribution

Climbing fern in forests.

Parts Used

Leaves

Medicinal Properties and Uses

Young leaves decoction used in dysentery. Leaves also applied in the form of poultices to skin diseases and swellings.

Ethnomedicinal Uses

Equal proportion of leaves mixed with leaves of *Andrographis paniculata* (Burm.f.) Wall.ex. Nees and rhizome of *Curcuma longa* L. are made into paste and applied for one week to get relief from joint pain.

Macaranga peltata (Roxb.) Muell.-Arg.

Family

Euphorbiaceae

Vernacular Names

Oriya : Piania, Gondaguria; **Ko** : Dau

The Plant

Moderate sized tree, bark pale. Leaves large, peltate, entire, acuminate, more or less hairy on the nerves beneath and glandular. Female flowers simple racemes or branched at base, bracts large, rusty tomentose. Fl. March, Fr. April.

Distribution

Common near streams.

Parts Used

Leaves

Medicinal Properties and Uses

Paste of leaves applied to veneral sores. Decoction of leaves and bark used as a vulnerary.

Madhuca longifolia (Koenig) Macbride

Family

Sapotaceae

Vernacular Names

Oriya : Mahula; **Hindi :** Mauwa, Mahva; **Sans :** Madhukah; **K :** Natkam.

The Plant

A large or moderate sized tree, bark brown, nearly smooth. Leaves clustered near the ends of the branches. Flowers cream, fleshy, on rusty tomentose pedicles, clustered at the ends of the usually leafless branches. Fruits ovoid berry, yellow when ripe. Fl. Feb.-April, Fr. May-July.

Distribution

Common in forests.

Parts Used

Bark, heartwood, flowers, fruits, seeds.

Medicinal Properties and Uses

The bark is sweet, bitter, astringent and emollient and is good for inflammatins, sprains. The heartwood is recommended for epilepsy. Flowers are stimulant, sweet, refrigerant and anthemintic and are useful in strangury, verminosis. The fruits are sweet, refrigerant, aphroidisiac and tonic and are useful in dipsia, bronchitis consumption. The oil obtained from the seed Mahua oil is emolient and laxative and is useful in dermatopathy, rheumatism and haemorrhoids.

Ethnomedicinal Uses

Flowers (corolla) are boiled in water with a pinch of salt for half-an-hour; 5-10ml of this decoction is given with honey, thrice a day for seven days in piles and fistula. Nectary honey collected from flowers is taken continuously for 7-days for cure of piles. Gum is used to prevent boil. Stem bark is boiled in water, teeth and gums washed with this water prevents cavities and allied dental troubles.

Mallotus philippensis (Lam.) Muell.- Arg.

Family

Euphorbiaceae

Vernacular Names

Oriya : Kamalagundi, Sinduri; **Hindi** : Kamela, Senduri, Rohini; **Sans** : Senduri, Kamela; **Ko** : Gara sindur

The Plant

A small sized tree with thin, grey bark. Leaves ovate-elliptic, reddish-glandular beneath. Flowers in spikes, small. Capsule globose, covered with reddish-brown glandular pubescence. Fruit roundish, 3 lobed, densely covered with a reddish brown, powdery substance and minute hair, which are easily rubbed out. Fl. Oct.-Nov, Fr. Feb-March.

Distribution

Common in forests.

Parts Used

Fruit

Medicinal Properties and Uses

Fruit contains cardenolides, rottlerin and isorottlerin. Seed contains corotoxigenin. Plant is used externally in treatment of skin diseases like ring worm and scabies. They are also useful in constipation, poisonous affection, and vesical calculi.

Ethnomedicinal Uses

The red seed powder is used by women. The wood is used for making implements and for fuel. 3 gms fruit powder mixed with 10 gms of molasses and used to remove thread-worms.

Mangifera indica L.

Family

Sapindaceae

Vernacular Names

Oriya : Ambo; **Hindi :** Aambaa, Aamra, Aam, Amb.; **Sans:** Amra; **Ko :** Maska, Uli

The Plant

Large tree. Leaves variable in size & shape, lanceolate, elliptic, entire, acute to acuminate. Flowers greenish–yellow, polygamous, small. Drupe very variable in size, shape and colour, usually ovoid, yellow when ripe, with large stone, thin epicarp and yellow or orange coloured fleshy and juice mesocarp. Seed with testa free from the endocarp. Fl. Jan.-March, Fr. Apr.-May.

Distribution

Common in deciduous forests.

Parts Used

Fruit, bark, seed, bud, leaves.

Medicinal Properties and Uses

Fruit laxative, diuretic. Unripe fruit is acrid, astringent, tasty and stomachic, cures vaata, *kapha* and tridosha and biliousness. Useful in throat troubles, ulcers and vaginal troubles. Bark used for uterine hemorrhage. Seeds used in asthma.Bud is used to care chronic dysentery. Leaves are astringent, refrigerant, styptic, vulnerary and constipating. They are useful in hyperdipsia, burning sensation, hemorrhages, haemoptysis, wounds, ulcers, diarrhoea and dysentery. Flowers are astringent, refrigerant, styptic, constipating and haemanic. They are useful in vitiated conditiond of *pitta*, haemorrhages, haemoptysis, wounds, ulcers and dyspepsia.

Ethnomedicinal Uses

Stem bark decoction (15ml) is taken in empty stomach twice a day continuously for three days as a cure for blood dysentery and pasty mass of cotyledons is applied on heads as a cure for falling of hairs. Buds of *Punica granatum* (Dalimbo) and bark of *Terminalia arjuna* (Arjuna) mixed with milk is given in chronic dysentery. The gum of it is used to keep soft in the cracks of foot during winter. Seven petioles grounded and given internally for urinary troubles in summer. Seven leaves rolled and tied on the navel for half hour for urinary troubles. The seed is given as paste internally as cure for diarrhoea.

Marsilea minuta L.

Family

Marsileaceae

Vernacular Names

Oriya : Sunusunia

The Plant

Rhizome widely creeping, branched. Stipes variable, slender, glabrous. Leaflets cruciform, obovate, variable in size, outer margin rounded. Sporocarps 2-4, variable in shape and size, rounded in front. Fr. Nov.-March.

Distribution

Common in wet places.

Parts Used

Whole plant.

Medicinal Properties and Uses

The plant is sweet, astringent, emillent, ophthalmic diuretic and febrifuge. It is useful in psycopathy, opthalmia, diarrhoea, caugh, leprosy, fever and insomnia.

Ethnomedicinal Uses

About 10 g whole fresh plant paste is mixed with 100g of curd prepared from black cow's milk. The dosage is given orally once a day in empty stomach for one month against epilepsy.

Melaleuca leucadendron L.

Family

Myrtaceae

Vernacular Names

Hindi : Kayaputi

The Plant

A middle size tall tree with white or ashy bark peeling of in large, branches pendulous. Leaves alternate, entire, thick, incurvedly nerved with whitish willi when young. Flowers small, creamy white, odorless in erect axillary spikes. Capsules loculicidally dehiscent at the apex. Seeds many, very small.

Distribution

Frequent in garden.

Parts Used

Leaves

Medicinal Properties and Uses

The leaves possess antibacterial, anti-inflammatory and

anodyne properties. They are effective for influenza, cough, asthma, dyspepsia, earache, toothache, osteodynia, wounds, burns and post-partum haematometra and rheumatism. An essential oil solution is prescribed for massage and for oral administration, parenteral injection or nasal instillation.

Merremia umbellata (L.) Hall. f.

Family

Convolvulaceae

Vernacular Names

Oriya : Paninoi

The Plant

Stems long, herbaceous, prostrate and rooting at the nodes or sometimes twining, slightly angular. Leaves ovate, elliptic or lanceolate. Flowers white or cream in axillary. Capsule globose. Seeds long. Fl. & Fr. Jan.-April.

Distribution

Common in mixed forests.

Parts Used

Plant, seed.

Medicinal Properties and Uses

Plants used for fistulae, pustules and tumours. Poultice of leaves applied to burns, scalds and sores. Seeds yield mucilage used as an aperient's, and also in cutaneous diseases.

Mesua ferrea L.

Family

Clusiaceae

Vernacular Names

Oriya : Nageswar; **Hindi :** Nagakesar; **Sans:** Nagakeshara.

The Plant

A medium sized to large handsome, glabrous, evergreen tree. Leaves simple, opposite, thick, lanceolate, coriaceous covered with waxy bloom underneath. Flowers white, very fragrant, axillary ot terminal. Fruits ovoid with a conical point surrounded by the enlarged sepals. Fl. Mar.-July, Fr. Oct.-Nov.

Distribution

Occasional in evergreen forests near streams.

Parts Used

Root, flowers, leave, oil.

Medicinal Properties and Uses

Root bark is astringent and aromatic used in rheumatism. Leaves are used as poultice for pustular eruptions, applied on forehead in severe cold. The flowers are astringent, bitter, acrid, stomachic, used in cough attended with expectoration. Made into a paste with butter and sugar used in bleeding piles and burning of feet. The seed oil is used in vitiated conditions of *vata* and skin diseases.

Ethnomedicinal Uses

One teaspoonful of dust of dried flower buds and flowers are soaked overnight. Next day taken with pinch of salt in order to control stomach disorder. Stamen paste is mixed with butter milk and taken in rice in case of ascitis (Pradar).

Michelia champaca L.

Family

Magnoliaceae

Vernacular Names

Oriya : Champa, Champoko; **Hindi** : Champaka; **Sans:** Champaka

The Plant

A large or middle sized evergreen tree with straight stem and smooth grey or brown black. Leaves simple, alternate, oblong-lanceolate, entire and glabrous. Flowers yellowish to orange, very fragrant, solitary and axillary. Fruits 5-10 cm long, ovoid, dark brown. Seeds 1-12, brown rounded on the back with pink fleshy aril. Fl. March-April, Fr. July.

Distribution

Common in cool valleys.

Parts Used

Roots, bark, leaves, flowers and fruit rind.

Medicinal Properties and Uses

Dried root and root bark of champaka are purgative; in the form of infusion, useful as an emmenagogue; mixed with curdle milk useful as application to abscesses. Juice of leaves is given with honey in colic. Bark is bitter, tonic, febrifuge, stimulant, expectorant and astringent. Flowers and fruits are stimulant, antispasmodic, tonic, stomachic, carminative and bitter, used in dyspepsia, nausea and fever and also useful in renal diseases and gonorrhoea. Oil from flowers is useful application in cephalgia and gout. Seeds and fruit are used for healing cracks in feet.

Ethnomedicinal Uses

The bark is aromatic and used for bitter tonic in fever. The bark and leaves are considered as febrifuge. Extract of flower oil is applied on forehead in case of headache.

Mimosa pudica L.

Family

Mimosaceae

Vernacular Names

Oriya : Lajkuli, Sensitive plant; **Hindi :** Lajawanti, Lajwati; **Sans :** Lajallu, Lajja.

The Plant

A diffuse prickly undershrub. Leaves bipinnately compound, pinnae–4, digitately arranged with 10-20 pairs of leaflets. Flowers pink, in globose heads, pendunclеs prickly. Fruits bristly pods, flat, straw coloured. Fl. & Fr. Aug.-May.

Distribution

Common weed.

Parts Used

Root, leaves.

Medicinal Properties and Uses

The roots are bitter, astringent, acrid, cooling, vulnerary, alexipharmic, resolvent, diuretic, antispasmodic, emetic, constipating and febrifuge. They are useful in vitiated conditions of *pitta*, leucoderma, vaginopathy, metropathy, ulcers, dysentery, inflammations, burning sensation, haemorrhoids, jaundice, asthma, fistula, smallpox and fevers. Decoction of root used in gravel and other urinary complaints. The leaves are bitter, sudorific and tonic and are useful in hydrocele, haemorrhoides, fistula, scrofula, conjunctivitis, cuts and wounds and haemorrhages. internal and external haemorrhages, dental caries, oral ulcers and intermittent fevers. Juice of leaves used in dressing for sinus and also for sores and piles.

Ethnomedicinal Uses

Decoction of root (3ml) mixed with paste of *Piper longum*

(2gm) is taken in empty stomach once in the morning up to fifteen days for the treatment of chylous urine. Leaves are grinded with 11 nos. of black peper and taken for 3 days in smallpox.

Mitragyna parvifolia (Roxb.) Korth.

Family

Rubiaceae

Vernacular Names

Oriya : Godi Koima, Keli Kadamba, Mundi, Mur; **Hindi:** Kayim; **Ko :** Sande kuma

The Plant

A medium sized to large deciduous tree with rounded crown and light grey smooth bark exfoliating in small scales. Leaves simple, opposite, broadly elliptic or obovate, obtuse, sometimes rounded. Flowers white, fragrant, in globose heads. Fl. May-June. Fr. Mar.-April.

Distribution

Common in deciduous and evergreen forests.

Parts Used

Bark, root, leaves.

Medicinal Properties and Uses

Bark and roots are acrid, bitter, stomachic and febrifuge and are useful in gastropathy, colic and fever. The leaves are acrid, bitter, sweet, styptic, vulnerary, stomachic, anti inflammatory, anodyne depurative and febrifuge. They are useful in vitiated conditions of *vata* and *kapha*, internal and external haemorrhages, wounds, colic, flatulence, dyspepsia, inflammations, myalgia, skin diseases, leprosy, erysipelas and fever.

Morinda citrifolia L.

Family

Rubiaceae

Vernacular Names

Oriya : Pindra, Achu; **Hindi :** Al, ach, surangi, bartundi; **Sans :** Ashyuka

The Plant

Medium sized tree. Young twigs angular, slightly compressed and grooved. Leaves opposite, stipuliferous, shining green above, pale below margins undulate. Flowers white, then yellow. Fruit ovoid including many drupelets, yellow when ripe. Seeds numerous, embedded in the pulp. Fl. Apr.-May.

Distribution

Commonly found in forests.

Parts Used

Roots, fruit and leaves

Medicinal Properties and Uses

The root bark has a beneficial effect in hypertension, osteodynia and lumbago. A decoction of the leaves taken by mouth in effective foe fever, dysentery and diarrhoea. A poultice of pounded fresh leaves cures furunculosis. The fruit, taken together with a little salt is stomachic, aperient, and active on dysentery, uterine haemorrhage, metrorrhoea and cough.

Morinda pubescens Sm.

Family

Rubiaceae

Vernacular Names

Oriya : Aacchu, Achchu; **Hindi :** Acc, Al.; **Ko :** Chaili

The Plant

A moderate sized deciduous tree, brown or grey, corky, branchlets glabrous or pubescent. Leaves ovate, obovate, elliptic, base often unequal. Flowers white, scented, in dense ovoid leaf opposed heads. Fruits multiple globose drups about 2 cm in diameter. Fl. Apr.-July, Fr. Nov.-April.

Distribution

Commonly found in forests.

Parts Used

Root, leaves.

Medicinal Properties and Uses

The roots are styptic, constipating, anti-inflammatory, alexteric and tonic, and are useful in haemorrhages, dysentery, inflammations, boils and general debility. The leaves are digestive, carminative, febrifuge and tonic. They are useful in gastropathy, dyspepsia, diarrhoea, ulcerative stomatitis, wounds, gout, inflammation, hernia, sarcocele and fever.

Ethnomedicinal Uses

Root bark paste is applied on soft portion of head of new born child. Tree bark yields dye.

Morus australis Poir.

Family

Moraceae

Vernacular Names

Oriya : Tutkuli, Chuch koli; **Hindi :** Tut

The Plant

Shrub or small tree, bark light grey. Leaves ovate or ovate-oblong, serrate or sharply serrate, often deeply lobed. Male spike rather lax-flowered, broadly cylindric or ovoid. Female spikes short, ovoid. Fruit ovoid or subglobose, red, turning black. Planted. Fl. & Fr. Nov.-May.

Distribution

Planted.

Parts Used

Leaves, fruit, bark.

Medicinal Properties and Uses

Fruits eaten, refrigerant, used also for sore throat, dyspepsia and melancholia. Leaves diphoretic, roots anthelmintic. Bark purgative and vermifuge.

Mosla dianthera
(Buch.-Ham. ex Roxb.) Maxim

Family

Lamiaceae

The Plant

Erect, slender aromatic herb, stems quadrangular, pubescent. Leaves petioled, ovate, serrate, acute, pubescent, and glandular beneath. Racemes slender, lax flower. Flowers bluish, purplish or white. Nutlets minute, brown or black. Fl.& Fr. August–November.

Distribution

Common near streams.

Parts Used

Whole plant

Medicinal Properties and Uses

Plant is useful in the treatment of hyperthyreosis. It inhibits the action of thyrotropic hormone and thyroxin output of thyroid.

Mucuna nigricans (Lour.) Steud.

Family

Fabaceae

Vernacular Names

Oriya : Baidonko; **Ko :** Itika, Etka, Marang atkir.

The Plant

Large climber, branches slender. Leaflets lanceolate, ovate or elliptic, acuminate, glabrous. Flowers dark purple. Seeds large, flat. Fl. July-September, Fr. December-February.

Distribution

Occasional in forest.

Parts Used

Stem

Medicinal Properties and Uses

Watery sap from stem is used for cough and fevers, tricomes on pots produce dermatitis.

Ethnomedicinal Uses

The paste made of powdered root is employed in dropsy and leaves paste is used on boils, blisters and ulcers.

Mucuna pruriens (L.) DC

Family

Fabaceae

Vernacular Names

Oriya : Baidonko; **Hindi** : Gonca, Kaunc; **Sans** : Kapikachhu; **Ko** : Itika

The Plant

Annual twiner, densely clothed with rigid hairs. Leaves trifoliate, leaflets broadly ovate, elliptic or rhomboid ovate, membranous, unequal at base, pubescent above and densely clothed with silvery grey hairs beneath. Flowers dark purple. Pods turgid. Seeds 5-6, black, shinning. Fl. Sept.-November, Fr. Jan.-April.

Distribution

Common in forests, hedges and bushes.

Parts Used

Root, leaves, seeds.

Medicinal Properties and Uses

Roots are bitter, sweet, thermogenic, emollient, stimulant, purgative, aphrodisiac, diuretic and tonic. They are useful in fever, nervous system, renal affections and dropsy. An ointment prepared from the roots is used in elephantiasis. The leaves are aphrodisiac, anthelmintic and tonic, and are useful in ulcers, inflammation, helminthiasis and general debility. The seeds are astringent, laxative, anthelmintic, aphrodisiac and tonic. They are useful in gonorrhoea, sterility and general debility.

Ethnomedicinal Uses

Paste of the seeds is applied to the ulcers of the genital

organs of both sexes. Paste of the seeds is applied to the ulcers of the genital organs of both sexes. Meat preparations are restricted in the diet during the period of treatment.

Murraya koenigii (L.) Spreng.

Family

Rutaceae

Vernacular Names

Oriya : Ban mallika, Kamini; **Hindi** : Mithanim, Katnim; **Sans** : Kaidarya; **Ko** : Mirsinga.

The Plant

An unarmed, small, aromatic tree with dark grey bark and closely crowded, spreading dark green foliage. Leaves imparipinnate, alternate, shining. Flowers white, fragrant, terminal cymes. Fruits subglobose or ellipsoid berries, purplish black when ripe. Fl. mainly Feb.-April, Fr. May-September.

Distribution

Common.

Parts Used

Root, bark, leaves.

Medicinal Properties and Uses

Root is slightly purgative. Bark and root are stimulant, externally used to cure eruptions and bites of poisonous animals. Leaves promote appetite and digestion, destroy pathogenic organisms. It is acrid, bitter, astringent, cool and light and is useful in emaciation or wasting conditions, skin diseases, worm troubles, neurosis and poisons in the system. Green leaves are eaten raw as cure for dysentery, bruised and applied externally to cure eruptions, given in decoction with bitters as febrifuge and used in snake-bite.

Ethnomedicinal Uses

The green leaves are used in curries to check gastric troubles. The decoction of green leaves (20ml) is taken internally in stomach disorders.

Mussaenda incana Wall.

Family

Rubiaceae

The Plant

Undershrub, densely hairy. Leaves subsessile or very shortly petiolate, ovate, acute, pale beneath, densely hairy beneath. Flowers yellow with the foliaceous sepals, cream or yellowish. Berry depressed globose. Fl. & Fr. Aug.-October.

Distribution

Occasional in open grassy ground or in open forests.

Parts Used

Root

Medicinal Properties and Uses

Root useful for cough, also chewed as an appetizer.

Nyctanthes arbor-tristis L.

Family

Oleaceae

Vernacular Names

Oriya : Gangasioli, Singharharo, Sephali, Gantha khelika, Singhara; **Hindi :** Harsimgar; **Sans :** Parijata.

The Plant

A hardy large shrub or small tree upto 10m in height with grey or greenish white rough bark and sharply quadrangular strigose young branches. Leaves simple, opposite, ovate, entire or coarsely toothed, acute or acuminate. Flowers small, white with bright orange corolla tubes, 3-7 in each head, in trichotomous cymes. Capsule elliptic or obovoid. Seeds orbicular. Fl. Sept.-October, Fr. Dec.-January.

Distribution

Frequent in open forests.

Parts Used

Bark, leaves, flowers, seeds.

Medicinal Properties and Uses

The leaves are bitter, acrid, thermogenic, antibacterial, anodyne, anti-inflammatory, digestive, anthelmintic, expectorant, diuretic, laxative, trichogenous and tonic. They are useful in vitiated conditions of *kapha* and *vata,* obstinate sciatica, inflammations, dyspepsia, helminthiasis, pruritus, dermatopathy. Chronic fever, bronchitis, asthma, cough, greyness of hair and baldness.

The flowers are bitter, astringent, stomachic, carminative and trichogenous and are useful in inflammations, ophthalmopathy, flatulence, colic, dyspepsia, splenomegaly, greyness of hair and baldness. The bark is expectorant, contains two alkaloids, of these the water soluble one stimulates the ciliary movements of oesophagus. The powdered seeds used for baldness, scurvy and affections of the scalp.

Ethnobotanical Uses

Decoction of shoot tips mixed with honey is taken once in a day in empty stomach for 7 days to cure malaria fever. Three leaves each of this plant and those of 'tulsi' (*Ocimum sanctum* L.) and 'nimbo' (*Azadirachta indica* A. Juss) are made into paste with water and given twice daily for two days in fever. Decoction of stem (3ml) with common salt (2gm) is taken in empty stomach for cure of dysentery and decoction of leaf (10ml) with paste of *Piper longum* (2gm) & honey (1ml) is taken twice a day before food against cold, cough and fever.

Ocimum basilicum L.

Family

Lamiaceae

Vernacular Names

Oriya : Subasi, Kapur kanti, Sugandhi, Longa baguli; **Hindi:** Gulal tulsi, Kali tulsi

The Plant

Erect, branched herb. Leaves ovate or lanceolate, entire or cut, acute, glabrous. Racemes 10-15cm long. Verticillasters many flowered, flower white. Nutlets oblong or ellipsoid. Fl. & Fr. Sept.-June.

Distribution

Common in shady and waste places.

Parts Used

Leaves, seed.

Medicinal Properties and Uses

Plant is considered stomachic, alexipharmac, antipyretic, diaphoretic, expectorant, carminative, stimulant and anthelmintic. Juice of the leaves is used as a nasal douche and for ringworm. Seeds demulcent, stimulant, diphoretic and diuretic. It is used in case of habitual constipation and piles and in poultices for sores and sinuses.

Ethnomedicinal Uses

Leaf paste mixed with sugar candy and is taken for some days in excessive menstruation.

Ocimum gratissimum L.

Family

Lamiaceae

Vernacular Names

Oriya : Ban tulsi; **Hindi :** Ram tulasi; **Sans :** Vriddha tulasi.

The Plant

Shrub or under shrub. Leaves ovate, coarsely serrate or crenate, acute or acuminate. Flowers white, inconspicuous, verticillasters in racemes. Nutlets subglobose. Fl. & Fr. Aug.–April.

Distribution

Common in shady waste ground.

Parts Used

Plant, seed.

Medicinal Properties and Uses

Species is more strongly scented than other species of the genus. It is mosquito repellent. The oil shows antibacterial activity. The oil is used for relief from ear-ache, tooth-ache and abdominal colic in children. Plant is digestive, tonic, stimulant, demulcent, diuretic, anthelmintic, antiseptic and styptic employed in cough mixtures. Seeds are given in headache, neuralgia and dysentery, an infusion used in urinary disorders, decoction given in seminal weakness. Herb is also used in aromatic baths of fumigations for rheumatism and paralysis.

Ethnomedicinal Uses

Dried leaf powder is smoked as a cigarette for getting relief from asthma and leaf juice (3ml) with honey is given to babies once in the early morning continuously ten days for the treatment of common cold and cough.

Olax scandens Roxb.

Family

Olacaceae

Vernacular Names

Oriya : Bhadai, Boderia, Bhadobhadolia; **Hindi :** Dheniani.

The Plant

Shrub or small tree or subscandent (rarely spinous); branches pubescent, leaves ovate, oblong-elliptic, obtuse rounded pubescent. Flowers white in short racemes, pedicel short. Fruit yellow, or orange, fleshy more than half enclosed in the accrescent calyx. Fl. April-August; Fr. September-October

Distribution

Occasional in forests

Parts Used

Bark

Medicinal Properties and Uses

Bark is used in a medicine and given in anaemia due to fevers.

Operculina turpethum (L.) Silva Manso

Family

Convolvulaceae

Vernacular Names

Oriya : Tihudi, Dudhalum; **Hindi :** Nisoth; **Sans :** Trivrt.

The Plant

A large stout perennial twiner with milky juice, winged, twisted, pubescent, twining stems and long slender fleshy much branched roots; leaves simple, large, very variable in shape, subacute, mucronate, more or less pubescent on both sides especially when young, base cordate or truncate; flowers white, tubular-campanulate in few flowered cymes; fruits globose capsules, enclosed in enlarged brittle imbricate sepals, seeds 4 or less, glabrous dull black. Fl. Feb.-March.

Distribution

Occasional in forests.

Parts Used

Roots.

Medicinal Properties and Uses

The roots are bitter, acrid, sweet, thermogenic, purgative, carminative, anthelmintic, expectorant, antipyetic, hepatic, stimulant and hydragogue. They are useful in colic, constipation, dropsy, vitiated conditions of *vita,* paraltsis, my algia, arthralgia, pectoralgia, bronchitis, obesity, helminthiasis, gastropathy, ascites, inflammations, intermittent fever, leucoderma, pruritus, ulcers, erysipelas, haemorrhoids, tumours, jaundice, consumpation and ophthalmia.

Ethnomedicinal Uses

Leaf paste is applied externally in case of ring worm.

Ophioglossum reticulatum L.

Family

Ophioglossaceae

Vernacular Names

Oriya : Chunuri

The Plant

Rhizome cylindrical, narrow, short, erect, without persistent brown sheaths. Tropophyll ovate, acute to rounded at apex. Strobilus long on a slender stalk, venation of the barren segment reticulate with a more or less distinct central vein but no mid rib. Fertile: Aug.-December.

Distribution

Under shade in hill forests.

Parts Used

Leaves

Ethnomedicinal Uses

5g fresh leaf along with 100g rice is made into a cake and the boiled cake is taken orally in empty stomach for 15-20 days against menstrual disorders. Seed paste is applied to the mumps. Paste of seeds (three number) is given to children twice a day for stomach-ache. Decoction of stem bark (2ml) with common salt (1gm) is prescribed twice a day for one month against menorrhagia of women.

Oroxylum indicum (L.) Kurz

Family

Bignoniaceae

Vernacular Names

Oriya : Phimpinia, Phanphana; **Hindi :** Sonapatha, Syona, Arlu, Pharkhat; **Sans :** Syonaka; **Ko :** Ringevenam

The Plant

A small to medium sized deciduous tree with soft light

brown bark with corky lenticels. Leaves very large, 90-180cm long, 2-3 pinnate with 5 or more pairs of primary pinnate, rachis very soft, cylindric swollen at the junction of the branches, leaflets 2-4 pairs ovate or elliptic, acuminate, glabrous. Flowers lurid to reddish purple outside, dull or pale pinkish yellow within, numerous in large erect racemes. Fruits flat capsules. Fl. July-August, Fr. Dec.- March.

Distribution

Occasional in open mixed forests.

Parts Used

Roots, leaves, fruits, seeds

Medicinal Properties and Uses

The roots are sweet, astringent, bitter, acrid, refrigerant, anti-inflammatory, anodyne, aphrodisiac, expectorant, appetizing, carminative, digestive, diuretic, febrifuge and tonic. They are useful in vitiated conditions of *vata* and *kapha*, inflammations, dropsy, sprains, neuralgia, hiccough, cough, asthma, bronchitis, anorexia, dyspepsia, colic and fever. The leaves are stomachic and anodyne and are useful in flatulence, cephalgia, ulcers, splenomegaly and vitiated conditions of vata. The tender fruits are expectorant, carminative and stomachic and are useful in cough, bronchitis, dyspepsia, flatulence, colic and leucoderma. The mature fruits are acrid, sweet, anthelmintic and stomachic. They are useful in pharyngodynia, cardiac disorders.

Ethnomedicinal Uses

The bark grounded into a paste is locally applied and tied for 28 days in bone fracture.

Osyris wightiana Graham

Family

Santalaceae

The Plant

Evergreen shrub, bark greyish-brown. Leaves oblanceolate, obovate, elliptic, lanceolate. Flowers very small, yellowish green. Fl. Oct.-November; Fr. Feb.-April.

Distribution

Frequent

Parts Used

Leaves

Medicinal Properties and Uses

Infusion of leaves is powerful emetic. Leaves contain tannin (20%) and may prove a good substitute of stomach.

Oxalis corniculata L.

Family

Oxalidaceae

Vernacular Names

Oriya : Ambiliti, Kumari; **Hindi :** Tinpatiya, Amrulsak, Cukatripati; **Sans :** Cangeri

The Plant

Procumbent herbs, stem creeping, rooting at nodes, hairy. Leaves alternate, leaflets subsessible. Flowers yellow, axillary or subumbellate. Fruits loculicidal cylindrical capsules. Seeds numerous, dark brown, transversely striate. Fl. & Fr. all the year round.

Distribution

Common, cultivated fields and moist places.

Parts Used

Whole plant.

Medicinal Properties and Uses

The plant is sour, astringent, thermogenic, cooling to touch, anti-inflammatory, digestive, carminative, liver tonic, diuretic, constipating, antibacterial and antiseptic. Fresh juice of plant is given in dyspepsia, piles, anemia and tympanitis, fever, dysentery, diarrhoea and burning sensation. Infusion of leaves is used to cure opacity of the cornea. Leaf juice is given to counteract Datura poisoning. Leaves are also used to cure cough and indigestion. The ground leaves are eaten as chutney to help purify the blood. An infusion of the leaves is used to treat indurations of the breasts and watery vaginal discharges. It is used to treat wounds and sores and swelling beneath tongue.

Ethnomedicinal Uses

Roots are made into paste along with garlic and given 1 teaspoonful twice a day for cold. The leaves are eaten as vegetable to check burning sensation of soles.

Paederia foetida L.

Family

Rubiaceae

Vernacular Names

Oriya : Gandhali, Prasaruni; **Hindi** : Prasaruni; **Sans** : Prasaruni

The Plant

Foetid shrub, climbing by means of twining stems and twisted petioles. Leaves elliptic-ovate, narrow ovate acute, glabrous. Flowers purple, nearly sessile, tube funnel shaped. Fl. Aug.-October.

Distribution

Occasional in mixed forests near streams.

Parts Used

Fresh leaves

Medicinal Properties and Uses

The leaves are well known for their anti-dysenteric properties and are indicated in the treatment of bacillary dysentery. Fresh leaves which are fine cut and mixed with a hen egg then covered with banana leaves and grilled or fried in a frying pan, a decoction of the leaves is also used in treating urinary lithiasis, dysuria, rheumatism, dyspepsia, gastritis and enteritis. Juice of roots used in piles, inflammations of spleen and pain in chest and liver.

Ethnomedicinal Uses

Leaves cooked as curry is taken with food to get relief from joints pain. Stem is tied around waist for two to three days to get relief from waist pain.

Panicum sumatrense Roth ex R. & Schult.

Family

Poaceae

Vernacular Names

Oriya : Gundla, Gurunji; **Hindi :** Kungu, Kutki; **Ko :** Gundi.

The Plant

A slender erect, branched usually leafy up to the panicle. Leaves linear, tapering from a broad base, glabrous or finely hairy. Spikelets glabrous. Fl. & Fr. August.

Distribution

Cultivated

Parts Used

Grains

Medicinal Properties and Uses

The grains are astringent, sweet, emollient, cooling and constipating. They are useful in burning sensation, diarrhoea, dysentery wounds, ulcer and gonorrhoea

---

Parthenium hysterophorus L.

Family

Asteraceae

The Plant

Erect pubescent herb. Leaves oblong or obvate, acute. Head heterogamous. Capitula white. Fl. & Fr. mainly Oct.-April.

Distribution

Common in waste places, river sides and cultivated open land.

Parts Used

Plant, Root

Medicinal Properties and Uses

Plants used as tonic, febrifuge, emmenagogue and analgesic. Decoction of roots given in dysentery.

Paspalum scrobiculatum L.

Family

Poaceae

Vernacular Names

Oriya : Kodo, Kogue; **Sans. :** Kodravah; **Hindi :** Kodra; **Ko :** Garakode

The Plant

An annual grass with tufted on very short rhizome. Leaves glabrous or sometimes softly hairy, spikelets suborbicular, glumes glabrous. Fl. & Fr. October-November.

Distribution

Common in moist and wet places.

Parts Used

Grains, stem.

Medicinal Properties and Uses

The grains are sweet, bitter, astringent, cool, diuretic, sedative and tonic. They are useful in ulcers, flatulence, diarrhoea, hepatopathy, haemorrhages and general debility. Stem is useful in corneal opacity.

Peperomia tetraphylla (Forst.) Hook. & Arn.

Family

Piperaceae

The Plant

Small tufted glabrous herb. Leaves mostly 4 in whorl, obovate, obtuse or rounded, thick and flesh when fresh, coriaceous when dry. Spikes mostly terminal. Flowers sunk in cavities of the rachis. Fl. & Fr. Oct.-April.

Distribution

Occasional in damp forests on moss clad rocks and tree trunk.

Parts Used

Leaves

Medicinal Properties and Uses

Tonic prepared from leaves is used specially in kidney disorders.

Pergularia daemia (Forsk.) Chiov.

Family

Asclepiadaceae

Vernacular Names

Oriya : Utrali, Euturudi; **Hindi :** Utaran, Sagovani; **Sans.:** Kuruta kah

The Plant

A slender foul smelling perennial milky twining herb. Leaves opposite, cordate, acuminate and valvety pubescent beneath. Flowers greenish yellow or dull white in long peduncled umbellate or corymbose clusters. Fl. Aug.-December. Fr. Jan.-April.

Distribution

Common in hedges and also in forests.

Parts Used

Whole plant.

Medicinal Properties and Uses

The plant is astringent, acrid, expectorant, anthelmintic, antipyretic and laxative. It is useful in inflammations, cough, asthma, amenorrhoea, fevers and leucoderma, The leaves are useful in leprosy and haemorrhoids. Fruits are digestive and thermogenic. Plant extract is useful in uterine and menstrual disorders and in facilitating parturition.

Ethnomedicinal Uses

Leaf (500 g) and root (500 g) of the plant, root of *Cyperus rotundus* (500 g) are boiled in mustard oil (250 ml). The residue is applied on leprotic wound.

Petalidium barlerioides (Roth)Nees

Family

Acanthaceae

Vernacular Names

Oriya : Drakappa, Malpi.

The Plant

Straggling shrub. Leaves ovate, crenate, and serrate. Flowers white, sub-solitary or in opposite decussate pairs in dense or subcapittate spikes. Capsule cuspidate, glabrous. Seeds usually 2. Fl. Feb.-April, Fr. April-May.

Distribution

Occasional in forests.

Parts Used

Root.

Medicinal Properties and Uses

Roots used in renal affections.

Phoebe lanceolata Nees

Family

Lauraceae

Vernacular Names

Hindi : Haulia.

The Plant

Small tree, bark grey, nearly smooth, twigs brown, with persistent leaf scars and lenticels. Leaves lanceolate, narrowly oblong, long acuminate or caudate, glabrous, secondary nerves 6-11, fine, distinct.. Fl. March-May. Fr. May–July.

Distribution

Common in shady valleys.

Parts Used

Berry

Medicinal Properties and Uses

Ash of the berries is applied in wounds and sores.

Phyllanthus emblica L.

Family

Euphorbiaceae

Vernacular Names

Oriya : Anola, Amla; **Hindi :** Aonla, Amlika; **Sans :** Amlika; **Ko :** Aura

The Plant

Small or moderate sized deciduous tree; bark light grey. Leaves linear or linear oblong, margined, apiculate, glabrous. Flowers monoecious, yellowish minute in axillary fascicles. Male and female flowers mixed or frequently female in the lower and males in upper axils of present or fallen leaves. Drupe globose, succulent, yellow or tinged with pink when ripe, with a 6 ridged putamen which is tardily dehiscent at the ridges. Fl. Feb.- May. Fr. Oct.-April. Deciduous: March–April.

Distribution

Common in forest.

Parts Used

Root, bark, leaves, fruits.

Medicinal Properties and Uses

The root bark is astringent, and is useful in ulcerative stomatits and gastrohelcosis. The bark is useful in gonorrhoea, jaundice, diarrhoea and myalgia. The leaves are useful in conjuctivitis, inflammation, dyspepsia, diarrhoea and dysentery.

The fruits are sour, astringent, bitter, acrid, sweet, cooling, anodyne, ophthalmic, carminative, digestive, stomachic, laxative, antipyretic, tonic and trichogenous. They are useful in vitiated conditions of tridosa, diabetes, cough, asthma, bronchitis, dyspepsia, diarrhoea, dysentery, hemorrhages, menorrhagia, cardiac disorders and greyness of hair. The fruit is rich in vitamin C.

Ethnomedicinal Uses

Fresh leaf juice (2ml) with diluted solution of common salt (1ml) used as a drop in eyes for improving weak eyesight.

Phyllanthus fraternus Webster

Family

Euphorbiaceae

Vernacular Names

Oriya : Bhuianla, Bariamla, Bhui amla; **Hindi :** Jangli amli; **Sans :** Amalaki.

The Plant

Erect annual herb. Leaves ellipitic-oblong, rounded, dark green above paler beneath, with prominent midrib. Flowers in axillary, unisexual cymules on deciduous branchlets, whitish green. Capsule rounded. Seeds with 6-7 longitudinal ribs and many fine transverse striae on the back. Fl. & Fr. April-January.

Distribution

Common weed.

Parts Used

Whole plant.

Medicinal Properties and Uses

Plant is astringent, deobstruent, stomachic, diuretic, and febrifuge, used for stomach trouble such as diarrhoea, dysentery, dyspepsia and colic. It is also used in dropsy and diseases at urino-genital system. Fresh roots are given in jaundice and also used as a galactagogue and viral hepatitis. Latex is applied to sores.

Ethnomedicinal Uses

3 gms root powder is taken with milk for 3-4 days in case of ascitis (rakta pradar).

Piper trioicum Roxb.

Family

Piperaceae

Vernacular Names

Oriya : Chaikatho; **Ko :** Rali.

The Plant

Rambling or climbing by adventitious roots, branches glabrous. Leaves broadly ovate, membranous or coriaceous, pale or glaucous, glabrous above, especially on the nerves beneath. Spikes, bracts adnate, cupular, rounded at apex. Female spikes, on slender penduncles. Berries globose.

Distribution

Frequent in damp valleys.

Parts Used

Fruit.

Medicinal Properties and Uses

The berries are well known for their stomachic, anodyne and antibacterial properties. They are prescribed for treating dyspepsia, vomiting, diarrhoea and colic, resulting from cold. The powdered berries are applied topically to cure toothache. Pepper is employed as an aromatic stimulant and as an anti-periodic in malaria fever.

Ethnomedicinal Uses

Paste of bark mixed with raw tea (tea and sugar in hot water) is given in cough and asthma. Fresh stem piece is dipped in water and a drop of water is poured in redness of eyes. For eye troubles, especially when they turn reddish a fresh stem piece of this plant is taken and dipped in water and a drop of water is poured in each eye. A decoction of stem is given in asthma. The nodal portion of stem (2-5 cm long) is made into paste with black peppers and garlic, heated and given thrice a day for two days only for cold, tonsillitis and throat infection.

Plesmonium margaritiferum (Roxb.) Schott

Family

Araceae

Vernacular Names

Oriya : Jhumpagudi; **Hindi :** Jalulija, bansur; **Ko :** Had.

The Plant

Tubers large. Leaf solitary, digitately 3-foliolate. Spathe broadly ovoid or deltoid, green and leathery, deep purple at base within and often flushed purple above. Berries orange. Fl. May-June, Fr. Oct.-November.

Distribution

Common in open forests.

Parts Used

Tubers, seeds.

Medicinal Properties and Uses

Tubers pounded and used on swelling. Crushed seeds used for tooth ache and as an external application to bruises.

Plumbago zeylanica L.

Family

Plumbaginaceae

Vernacular Names

Oriya : Dhola chitaparu; **Hindi** : Chitra; **Ko** : Sitaparu

The Plant

A perennial, sub-scandent shrub, glabrous. Leaves ovate or oblong-ovate, glabrous. Flowers white, in elongated, terminal. Capsule oblong, acute with 5 furrows. Fl. & Fr. Sept.-April.

Distribution

Frequent in open places.

Parts Used

Root, leaves.

Medicinal Properties and Uses

Externally a paste of the leaves and root is applied to painful rheumatic areas or to chronic and itchy skin problems.

Paste of root applied for opening abscesses. Infusion of roots used in influenza and black–water fever. Root bark contains plumbagin, the active principle.

Ethnomedicinal Uses

About 5 g of root powder is given daily after menses to check conception. Two teaspoons of root infusion is given twice daily for 10 days to treat spleen enlargement.

Pogostemon benghalensis (Burm. f.) Kuntze

Family

Lamiaceae

Vernacular Names

Oriya : Poksunga

The Plant

Erect herb or shrub. Leaves ovate, lanceolate, serrate, acute. Flowers bluish, purple in capitate. Fl. & Fr. February to April.

Distribution

Common in forests and shady places.

Parts Used

Leaves, root.

Medicinal Properties and Uses

Leaves used as a stimulant and styptic. Juice used in colic and febrifuge. Leaves contain an essential oil. Roots are stimulant and antihaemorrhagic.

Polyalthia longifolia (Sonn.) Thw.

Family

Annonaceae

Vernacular Names

Oriya : Debdaru; **Hindi :** Asoka, Debdari

The Plant

Tall evergreen tree, young branches, slender, glabrous. Leaves narrowly lanceolate, shining, margin undulate. Flowers yellowish green. Seeds smooth, shining. Fl. Mar.-April, Fr. July-August.

Distribution

Commonly planted in gardens and as avenue trees.

Parts Used

Bark

Medicinal Properties and Uses

Bark is febrifuge, bitter, acrid and anthelmintic. It is useful in fever, skin diseases, diabetes, hypertension and vitiated conditions of *vata* and *pitta*.

Ethnomedicinal Uses

The dry and old seed rubbed against stone with water is applied in reptile-bites and scropion stings.

Polygonum hydropiper L.

Family

Polygonaceae

The Plant

Decumbent, ascending or rarely erect, glabrous herb. Leaves linear, lanceolate, gland dotted, stipules glabrous. Flowers pink, in rather lax, very slender or filiform racemes with lower bracts distant. Nut usually triquetrous. Fl. & Fr. Sept.-Jan.

Distribution

Common along stream banks.

Parts Used

Root

Medicinal Properties and Uses

Plant is stimulant, diuretic, styptic, emmenagogue and lithontriptic. Liquid extract of herb is used as an oral contraceptive. Infusion is used in uterine disorders and as a hemostatic. Root is stimulant, diuretic, carminative, tonic and anthelmintic. Their juice is used for skin affections. Powder of the dried herb is used as a fish poison. Yields a dye and an essential oil.

Ethnomedicinal Uses

The inflorescence and upper leaves are made into paste and applied over affected parts in ringworm.

Polygonum strigosum R. Br.

Family

Polygonaceae

The Plant

Suberect herb, widely creeping at the base, stem angular. Leaves oblong or liner oblong, base rounded or sub cordate. Flowers pink, in very short, sub globose heads or racemes. Nut globosely trigonous. Fl. November.

Distribution

Frequent along streams

Parts Used

Leaves

Medicinal Properties and Uses

Infusion of leaves is used as fish poison. Cases of poisoning in livestock are reported.

Ethnomedicinal Uses

Leaves are used in gastric disorders.

Pongamia pinnata (L.) Pierre

Family

Fabaceae

Vernacular Names

Oriya : Karanjo; **Hindi :** Karanj, Karanja; **Sans :** Koranja; **Ko :** Karanj

The Plant

Moderate to large sized tree, sometimes flowering in shrubby form on the sea coasts, bark smooth, thin grey. Leaves 20-35 cm long, leaflets 5-7, ovate or oblong, entire, acuminate. Flowers purplish white or pinkish white. Pods woody. Seed reddish–brown. Fl. May-June, Fr. Dec.-January.

Distribution

Common along streams.

Parts Used

Root, bark, leaves, flowers, seed oil.

Medicinal Properties and Uses

Medicinally it is applied in scabies, herpes, leucoderma and other cutaneous diseases. Internally it is used in dyspepsia with sluggish liver. The roots are good for cleaning foul ulcers, cleaning teeth, strengthening gums and gonorrhoea. A root paste is used for local application of scrofulous enlargements. The fresh bark is sweet and mucilaginous to taste, soon becoming bitter and acrid. It is anthelmintic and alexeteric and is useful in haemorrhoides, beriberi, ophthalmopathy, dermatopathy and ulcer. Fresh bark given for piles. Decoction of bark used in beri beri. Leaves are digestive laxative and anthelmintic and are good for flatulence, dyspepsia, diarrhoea, leprosy, gonorrhoea and cough. Flowers are useful to quench dipsia in diabetes and for alleviating *vata* and *kapha.* The seeds are anthelmintic, haematinic, bitter, acrid and carminative. They are useful in inflammation, otalgia, lumbago, chronic fever and anaemia. The oil is anthelmintic, stypic and depurative and is recommended for scabies, opthalmia, leprosy, haemorrhoides, ulcers, herps and lumbago.

Ethnomedicinal Uses

Stem is used as tooth brush. The juice from the bark is touched with an hot iron rod and then the juice is orally given to mother immediate as a precautions to tetanus. Seed oil is used in skin diseases and rheumatism. The dried flower powder mixed with honey is used to cure diabetes.

Pothos scandens L.

Family

Araceae

The Plant

Much branched scandent herb. Leaf blade elliptic, ovate, oblong, acute. Spathe peduncled cymbiform. Spadix ellipsoid, globose. Fl. September.

Distribution

Occasional in shady valleys.

Parts Used

Leaves, fruits.

Medicinal Properties and Uses

Powdered leaves are applied to small pox pustules. Root is bruised and fried in oil for application to abscesses.

Premna coriacea C.B.Cl.

Family

Verbenaceae

The Plant

Large woody climber. Leaves ovate-oblong, caudate, glabrous or minutely pubescent coriaceous. Flowers very small, white fragrant, in pubescent, corymbose panicles. Drupe narrowly obovoid. 1 seed. Fl. & Fr. May–June.

Distribution

Common in forests.

Parts Used

Root, leaves.

Medicinal Properties and Uses

Roots are laxative, stomachic, cordial and tonic and form a constituent of Ayurvedic medicine. Leaves are carminative and galactagogue and are used in the preparation of soups and given as a stomachic. Decoction of leaves is given in flatulence and colic.

Ethnomedicinal Uses

Leaf juice is applied externally to cure headache.

Prunus ceylanica (Wight) Miq.

Family

Rosaceae

The Plant

Tree, twigs brown. Leaves ovate, elliptic or oblong, acute or shortly acuminate, shining base. Flowers yellowish green. Drupes transversely ellipsoid. Fl. August. Fr. April–June.

Distribution

Common along stream.

Parts Used

Bark

Medicinal Properties and Uses

Bark is used for stomach-ache. Kernels used for the fish poison.

Pteris pellucida Presl.

Family

Pteridaceae

Vernacular Names

Ko : Saloi

The Plant

Larger and stout plant. Stipes 30 cm or more. Fronds long, simply pinnate or occasionally lowest forked. Pinnae usually 3-6 sessile pairs, entire or serrate. Young fronds often digitate. Fertile : Nov.-December.

Distribution

Occasional in moist hill sides.

Parts Used

Leaves.

Medicinal Properties and Uses

50g fresh leaf paste mixed with 5ml of cow ghee is administered thrice a day for 7 days for early maturation of boils.

Pteris quadriaurita Retz.

Family

Pteridaceae

Vernacular Names

Ko : Sunkia

The Plant

Stipe glabrus. Fronds variable in size, texture, lanceolate or ovate, acute, entire or serrate. Sori generally partial on the segment rarely continued to the apex. Fertile: Nov.- March

Distribution

Common in forests along streams.

Parts Used

Leaves.

Medicinal Properties and Uses

10 ml of fresh leaf juice is taken with 200ml toddy (sap) obtained from *Phoenix sylvestris* Roxb. in the early morning on empty stomach and at noon for 2-3 days for irregular menstrual cycle.

Pterocarpus marsupium Roxb.

Family

Fabaceae

Vernacular Names

Oriya : Bija, Piasala; **Hindi :** Bijasala, Bija; **Sans :** Asana

The Plant

A medium sized to large tree with dark brown of grey bark having shallow cracks. Leaves compound, imparipinnate, leaflets 5-7 coriaceous, oblong, obtuse, glabrous on both surfaces. Flowers yellow in terminal panicles. Fruits nearly circular, glabrous flat winged pods. Fl. Apr.-July, Fr. Aug.-October.

Distribution

Frequent in deciduous and evergreen forests.

Parts Used

Heartwood, leaves, flowers, gum.

Medicinal Properties and Uses

The heartwood is astringent, bitter, acrid, anti-inflammatory, depurative, urinary astringent and useful in leprosy, skin diseases, leucoderma, diabetes, haemorrhages. The leaves are useful in boils, sores and skin diseases. The flowers are bitter, sweet, cooling, appetizing and febrifuge, and are useful in vitiated conditions of *pitta,* anorexia and fevers. The gum is bitter, styptic, vulnerary, antipyretic, anthelmintic and liver tonic. It is useful in spasmodic gastralgia, vitiated conditions of *pitta,* boils, urethrorrhoea, diarrhoea, psoriasis, wounds and ulcers.

Ethnomedicinal Uses

Juice of bark (10gms) is given two to three times for cure of mouth sores. The small heart wood pieces dipped in water in night and that water is taken in morning every days in diabetes.

Pueraria tuberosa (Willd.) DC.

Family

Fabaceae

Vernacular Names

Oriya : Bhuikakharu, Patal kumra; **Hindi :** Viddari kand, sural.

The Plant

A large woody deciduous climbing shrub with huge tuberous root. Tubers white inside, starchy and mildly sweet. Leaves alternate, 3-foliolate, leaflets egg-shaped. Flower bisexual with bluish purplet pale violet. Fl. Feb.-April, Fr. May-June.

Distribution

Occasional in forests

Parts Used

Tubers

Medicinal Properties and Uses

Tubers used for treatment of dysuria, cough, rheumatism and malaria fever. The roots are said to be used in medicine as a demulcent and refrigerant in fevers for swellings of joints and as lactagogue.

Ethnomedicinal Uses

The tuber and other parts of the plant pounded in water and taken in body swellings.

Punica granatum L.

Family

Punicaceae

Vernacular Names

Oriya : Dalimba, Dalim; **Hindi :** Anar; **Sans :** Dalima.

The Plant

Shrub to small tree up to 6m high. Leaves mostly opposite, short petiolate, blades oblong-elliptical upto 8cm long. Flowers showy, bisexual, 5-8 petals, reddish, numerous stamens surrounding a conspicuous hypanthial tube, the flowers usually occurring terminally or in axis. Fruit a red spherical berry. Flowers available during the summer. Fl. chiefly April-May, Fr. July-September.

Distribution

Commonly cultivated as an ornamental and fruit tree.

Parts Used

Seeds, flowers.

Medicinal Properties and Uses

Root and stem bark of Dalimbo are astringent, anthelmintic, specific in tapeworm. Grains and its alkaloids are astringent, anthelmintic and taenifuge. Flowers, bark of the tree and rind of fruit are astringent and stomachic. Fresh juice is cooling and refrigerant. Rind of fruit combined with aromatics like cloves etc. useful in diarrhoea and dysentery. Seeds are stomachic, pulp is cardiac and stomachic.

Ethnomedicinal Uses

Leprosy patients get benefit from fruit juice. Tannin is obtained from fruit rind, stem, root bark and leaves. The flowers yield red dye which is used for dyeing cloth. Fruit juice with molasses is used in case of indigestion.

Quisqualis indica L.

Family

Combretaceae

Vernacular Names

Oriya : Rangani, Baramasi; **Hindi :** Rangoon, Laata chameli; **Sans :** Madhumalati

The Plant

Large sarmentose or climbing shrubs, young parts brown–villous or pubescent. Leaves elliptic or obovate, entire, shortly acuminate. Flowers scented, showy pink- white or reddish–white. Fl. & Fr. most part of the year.

Distribution

Commonly cultivated in gardens.

Parts Used

Leaves, seeds.

Medicinal Properties and Uses

Leaves are given in a compound decoction for flatulent distension of abdomen. Fruits and seeds are used as children's anthelmintic for ascaris. Roasted seeds used in diarrhoea and fever. They are also used for rickets in children. Oil is used in parasitic skin troubles. Macerated in oil seeds are used as an external application to parasitic skin diseases. Oil from seeds is purgative.

Ranunculus pennsylvanicus L.f.

Family

Ranunculaceae

The Plant

Annual hairy herb. Leaves long petiolate, 3 foliolate with 3 sect. leaflets, upper most leaves sessile on a short sheath. Flowers corymbose, yellow, achenes smooth and glabrous. Fl. April-July. Fr. June-August.

Distribution

Along streams and water courses in wet places.

Parts Used

Whole plant.

Medicinal Properties and Uses

Plant is used to raise blisters. It is also used as a vesicant and shows antibacterial activity.

Rauvolfia serpentina (L.) Benth.ex Kurz.

Family

Apocynaceae

Vernacular Names

Oriya : Patal garura, Patalgaruda, Bhuin karua; **Hindi :** Chota chand, Sarpagandha; **Ko :** Chhedabag

The Plant

Glabrous undershrub. Leaves 3-4-nately whorled, opposite, elliptic-oblong, glabrous, bright green and shining above. Flowers small, white with pink tube, in terminal, peduncled bright red cymes. Drupes black when ripe, globose. Fl. & Fr. May-November.

Distribution

Scarce, in miscellaneous forests, rare.

Parts Used

Root

Medicinal Properties and Uses

The chief use of the drug is as sedative and hypnotic and for reducing blood pressure. The drug is now largely used in insanity and high blood pressure. The alkaloids stimulate the central nervous system. It is more suitable for chronic mental illness. The drug has tranquillizing effect. Root is also considered as anthelmintic and an antidote to snake venom. Its decoction is given during labour pains to increase uterine contraction. Juice of the leaves is used for the cure of corneal opacity of the eyes.

Ethnomedicinal Uses

The root made into poultice is applied externally in eczema. The drug is suitable for mild anxiety cases or patients of cronic mental illness. Root powder mixed with 21 nos. of *Piper nigrum* and is taken with water at every half an hour as antivenus.

Rhinacanthus nasutus (L.) Kurz

Family

Acanthaceae

Vernacular Names

Oriya : Kaura sago; **Hindi :** Palak juhi

The Plant

Slender, divaricately branched under shrub. Leaves large, ovate, elliptic, acute, flowers white, in clusters at the ends of the branches of large spreading nearly marked. Capsule, seeds 4-2. Fl. & Fr. Sept.–April.

Distribution

Frequent in shady places in forests.

Parts Used

Root, leaves.

Medicinal Properties and Uses

Fresh roots and leaves bruised and mixed with lime, are

used externally in eczema, ringworm and dhobi's itch. Leaves are used against cancer. Roots are boiled in milk and used as an aphrodisiac. Roots contain rhinacanthin accredited with antiseptic and anti-parasitic properties.

Rhus chinensis Miller

Family

Anacardiaceae

Vernacular Names

Hindi : Tatri.

The Plant

Small tree, bark rough, twigs, rachis and leaves beneath densely pubescent. Leaves imparipinnate, narrowly margined or winged towards the end. Flowers white or yellowish green. Drupe red, shining, subglobose compressed. Fl. June–Sept., Fr. December.

Distribution

Found in south Similipal.

Parts Used

Gallnut

Medicinal Properties and Uses

Astringent, haemostatic, antibacterial, antifungal, antiviral. Used in colic, diarrhoea, dysentery, abnormal sweating and haemorrhage.

Rhynchostylis retusa (L.) Bl.

Family

Orchidaceae

Vernacular Names

Oriya : Pumam

The Plant

Stem stout, closely covered with half sheaths. Leaves jointed at the base above the sheath, linear, curved. Flowers pink-purple, in drooping racemes. Capsules clavate, reflexed. Fl. May-June, Fr. July-December.

Distribution

Common epiphyte in open forests.

Parts Used

Leaves.

Medicinal Properties and Uses

Leaves of these plants are used to treat rheumatic diseases.

Ethnomedicinal Uses

Plant paste is applied in the treatment of bone fracture. Leaf paste is applied over the body during fever.

Rubia cordifolia L.

Family

Rubiaceae

Vernacular Names

Oriya : Rango chireta; **Hindi** : Manjeet, Majith.

The Plant

A very variable prickly or scabrous climbing perennial herb with long cylindric, flexuose, smooth reddish, roots and 4-angled rough stems and branches. Leaves very variable 2-8 in a whorl often only 4, cordate-ovate-lanceolate, base rounded or slightly cordate, petioles very long, provided with sharp recurved prickles on the edges, stipules absent. Flowers white, greenish yellowish or reddish, sweet scented, small, in terminal panicled glabrous cymes. Fruits globose or slightly 2-lobed, fleshy, smooth, purplish black when ripe. Seeds two, small. Fl. Oct.-November, Fr. Dec.-February.

Distribution

Commonly found in forests.

Parts Used

Root

Medicinal Properties and Uses

The roots are sweet, bitter, astringent, thermogenic, anti-inflammatory, antiseptic, digestive, carminative, constipating, anthelmintic, depurative, vulnerary, diuretic, galacto-purifier, alterant, ophthalmic, febrifuge and tonic. They are useful in vitiated conditions of *kapha* and *pitta*, rheumatoid arthritis, neuralgia, cephalagia, dyspepsia, flatulence, colic, diarrhoea, dysentery, helminthiasis, leprosy, skin diseases, leucoderma, wounds, ulcers, diabetes and general debility.

Ethnomedicinal Uses

Root along with that of *Cissampelos pareira* L. is used in the preparation of wine to give it more intoxicating effect.

Rungia pectinata (L.) Nees

Family

Acanthaceae

Vernacular Names

Ko : Sankh sago.

The Plant

Diffuse or erect herb. Leaves ovate lanceolate, linear or narrowly lanceolate to narrowly elliptic. Flowers very small, blue, in clustered secund spikes. Capsule 2mm. compressed. Fl. & Fr. most part of the year.

Distribution

Fairly common weed.

Parts Used

Leaves.

Medicinal Properties and Uses

Juice of leaves are refrigerant and aperients. Bruised leaves are applied to contusions. Roots are used as febrifuge. Herb is used as an adulterant of the drug fumitory.

Salix tetrasperma Roxb.

Family

Salicaceae

Vernacular Names

Oriya : Panibegunia, Panijamo; **Hindi :** Jalmala, Luila, Bains; **Ko :** Nachal.

The Plant

Small tree or large shrub with often silky pubescent branchlets, bark rough leaves, linear-lanceolate, entire, acuminate. Flowers creamy white. Fl. October. Fr. Feb–May.

Distribution

Common along rivers and streams.

Parts Used

Leaves, Bark.

Medicinal Properties and Uses

Dried leaves, mixed with sugar, are given in rheumatism, epilepsy, veneral diseases, stone in the bladder, piles and swellings. Bark is used as a febrifuge.

Saraca asoca (Roxb.) de Wilde

Family

Caesalpiniaceae

Vernacular Names

Oriya : Ashok; **Hindi :** Ashok; **Ko :** Usangid-ba; **Sans:** Ashoka.

The Plant

Small tree, leaves subsessile, dark green, leaflets 3-6 pairs, large, oblong, lanceolate, acute or acuminate. Flowers bright orange–scarlet. Pods slightly oblique both ends. Fl. March-April, Fr. September.

Distribution

Occasional in valleys along stream.

Parts Used

Bark, leaves, flowers.

Medicinal Properties and Uses

The plant is known as uterine tonic. It imparts a healthy tone and strength to uterus. In bloody leucorrhoea whether acute or chronic, it exerts an exhilarating and permanent curative action. It is an excellent remedy in suppressed menses for which colicky abdominal pains supervine, also useful for complaints of menopause and barrenness. Bark is astringent, bitter, sweet, styptic, febrifuge and used in uterine affection, dyspepsia, fever, dipsia, visceromegaly, colic, ulcers and menorrhagia. Leaves are depurative and their juice mixed with cumin seeds is used for treating stomachalgia. Flowers used as a uterine tonic and also used in biliousness, hemorrhagia, dysentery and diabetes.

Ethnomedicinal Uses

Alcoholic extract of the flower bud effectively useful in the case of late menstruation in case of domestic animals like cow, buffalo etc. Pounded flowers mixed with water is given for haemorrhagic dysentery.

Sauropus quadrangularis (Willd.) Muell. - Arg.

Family

Euphorbiaceae

The Plant

Glabrous undershrub, stems more or less angled. Leaves elliptic, obovate, apex rounded, obtuse, acute. Male flowers greenish yellow, minute, stellate. Fruit globose, depressed. Fl. & Fr. Most part of the year.

Distribution

Frequent in forests.

Parts Used

Leaves.

Medicinal Properties and Uses

Dried leaves smoked as a cure for tonsillitis.

Schleichera oleosa (Lour.) Oken

Family

Sapindaceae

Vernacular Names

Oriya : Kusum; **Hindi :** Kasma, Kausum; **Ko :** Kohumu, Baru

The Plant

A medium sized to large tree with a dense spreading crown and smooth pale brown bark exfoliating in small irregular flakes. Leaves paripinate, alternate, leaflets 2-4 pairs, large, elliptic or oblong. Flowers small, greenish yellow. Fruits ovoid or globose. Seeds 1-2 brown, oily. Fl. Feb.-March, Fr. June-August.

Distribution

Frequent in forests especially in valleys.

Parts Used

Bark, oil.

Medicinal Properties and Uses

The bark is astringent and antipyretic and is useful in pruritus, adenitis, ripening boils, malaria, inflammations and ulcers. The seed oil is bitter, sour, sweet, stomachic, anthelmintic, purgative and tonic. It is useful in pruritus, burns, acne, dermatopathy, scald, ulcers and vitiated conditions of *vata.*

Ethnomedicinal Uses

Stem bark paste is applied on skin before bed as curative against for itching and seed oil are used for treatment of gout and scabies. Seed-paste is heated and applied warm to the cuts. White patches on the skin are cured by applying seed-paste.

Flowers and flower buds yield an oil, applied both on hair and skin. The oil extract of seeds is used in leg swelling.

Schrebera swietenioides Roxb.

Family

Oleaceae

Vernacular Names

Oriya : Eksira; **Hindi :** Moka, Banpalas

The Plant

A moderate sized deciduous tree upto 20m in height with thick grey bark. Leaves imparipinnate, leaflets opposite, 3-4 pairs, ovate, entire, unequal-sided, petioles thickened at the insertion of leaflets. Flowers yellowish brown in terminal trichotmous, corymbose, compound cymes. Fruits pendulous, pear shaped, 2-valved capsules. Seeds 8, ending in long wings. Fl. May-June with the new leaves, Fr. Oct.-March. Deciduous Feb.-March.

Distribution

Frequent in mixed forests.

Parts Used

Roots, bark, leaves, fruits

Medicinal Properties and Uses

The roots, bark and leaves are bitter, acrid, appetizing, digestive, thermogenic, stomachic, depurative, constipating, urinary astringent and anthelmintic. They are useful in vitiated conditions of *kapha,* dyspepsia, colic, flatulence, skin diseases, leprosy, diarrhoea, urethrorrhoea, anaemia, helminthiasis, boils, burns and rectal disorders. The fruits are reported to be useful in curing hydrocele. It is digestive, purgative and stomachic, and is useful in flatulence, anorexia, colic, anaemia, haemorrhoides, vesical calculi and diabetes.

Scindapsus officinalis (Roxb.) Schott

Family

Araceae

Vernacular Names

Oriya : Girudhuni, Gajapippali, Panchamula; **Hindi:** Gajapipal; **Sans :** Gajapippali

The Plant

A large epiphytic climber with adventitious aerial roots growing on trees and rocks. Leaves large, up to 25cm long, leathery. Flowers densely arranged in the spadix which is cylindric, spathe green outside and yellow within. Fruit berries. Fl. June-July, Fr. January.

Distribution

Occasional in forests.

Parts Used

Fruits, inflorescence.

Medicinal Properties and Uses

Fruits stimulant, diaphoretic, carminative and anthelmintic. It is given in diarrhoea. Decoction given as an expectorant in asthma. Fruits as well as shoots show hypoglycaemic activity and the former also show antiprotozoal activity. Fruits yield a fatty oil. Mature inflorescence powder with jaggery is given twice a day before meal for 15 days to cure diabetes.

Ethnomedicinal Uses

Roots of the plant is used in cough and fever.

Scoparia dulcis L.

Family

Scrophulariaceae

Vernacular Names

Oriya : Chirarita, Khelopapada; **Sant :** Jastimadhu

The Plant

Annual herbaceous plant. Stems woody at the base, much branched, quadarangular when young. Leaves small or opposite, coarsely toothed-serrate. Flowers white. Capsule small, globose, many seeded. Fl. & Fr All the year round.

Distribution

Common weed.

Parts Used

Whole plant.

Medicinal Properties and Uses

The entire plant, including the roots, possesses anti-inflammatory, antifertile and diuretic properties. It is used in treating coryza, hyperthermia, sore throat, cough, erythema, measles, boils, impetigo, manioc and other poisoning and menorrhagia. The fresh plant is especially active against dry cough.

Ethnomedicinal Uses

Few drops of plant juice is mixed with the urine of a woman, any change in colour suggests that the woman is pregnant. A handful of leaves are chewed twice daily to cure diarrhoea and excessive and irregular mensturation.

Selaginella repanda (Desv. ex Poir.) Spring

Family

Selaginellaceae

Vernacular Names

Oriya: Muli saga

The Plant

Stems suberect to erect, pale brown with age. Branched from the base. Pinnately compound. Rhizophores restricted at the base only. Leaves heteromorphic. Strobili tetragonous, single at the apex of branchlets. Sporophylls uniform, ovate, acuminate. Fertile; most part of the year.

Distribution

Fairly common in damp places.

Parts Used

Root.

Medicinal Properties and Uses

Decoction given as a protective medicine after parturition.

Ethnomedicinal Uses

About 10g of the root powder is mixed with boiled water and made a paste. The paste is applied externally on the white patches in case of leprosy. Care should be taken to remove the paste after 5-7 minutes, otherwise there is a chance of irritation.

Semecarpus anacardium L.f.

Family

Anacardiaceae

Vernacular Names

Oriya : Bhalia; **Hindi :** Bhela, Bhilava; **Ko :** Soso; **Sans:** Bhallataka

The Plant

Small tree, young branchlets pubescent or tomentose.

Leaves obovate or oblong, clustered at the ends of the branches. Flowers dull greenish – yellow. Drupe oblong or obliquely ovoid, black when ripe. Fl. June-September, Fr. Nov.-December, Deciduous March-May.

Distribution

Common in forests.

Parts Used

Fruits

Medicinal Properties and Uses

Fruit is astringent. Gum–resin used in leprosy and nervous debility. Fruits used for rheumatism, asthma, neuralgia, epilepsy and psoriasis and also for warts and tumours. A seed oil is taken internally for cough and cold. It is applied over finger tips to cure malaria fever. Oil also applied over cattle tail to check the spread of epidermis. Gum from the nuts is used in scrofulous, venereal and leprous affections and nervous debility.

Ethnomedicinal Uses

Seed oil taken orally in cough and cold and applied over finger tips to cure malarial fever.

Sesamum indicum L.

Family

Pedaliaceae

Vernacular Names

Oriya : Rasi, Khasa, Rasa; **Hindi :** Til; **Sans :** Tilah; **Ko:** Tilming

The Plant

An erect pubescent annual herb. Leaves large, thin, hairy,

usually ovate and toothed. Fowers white, pink or purplish with yellow marks in racemes in the leaf axils. Fruits quadrangular. Seeds black or white obovate, smooth, glabrous. Fl. & Fr. July-December.

Distribution

Found in open field and in road sides at lower elevation.

Parts Used

Roots, leaves, seeds and oils

Medicinal Properties and Uses

Roots and leaves are emollient and a decoction of them forms a good hair-wash which promotes hair growth. Leaves are useful in dysentery, cholera, cough, nephropathy and opthalmopathy. Seeds are useful in ulcers, migrane and obesity. The oil is bitter, astringent, digestiver, constipating and good for opthalmopathy.

Sesbania bispinosa (Jacq.)W.F. Wight

Family

Fabaceae

Vernacular Names

Oriya : Sheweree, Tentua; **Hindi :** Janjan; **Sans :** Jayanti; **Ko :** Chaipijan

The Plant

Erect shrubs, Leaves 15-40 pairs, linear, obtuse, glabrous. Flowers yellow. Pods ascending, very slender. Fl. & Fr. Aug.-October.

Distribution

Common in wet places.

Parts Used

Roots, bark, leaves, flowers, seeds.

Medicinal Properties and Uses

Root is hot, bitter, anthelmintic, carminative. Cures fever, ulcers, diabetes, leucoderma, relieves throat troubles. Seeds are stimulant, astringent, heal chronic ulcers and remove smallpox eruptions. Plant is considered a cure for wounds.

Setaria palmifolia (Koenig) Stapf

Family

Poaceae

Vernacular Names

Oriya : Kangu.

The Plant

Perennial grass, erect from a short woody stock. Leaves plicate, lower elliptic-oblong, the upper gradually more linear. Spikelets alternate, shortly pedicelled, spikes yellowish green or brown. Fl. & Fr. August-December.

Distribution

Occasional in hill forests and in moist shady valley.

Parts Used

Whole plant.

Medicinal Properties and Uses

Herb is emollient and diuretic. Tender shoots are eaten as vegetable. Leaves enter into a compound decoction used in irregular menstruation.

Shorea robusta Gaertn. f.

Family

Dipterocarpaceae

Vernacular Names

Oriya : Sal, Sekura, Rengal; **Hindi** : Sal; **Ko** : Sarjam

The Plant

A large deciduous tree upto 45m, bark dark, conspicuously vertically fissured. Leaves simple, ovate-oblong. Flowers white, cream coloured in lax axillary or terminal panicles. Fruits ovoid, beaked, wings linear oblong. Seeds ovoid with fleshy unequal cotyledons. Fl. March-April, Fr. May-June.

Parts Used

Bark, leaves, fruits, resin.

Medicinal Properties and Uses

The bark and leaves are astringent, acrid, cooling, anthelmintic, anodyne, constipating, and urinary astringent. They are useful in vitiated conditions of *Kapha* and *Pitta*, ulcers, wounds, bacterial affections, diarrhoea, dysentery, gonorrhoea, leprosy, cough and anaemia. The fruits are sweet, astringent, cooling and tonic which, are useful in dipsia, burning sensation, tuberculosis, ulcers and seminal weakness. The resin is astringent, sweet acrid, cooling, anodyne, vulnerary, antibacterial, deodorant, carminative. It is useful in hyperhidroses, vitiated conditions of *pitta*, wounds ulcers, burns, fever, diarrhoea, dysentery and burning of eyes. Fruits are used in diarrhoea. Flowers are good source of honey. The resin (*Jhuna*) is used in medicine.

Ethnomedicinal Uses

Seed paste is applied with slight boiling before bed for the treatment of carbuncle. The powder of resin is taken internally followed by cold water to check diarrhoea due to indigestion. Resinous exudates is used as insect repellent. The resin powder is taken three times a day for 20 days in dysentery.

Sida acuta Burm. f.

Family

Malvaceae

Vernacular Names

Oriya : Bajarmuli, Sunakhadika; **Hindi :** Naagabalaa, Kareta, Kharenta; **Ko :** Nelakuturi, Ipirpijon.

The Plant

Erect herb, stem rigid. Leaves lanceolate, obovate-lanceolate, margin serrate. Flowers solitary, axillary or clustered, flowers yellow. Seeds triangularly ovoid. Fl. & Fr. Sept.-May.

Distribution

Common weed.

Parts Used

Roots, leaves, seeds.

Medicinal Properties and Uses

Root is astringent, cooling, bitter tonic, useful in nervous and urinary diseases and in disorders of blood and bile. Leaves are demulcent and diuretic. Leaves are boiled in oil and are applied in testicular swellings in elephantiasis. Decoction of leaves and roots is emollient and tonic and is used in the treatment of haemorrhoieds and impotence. Juice of leaves is useful for relief in chest pain and as anthelmintic. Root is used as tonic, stomachic, diaphoretic, and antipyretic. It is used in nervous and urinary disorders.

Ethnomedicinal Uses

Decoction of leaf (3ml) mixed with paste of (2gm) *Piper*

nigrum and lime water (1ml) is taken twice a day after food for a week as a cure for swellings of scrotum.

The leaves and root are grounded and placed in the cavities of teeth for the relief of toothache. The leaves are eaten as vegetable during drought.

Sida cordata (Burm. f.) Borssum

Family

Malvaceae

Vernacular Names

Oriya : Bajramuli; **Hindi :** Bonaniyar

The Plant

Procumbent herb, 30-90cm. Stems and petioles hairy. Leaves ovate to suborbicular, cordate, crenate or serrate, 5-7 nerved at base. Flowers axillary, yellow. Seeds ovoid, brownish and glabrous.

Distribution

Common weed on road sides and other waste places.

Parts Used

Whole plant.

Medicinal Properties and Uses

The roots are sweet, sour, astringent, bitter, acrid and tonic. They are useful in fever, uropathy and arthritis. The bark of the root is used for the treatment of leucorrhoea, gonorrhoea and hyperdiuresis. The leaves are used in diarrhoea. The flowers and ripe fruits are refrigerant and are useful in relieving burning sensation, hyperdiuresis and promoting strength. The seeds make general tonic for improving sexual strength.

Ethnomedicinal Uses

Roots are boiled in water, filter it and is drunk for few days in enuresis.

Sida rhombifolia L.

Family

Malvaceae

Vernacular Names

Oriya : Bajramuli, Sahabeda; **Hindi :** Sahadevi, Lal berela; **Ko :** Ipirpijon

The Plant

Herb or undershrubs, 1-4 ft high. Leaves broadly rhomboid or obovate, always cuneate at the 3 nerved base. Flowers axillary, solitary or in clusters, flowers yellow. Seeds flattened. Fl. & Fr. Aug.-February.

Distribution

Common weed of waste places.

Parts Used

Root, stems.

Medicinal Properties and Uses

The stems are diuretic, febrifuge, demulcent and emollient and are used internally in dermatopathy. The roots are bitter, sweet, and aphrodisiac and promote sexual vigour. It is useful in rheumatic pains and pulmonary tuberculosis. Plant is good for colic, seminal weakness, arthritis and diarrhoea.

Ethnomedicinal Uses

Plant is pounded, warmed and applied on boils. Root decoction is applied externally twice a day for one month to get relief from rheumatic pain.

Sigesbeckia orientalis L.

Family

Asteraceae

The Plant

Branched coarse annual herb. Stem stiff, erect with branches horizontal below and dichotomously branched above. Leaves opposite, petiolate, ovate, coarsely irregularly dentate, and acute. Heads small, penduncled, in leafy panicles. Flowers yellow. Achenes each enclosed in a boat shaped bract, glabrous, slightly rough, black. Fl. & Fr. Oct.-January.

Distribution

Occasional in forest.

Parts Used

Whole plant.

Medicinal Properties and Uses

The leaves taste slightly bitter. Said to possess healing properties in gangrenous ulcers and sores. Tincture of plant used externally with glycerin to cure ringworm and other parasitic infections. Herb considered diaphoretic, cardiotonic, antiscorbutic and sialagogue. It is used in rheumatism and renal colic. Roots contain an essential oil.

Smilax perfoliata Lour.

Family

Smilacaceae

Vernacular Names

Oriya : Ramdantuni, Mutri; **Hindi :** Jangli aushbah; **Ko:** Atukiri

The Plant

Stout prickly climber, stems upto 2.5 cm. diameter, branches mostly terete, armed. Umbels in axillary and terminal panicles. Berry ovoid or sub globose, red to black. Seed usually 1, rarely 3, pale yellow, shining, rounded with a basal umbo.. Feb.-April. Fr. Nov.-Dec.

Distribution

Common in forests.

Parts Used

Root.

Medicinal Properties and Uses

Root is used for the treatment of rheumatism and employed for urinary complaints and dysentery. Root is also eaten in venereal and skin diseases. Decoction is given for sores, swellings and abscesses. The root powder is given once a day for 15 days after meal in piles.

Ethnomedicinal Uses

Root powder with sugar candy is given to increase blood.

Solanum erianthum D.Don

Family

Solanaceae

Vernacular Names

Oriya : Donka bejji; Orso; **Hindi :** Asheta

The Plant

Large unarmed shrub, branchlets densely stellate tomentose. Leaves alternate, entire, velvety-pubescent on both sides.

Inflorescence in axillary or terminal cyme. Flowers white. Berry globose, many–seeded, yellow when ripe. Fl. & Fr. Aug.-June.

Distribution

Occasional in the forests.

Parts Used

Leaves, root.

Medicinal Properties and Uses

A locally applied poultice of pounded and heated fresh leaves is indicated for the relief of hemorrhoids and scrofula. It is better to apply poultice during the night. A plaster made of concentrated fresh leaf juice cures dermatomycosis and impetigo. An internally applied decoction of the leaves is used as a taeniafuge in buffaloes and oxen. Leaves given in vaginal discharges. Decoction of roots used for body pains; vertigo and urinary troubles.

Ethnomedicinal Uses

A paste of the root and few grains of black pepper is applied externally in chest pain.

Solanum torvum Sw.

Family

Solanaceae

Vernacular Names

Oriya : Kantua, Dengabheji, Kathakoli; **Hindi :** Makoi

The Plant

Tomentose shrub, branches prickly. Leaves ovate or oblong, sinuate or coarsely lobed. Flowers white. Berry yellow, turning orange, globose. Fl. & Fr. most of the year.

Distribution

Common in moist places in forests, especially near streams.

Parts Used

Fruit, leaves.

Medicinal Properties and Uses

Fruits cooked and eaten as a vegetable, also dried and pressed. Useful in liver as well as spleen enlargement and their decoction given for cough. Herb is used as a sedative, diuretic and digestive. Leaves homeostatic, but do not contain vitamin K. Roots used in poultice and for cracks in the feet.

Ethnomedicinal Uses

Fruits are fried in oil and given in cough.

Solanum virginianum L.

Family

Solanaceae

Vernacular Names

Oriya : Ankaranti, Ankuranti, Beji begun, Bejari.

The Plant

Diffuse herb or under shrub, very copiously armed all over with straight, yellow, very sharp prickles. Leaves ovate, oblong or elliptic, glabrescent. Flowers deep blue. Berry yellow or white, blotched with green, globose. Fl.&Fr. all the year round.

Distribution

Common in waste places, roadsides.

Parts Used

Whole plant

Medicinal Properties and Uses

The plant is bitter, acrid, thermogenic, anthelmintic, anti-inflammatory, anodyne, digestive, carminative appetizer, stomachic, depurative, febrifuge, expectorant, stimulant, diuretic and aphrodisiac. It is useful in vitiated conditions of *vata* and *kapha,* helminthesis, dental caries inflammations, flatulence, colic, constipation, dyspepsia, leprosy, skin diseases, hypertension rheumatoid fever, cough, asthma bronchitis, pharyngitis, strangury, dysmenorrhoea, lumbago, cardiac disorder, epilepsy and catarrh.

Ethnomedicinal Uses

22 gms. of whole plant juice mixed with honey and is taken one teaspoonful daily for few days in case of urinary disorder.

Solena heterophylla Lour.

Family

Cucurbitaceae

Vernacular Names

Oriya : Bankundri, Matka, Makirla; **Hindi :** Tarali, Ban kundari; **Sans :** Amlavetasah; **Ko :** Chengo

The Plant

A scandent dioecious perennial with several tuberous roots and with slender branched furrowed stems bearing simple tendrils. Leaves polymorphous, ovate, sub orbicular, oblong, usually cordate at base. Flowers small, yellow, males in sub umbellate racemes or fascicled, females solitary. Fruits oblong ovoid, cylindric, brown ribbed, bright red when ripe. Fl. April.

Distribution

Occasional

Parts Used

Tuberous roots, leaves, seeds

Medicinal Properties and Uses

The tuberous roots are sour, astringent, thermogenic, appetizer, carminative, digestive, stimulant, cardio tonic and expectorant. They are useful in vitiated conditions of *kapha* and *vata*, dyspepsia, flatulence, colic, cardiac disorder, asthma, hepatosplenomegaly, gonorrhoea and spermatorrhoea. The leaves are useful in allergic inflammations and the seeds are used for their purgative action.

Soymida febrifuga (Roxb.) A. Juss.

Family

Meliaceae

Vernacular Names

Oriya : Sawan, Rohini; **Hindi :** Rohan, Rohin; **Ko :** Rohini; **Sans :** Mamsarohini

The Plant

Large or medium sized tree, bark dark brown, splitting into oblong flakes on old trees. Leaves long, leaflets 3-6 pairs, elliptic, apex obtuse or rounded, glabrous. Flowers white. Capsules large, seeds oblong, compressed. Fl. Feb.-April, Fr. May-June.

Distribution

Frequent in mixed deciduous forests.

Parts Used

Bark.

Medicinal Properties and Uses

Bark is astringent, bitter, tonic, febrifuge, particularly

prescribed in malaria, used in general debility, intermittent fevers, diarrhoea and dysentery. It is applied to rheumatic swelling and used as a gargle in stomatitis. Decoction is used as vaginal douche leucorrhoea.

Ethnomedicinal Uses

The bark juice mixed with water is taken internally for Kala-a-jar (Blackwater fever). Bark is boiled and mashed with turmeric and applied on affected parts in orthopedic troubles. Bark is boiled and a bath with this water relieves pain after child birth.

Spermacoce hispida L.

Family

Rubiaceae

Vernacular Names

Oriya : Solaganthi, Sanaghar-podia, Jibakata.

The Plant

A hispid procumbent with long branches and quadrangular stems. Leaves simple, opposite and oblong. Flowers pale mauve usually long tube. Fruits capsule. Seeds black. Fl. & Fr. April to November.

Distribution

Common.

Parts Used

Whole plant

Medicinal Properties and Uses

The plant is acrid, sweet, astringent, mildly thermogenic, emollient and stomachic. It is useful in vitiated conditions of *pitta* and *vata*, dyspepsia, colic. flatulence and general debility.

Sphaeranthus indicus L.

Family

Asteraceae

Vernacular Names

Oriya : Bhuinkadam, Halamundi; **Hindi :** Mundi; **Sans:** Mudi, Sravani.

The Plant

A spreading aromatic herb with glandular hairy stem and branches with purple or pink flowers. Leaves alternate, toothed. Clusters of heads terminal and leaf-opposed, purple. Fl. & Fr. Nov.-March.

Distribution

Frequent in moist places along streams.

Parts Used

Whole plant.

Medicinal Properties and Uses

The juice is used in epilepsy, jaundice, hepatopathy and gastropathy. The roots are bitter, acrid, sweet, diuretic and stomachic. They are useful in diabetes, leprosy, fever and dyspepsia. The powered leaf is good for skin diseases and used as nervine tonic.

Sphenomeris chinensis (L.) Maxon

Family

Lindsaeaceae

Vernacular Names

Oriya : Rukuna.

The Plant

Fronds tufted on the creeping rhizome. Stipes glabrous, shinning brown. Lamina ovate or lanceolate, tripinnate. Sori at the expanded tips of pinnules. Rachies flattened and grooved above. Fertile : Feb.-May.

Distribution

Frequent in forests.

Parts Used

Leaves.

Medicinal Properties and Uses

Tender leaves are chewed for at least 5-10 minutes for treatment of toothache.

Spondias pinnata (L.f.) Kurz

Family

Sapindaceae

Vernacular Names

Oriya : Ambada, Ambota, Amta, Amra, Salma; **Hindi:** Amra, Jungli-am; Ko : Amra.

The Plant

A medium sized aromatic, deciduous, tree. Leaves compound, crowded at the ends of branches, leaflets large having parallel nerves meeting in an intra marginal nerve. Flowers white, many, in terminal spreading panicles. Fruits fleshy drupes with woody endocarp, usually 1-3 seeded. Fl. Feb.-March, Fr. ripen in the following January when the tree is leafless.

Distribution

Occasional near rivers.

Parts Used

Root, bark, leaves, fruits.

Medicinal Properties and Uses

The roots are useful in regulating menstruation. The bark is aromatic, astringent and refrigerant and is administered in dysentery, diarrhoea, vomiting and muscular rheumatism. The leaves and bark are aromatic, astringent and refrigerent, useful in dysentery and diarrhoea and given to prevent vomiting. Unripe fruit is acrid, refrigerant, tonic, aphrodisiac and astringent. Cures vaata, biliousness, ulcers, burning sensation and blood complaints. Fruit is antiscorbutic and the pulp astringent, used in bilious dyspepsia. Decoction of wood is used in gonorrhoea and leucorrhoea. Gum exuded from the tree is demulcent.

Ethnomedicinal Uses

Root bark paste (5gm) with mustard oil (1ml) used as massage for the treatment of muscular pain. Unripe fruits (3-4) are roasted, peeled and pulp is made into three pills. One pill is given three times a day for two days for blood dysentery.

Paste of leaf is used in itches and ringworms. Ripe fruits are eaten.

Stachytarpheta jamaicensis (L.) Vahl

Family

Verbenaceae.

Vernacular Names

Oriya : Jalajali, Jatia; **Hindi :** Kariyar tharani; **Sans :** Jalajal.

The Plant

Herb, stem terete, branches somewhat 4 sided, mostly dichotomous. Leaves elliptic ovate, crenate, serrate. Spikes elongating to 30 cm or more. Flowers blue sunk in the rachis of spike. Fruit 3-4, 3mm. long. Fl & Fr. April-Nov..

Distribution

Common along road waste places.

Parts Used

Leaves, bark.

Medicinal Properties and Uses

Herb used for intestinal worms, venereal diseases, ulcers, erysipelas, dropsy and stomach ailments. Juice employed to remove cataract and decoction as an abortifacient. Infusion of barks used in diarrhoea and dysentery. Leaves employed for cardiac troubles. Their decoction used for ulceration of the nose.

Ethnomedicinal Uses

Root-powder is applied to the deep and old wounds.

Stephania japonica (Thunb.) Miers

Family

Menispermaceae

Vernacular Names

Oriya : Okanobindi, Musakani; **Hindi :** Akanadi.

The Plant

Slender, glabrous, climber. Leaves ovate, base broadly rounded. Male flowers green, white or yellow. Drupes red. Fl. May-October. Fr. Oct.-December.

Distribution

Occasional.

Parts Used

Root

Medicinal Properties and Uses

Roots used for fever, diarrhoea, dyspepsia and urinary

diseases. The alkaloid akanadine shoes significant antispasmodic activity on uterine spasms, brought about by posterior pituitary lobe extract, and it may be useful in obstetrical practices.

Ethnomedicinal Uses

3 gms. root and 43 gms. dry rhizome of *Hedychium spicatum* grinded and is used for few days to cure piles.

Sterculia urens Roxb.

Family

Sterculiaceae

Vernacular Names

Oriya : Udal, Kudalo; **Hindi :** Kulu, Gulu, Karai; **Ko :** Sisi; **Sans :** Kateera

The Plant

A middle-sized deciduous tree, conspicuous in the forest by its white or greenish white, shining, smooth papery bark. Leaves crowded at the ends of branches. Flowers yellowish brown, small in large, very densely hairy erect bunches. Fruit of 4-5 large, thick, red carpels, densely covered with stinging hairs. Fl. Feb.-March.

Distribution

Occasional in deciduous forests.

Parts Used

Gum.

Medicinal Properties and Uses

The gum is used as a mechanical laxative. The mucilage when applied to skin has a softer action. It is also used in throat infection and in dental fixture powders.

Ethnomedicinal Uses

The stem bark and gums are made into paste and taken to allay heat of stomach and burning sensation in urinary tracks.

Streblus asper Lour.

Family

Moraceae

Vernacular Names

Oriya : Sahada, Sara; **Hindi :** Sora, Karchanua, Rusa; **Ko:** Sukri–jang.

The Plant

Rigid, much branched shrub or small tree, bark rough, stringy, light grey. Leaves very shortly petioled, obovate or rhombic elliptic, obscurely toothed flowers green. Fruits yellow, succulent, and globose. Fl. March-April. Fr. May-June.

Distribution

Common in open forests, near streams and wastelands.

Parts Used

Root, bark, seed.

Medicinal Properties and Uses

Poultice of roots is applied to ulcers, sinuses, swellings and boils. Pulverized roots are given in dysentery. Decoction of bark is used in fever, diarrhoea, and dysentery. Latex is astringent and antiseptic and applied to sore heals and glandular swellings. Seeds are used in epistasis, piles and diarrhoea. Externally their paste is applied in leucoderma.

Ethnomedicinal Uses

Stem bark paste (about 10gm) is taken once a day continuously one month for the treatment of elephantiasis. The root bark mixed with the tender leaves of *Zizyphus cenoplia* and kalajira powdered is given 10mg-daily for menstrual irregularities.

Strobilanthes auriculatus Nees

Family

Acanthaceae

Vernacular Names

Oriya : Painya; **Ko :** Hudid.

The Plant

Shrub, branches glabrous, angled. Leaves sessile, auricled at base, those in a pair usually unequal. Flowers blue in numerous axillary and terminal, linear spike. Capsule, glabrous. Fl. Nov.-Feb. Fr. Mar.-April.

Distribution

Frequent under shade places and under sal forests.

Parts Used

Leaves.

Medicinal Properties and Uses

Powdered leaves used externally as a febrifuge. Flowers contain a volatile oil.

Ethnomedicinal Uses

Flowers are favourite of honey-bees. Honey production is said to increase considerably in the flowering years.

Strychnos nux-vomica L.

Family

Strychnaceae

Vernacular Names

Oriya : Kochila, Kora; **Hindi :** Kuchla, Kajra.

The Plant

A medium sized deciduous tree with a fairly straight and cylindrical bole having dark grey or yellowish grey back and minute tubercles. Leaves broadly elliptic, coriaceous, glabrous. Flowers numerous, greenish white in terminal cymes. Fruits globose, orange-red when ripe containing many discoid, compressed coin like seeds in fleshy pulp. Seeds concave on one side and convex on the other covered with fine grey silky hairs. Fl. Mar.-April, Fr. Dec.-January.

Distribution

Common in open ground.

Parts Used

Bark, leaves, seeds.

Medicinal Properties and Uses

The root bark is bitter and useful in cholera. The leaves are applied as poultice in the treatment of chronic wounds and ulcers and the leaf decocotion is useful in paralytic complaints. The pulp of the ripe fruit is used in treating paralytic affections of paws and foot. The seeds are bitter, acrid, alexeteric, aphrodisiac, appetised, antiperiodic, anthelmintic, digestive, febrifuge, purgative, stimulant and stomachic. They are useful in anemia, asthma, bronchitis, constipation, diabetes, intermittent and malarial fevers, skin diseases, paralysis and weakness of limbs.

Ethnomedicinal Uses

Pasty mass of stem (3gm) with Kusum (*Schleichera oleosa*) Seed oil (1ml) is prescribed twice a day after food for ten days continuously for the treatment of Leucoderma. Seed are used in gastric trouble and dyspepsia.

Strychnos potatorum L.f.

Family

Strychnaceae

Vernacular Names

Oriya : Katako, Kaya; **Hindi** : Nirmali, Nelmal.

The Plant

A medium sized deciduous, glabrous tree with cracked and scaly black and irregularly fluted trunk. Leaves simple, opposite, elliptic, acute, chartaceous, upto 15cm long and 6.25 cm broad, transverse nerves about 4 pairs joining the second pair of ribs to the mid rib, glabrous shining. Flowers white, fragrant, in dense glabrous cymes. Berry globose. Seeds large. Fl. May, Fr. Oct.-December.

Distribution

Found in deciduous forests.

Parts Used

Root, leaves, seeds.

Medicinal Properties and Uses

The seeds are sweet, bitter, astringent, refrigerant, demulcent, emetic, diuretic, digestive, anthelmintic, aphrodisiac, ophthalmic, appetizer, tonic and water purifier. They are useful in vitiated conditions of *kapha* and *vata*, hepatopathy, nephropathy gonorrhoea, leucorrhoea, gastropathy, bronchitis, chronic diarrhoea and dysentery, strangury, renal and vesical calculi, diabetes, burning sensation, dipsia, ulcers and other eye diseases. The leaves are used as a poultice for maggot-infested ulcers. Powdered bark is useful in cholera. The roots are useful in leprosy.

Ethnomedicinal Uses

Paste is applied on scorpion bitten area.

Symplocos racemosa Roxb.

Family

Symplocaceae

Vernacular Names

Oriya : Lodho, Mudha; **Hindi :** Lodh; **Sans :** Lodhra; **Ko:** Ludum

The Plant

Large shrub or trees. Leaves elliptic-lanceolate or elliptic-oblong, glandular-dendate or denticulate. Flowers white, in axillary pubescent racemes. Drupe elipsoid. Fl. Oct.-Dec. Fr. Jan.-April.

Distribution

Frequent in forests.

Parts Used

Bark.

Medicinal Properties and Uses

It is a specific remedy for uterine complaints, vaginal and menstrual disorders. Bark is light, cooling, mild, astringent, antidiarrhoeal, antidysenteric. Useful in dropsy, elephantiasis, filarial, liver complaint, bowel complaints, eye diseases, ulcers and leucorrhoea. Decoction of bark is used as gargle for giving firmness to spongy and bleeding gums.

Ethnomedicinal Uses

Powdered bark is applied on face for medicinal purpose.

Syzygium cerasoides (Roxb.) Raizada

Family

Myrtaceae

Vernacular Names

Oriya : Pita jamu; **Hindi :** Dugdugia, Oiaman; **Ko :** Topa

The Plant

Tree, bark rough, twigs 4-angular. Leaves broadly elliptic obovate or rounded, acuminate. Flowers white, sessile, in ternate trichotomous lateral panicles mostly from old leaf-scars. Fl. May-June, Fr. August.

Distribution

Common in the forests.

Parts Used

Bark, fruit.

Medicinal Properties and Uses

Bark acrid and astringent. Used in dysentery, biliousness and bronchitis. Fruits given in rheumatism.

Ethnomedicinal Uses

Fresh bark juice mixed with milk is used in diarrhoea. The seed powder about 15gm is administered orally thrice a day for 3-4 months in diabetes.

Syzygium jambos (L.) Alston

Family

Myrtaceae

Vernacular Names

Oriya : Gulabjamun, Jamrul; **Hindi :** Gulabjamb

The Plant

A large shrub or small tree with spreading branches. Leaves simple, opposite, lanceolate, narrowed into short petioles. Flowers greenish white in short terminal racemose cymes. Fruits pale yellow to pinkish white. Fl. April, Fr. June-July.

Distribution

Planted.

Parts Used

Bark, root, seeds.

Medicinal Properties and Uses

The bark is astringent, bitter, sweet, depurative, antidiarrhoeal and anthelmintic. It is useful in gout, haemorrhages, leprosy, diarrhoea, colic, wounds, ulcers, stomatitis and vitiated conditions of *pitta*. Root diuretic also used in applications for itch. Bark astringent, employed in mouth-washes used in thrush. Dried and pulverized leaves are applied to cracked tongue. The seeds are used to treat diabetes.

Syzygium cumini (L.) Skeels

Family

Myrtaceae

Vernacular Names

Oriya : Jamu; **Hindi :** Jamun, Jambhal, Jaman; **Ko :** Kuda; **Sans :** Jambu

The Plant

Large glabrous tree, bark grey brown or nearly black, more

or less cracked when old. Leaves simple, opposite, variable in shape, oblong or elliptic oblong, acute or acuminate, shining. Flowers white, sessile. Seeds thick rounded fleshy. Fl. April-May, Fr. July-August.

Distribution

Common along streams and roadsides.

Parts Used

Bark, leaves, fruits.

Medicinal Properties and Uses

The bark is astringent, sweet, sour, carminative, diuretic, digestive, anthelmintic, febrifuge, constipating, fever, gastropathy and dermatopathy. The leaves are antibacterial and are used for strengthening the teeth and gums. The tender leaves are used for vomiting. The fruits and seeds are sweet, acrid, sour, tonic and cooling and are used in diabetes, diarrhoea, splenopathy, urethrorrhoea and ring worm.

Ethnomedicinal Uses

In case a child has eaten hairs by accident, the ripe fruits of this plant are given to him to eat in good quantity. This will help in the cleaning of the bowels and expelling out the hairs. The liquor brewed from ripe fruits is taken for chronic diarrhoea. The decoction of bark is given internally to regulate menstrual disorders.

Tamarindus indica L.

Family

Caesalpiniaceae

Vernacular Names

Oriya : Tentuli, Kaiyan; **Ko :** Jajo; **Hindi :** Imli, Titar; **Sans:** Amlika

The Plant

A large tree, leaves compound, leaflets 10-20 pairs, about 1cm long. Flowers yellowish with reddish streaks, in small erect clusters among the leaves. Fruits 8-20cm long, 2-3cm broad, fleshy, pendulous, brown in colour. Fl. usually Apr.-June & Fr. Dec.-March.

Distribution

Fairly common, planted or self sown.

Parts Used

Root, leaves, fruits, seeds.

Medicinal Properties and Uses

The root bark is astringent, constipating, emmenagogue and tonic, and is useful in diarrhoea, asthma, ammenorrhoea, gingivitis and ulcers. The leaves are sour, astingent, thermogenic, anthelmintic, anodyne, anti-inflammatory, diuretic and ophthalmic. Leaves reduce inflammatory swellings and are applied externally for inflammation of ulcers. Fruit refrigerant from the acids they contain, digestive, carminative, slightly laxative, antiscorbutic and antibilious. Useful in diseases caused by deranged bile. The seeds are astringent, cooling, aphrodisiac, stomachic, constipating and tonic. They are useful in diarrhoea, dysentery, dipsia, burning sensation, inflammation, chronic ulcers and general debility.

Ethnomedicinal Uses

Seeds are placed on the killing places as antidote of snake bite poison. Powder of dead bark is applied on wounds of cattles. Dried seeds mixed with Mahua (*Madhuca longifolia*) flower is prepared as curry and eaten by tribal. The leaves grounded with garlic is locally applied in rheumatic swellings.

Tectaria cicutaria (L.) Copel

Family

Aspidiaceae

Vernacular Names

Oriya : Rakta mahajal; **Ko** : Cingari

The Plant

Tufted fern. Stipes deep chestnut-brown. Fronds membranous, long. Pinnae bipinnate or more compound. Sori with a reniform or usually peltate, indusium in a raw each side of the vein of the final lobe. Fertile : Nov.-January.

Distribution

Common in hill forests.

Parts Used

Leaves.

Ethnomedicinal Uses

Tender leaves are mixed with fresh leaves of *Azadirachta indica* in equal proportion (5:5) by adding little mustard oil and is thoroughly grounded and applied 2-3 times per day for 15 days against eczema and scabies.

Tephrosia purpurea (L.) Pers.

Family

Fabaceae

Vernacular Names

Oriya : Banokultha, Gileri, Pokha; **Ko** : Uttar; **Hindi:** Sarponkha, Damasia; **Sans** : Sharpunkha

The Plant

A much branched undershurb. Leaves imparipinnate, leaflets 5-8 pairs, oblong cuneate. Flowers purple. Pods long, slightly curved with short oppressed hairs. 6-10 seeded. Seeds ovoid. Fl. & Fr. most part of the year.

Distribution

Common in wasteland, along roadsides.

Parts Used

Whole plant.

Medicinal Properties and Uses

The plant is bitter, astringent, acrid, thermogenic, anthelmintic, digestive, laxative, diuretic, uterine tonic, anti-inflammatory depurative, styptic and antipyretic, and used in bronchitis, bilious febrile attacks, boils, pimples and bleeding piles. Decoction of roots given in dyspepsia, diarrhoea, rheumatism, asthma and urinary disorders. Roots given with black pepper in colic. A liniment prepared from the roots is used in elephantiasis. Pulverized roots smoked for relief from asthma and cough. The leaves are useful in dyspepsia, pectrol diseases, haemorrhoides, gonorrhoea and bruises. Decoction of pods used as a vermifuge and to stop vomiting.

Ethnomedicinal Uses

Decoction of leaf (5ml) is mixed with honey (2ml) and given to women twice a day continuously for one month against post natal complications.

Teramnus labialis (L.f.) Spreng.

Family

Fabaceae

Vernacular Names

Sans : Mashaparni; **Hindi :** Mashoni, Mashparui.

The Plant

Very slender twiner, Leaflets very variable in size, elliptic or ovate, acute, glabrous, hairy beneath. Flowers pink or white, Seeds red when fresh, black when dry. Fl. & Fr. Sept.-March.

Distribution

Common in forests.

Parts Used

Leaves, fruits.

Medicinal Properties and Uses

Leaves are used in rheumatism, tuberculosis, nervous affection, hemoptysis and catarrh. Fruits astringent, stomachic and febrifuge.

Terminalia alata Heyne ex Roth

Family

Combretaceae

Vernacular Names

Oriya : Asan, Sahaja, Kala Sahaja; **Hindi :** Asan, Saj.

The Plant

Large tree, bark dark rough, cracked into oblong segments. Leaves opposite or sub opposite, elliptic–oblong, ovate, entire with distinct tertiary nerves. Flowers panicled spikes. Fruit 5 winged. Fl. May-June, Fr. Oct.-Feb.

Distribution

Common in forest.

Parts Used

Bark.

Medicinal Properties and Uses

Bark is styptic and cardio tonic.

Terminalia arjuna (Roxb. ex DC.) Wight. & Arn.

Family

Combretaceae

Vernacular Names

Oriya : Arjuna; **Ko :** Kowa, Gara Hatana; **Sant :** Kahua; **Hindi :** Arjun; **Sans :** Arjuna.

The Plant

Large tree, bark grey or pale green, smooth. Leaves opposite or subopposite, subsessile or shortly petioled, entire or crenate, glabrous with two glands near the base of the lamina beneath or on the potiole. Flowers white in shortly panicled spikes. Fruits 5 winged. Fl. May-July, Fr. Oct.-February.

Distribution

Occasional in valleys, usually near streams.

Parts Used

Bark.

Medicinal Properties and Uses

The bark is astringent, sweet, acrid, demulcent, cardio tonic, antidysenteric, urinary astringent, expectorant and tonic. It is useful in fractures, ulcers, urethrorrhea, leucorrhoea, diabetes, vitiated conditions of *pitta*, cadiopathy, anemia, asthma, bronchitis, dysentery, cirrhosis of the liver and hypertension.

Ethnomedicinal Uses

Decoction of stem bark (20 ml.) is taken once a day in empty stomach continuously five days for the treatment of malaria fever. Bark paste is mixed with ghee and applied on fracture. A kwath is prepared with the bark of *Anogeissus latifolia* and taken 1 cup in morning and evening for 10 days for the treatment of gonorohoea.

Terminalia bellirica (Gaertn.) Roxb.

Family

Combretaceae

Vernacular Names

Oriya : Bahada; **Ko :** Lupurg; **Sant :** Lopong; **Hindi :** Bahera, Bahaira; **Sans :** Bibhitaka

The Plant

A large deciduous buttressed tree with thick brownish grey bark having shallow longitudinal fissures. Leaves clustered towards the ends of branchlets, alternate, broadly obovate, entire, rounded. Flowers greenish – white or greenish yellow in solitary axillary or extra axillary spikes. Drupes sub-globose or pyriform. Fl. Mar.-May, Fr. Oct.-December.

Distribution

Common in sal and mixed forests.

Parts Used

Bark, fruits.

Medicinal Properties and Uses

The bark is diuretic and useful in anaemia and leucoderma. The fruits are astringent, acrid, sweet, anti-inflammatory. Digestive, antipyretic. They are useful in vitiated conditions of *kapha* and *vata*, cough, bronchitis, insomnia, dropsy, dyspepsia and skin diseases. The mature and dry fruit is constipating and is useful in diarrhoea and dysentery. The oil obtained from the seeds is trichogenous and is useful in dyspepsia and greyness of hair.

Ethnomedicinal Uses

Stem bark paste (2gm) is prescribed to women with boiled water twice a day after food continuously ten days as a cure for leucoderma.

Terminalia chebula Retz.

Family

Combretaceae.

Vernacular Names

Oriya : Harida; **Ko :** Rola; **Hindi :** Hara, Harara, Harad; **Sans :** Haritaki

The Plant

Tree, bark grey or dark grey, cracked in old tree. Leaves usually sub opposite, ovate or elliptic, entire, acute, silky hairy when young, glabrous and nearly so when mature. Spikes pubescent or tomentose. Flowers whitish, very densely white villous within. Drupes ellipsoid, often 5 ribbed. Fl. Mar.-April, Fr. Nov.-December.

Distribution

Common in sal and mixed forests.

Parts Used

Mature and immature fruits.

Medicinal Properties and Uses

The fruits are astringents, sweet, acrid, bitter, sour, anti-inflammatory, stomachic, laxative. purgative, carminative, digestive and cardio tonic, diuretic, febrifuge, depurative and tonic. They are useful in vitiated conditions of tridosa, wounds, ulcers, inflammations, gastropathy, haemorrhoides, jaundice, cough, uropathy, versical and renal calculi and general debility.

Ethnomedicinal Uses

Fruit infusion (15 ml) is taken in empty stomach once a day as cure for dysentery. Fruit cover powder mixed with 20 gms. honey and is given for 7 days in case of block of nose. Decoction of fruit is taken one cup at bed time for 7 days to cure from constipation.

Thevetia peruviana (Pers.) Merr.

Family

Apocynaceae

Vernacular Names

Oriya : Koniyari, Koniyar phul; **Sant** : Berenjo; **Hindi** : Pila kaner, Zard kunel, Kulkephul.

The Plant

Small, evergreen plant with milky juice. Stems scaled with scars of fallen leaves. Leaves alternate, linear-oblong, entire, only main nerve conspicuous. Inflorescence in axillary cyme of 2-3 flowers, bright yellow. Drupe angular, smooth. Seeds brown. Fl. & Fr. most part of the year.

Distribution

Commonly cultivated and naturalized in many places.

Parts Used

Bark, seed, root.

Medicinal Properties and Uses

The purified glucoside thevitin, extracted from the seed and root is prescribed as a cardio tonic drug. The crushed seeds can be used as an insecticide. Caution is needed because of their high toxicity. Kernel of seed used as acro-narcotic poison. Bark is bitter, tonic, cathartic, febrifuge and useful in different kinds of intermittent fevers.

Toddalia asiatica (L.) Lam.

Family

Rutaceae

Vernacular Names

Oriya : Tundpora; **Hindi :** Jangli-kalli-mirchi.

The Plant

Rambling or scandent very prickly shrub. Leaves 3 foliolate leaflets sessile, lanceolate. Flowers white or yellowish, small. Berry orange, globose, 3-5 grooved or hardly lobed. Fl. & Fr. Aug.-April.

Distribution

Common especially in the scrub forests and also in the hills.

Parts Used

Roots, barks, leaves.

Medicinal Properties and Uses

Root-bark diaphoretic and antipyretic. Infusion of fresh root bark is stimulating tonic and carminative. Root-bark is used also in diarrhoea and debility during convalescence. An infusion of fresh root bark is stimulating tonic and carminative. Plant is used as a febrifuge. Fresh leaves eaten for pain in the bowels.

Toona ciliata Roem.

Family

Meliaceae

Vernacular Names

Oriya : Mahanimba; **Ko :** Katangai, Rorongo; **Hindi :** Tun, Mahanim.

The Plant

A large tree. Leaves abruptly pinnate, leaflets 4-5 pairs, base oblique. Flowers white, fragrant in large terminal drooping panicles. Fruits capsules. Fl. March-April & Fr. June-October.

Distribution

Found in valleys.

Parts Used

Bark, flowers.

Medicinal Properties and Uses

The bark is bitter, acrid, astringent, tonic, aphrodisiac, expectorant, anthelmintic, depurative and antiperiodic. It is useful in chronic infantile dysentery, cough, bronchitis, intermittent fevers, leprosy and ulcers. The flowers are emmenagogue and are useful in menstrual disorders.

Ethnomedicinal Uses

Bark of stem used in gastric disorders.

Trapa natans L.

Family

Trapaceae

Vernacular Names

Oriya : Pani singda, Paniphala; **Hindi :** Singhara, Paniphal.

The Plant

Aquatic herbs. Leaves alternate, floating, rhomboid, irregularly inciso-serrate. Flowers white, few, axillary, solitary. Fruits obovoid, angular with short conical beak in the center and a spreading flattened very sharp spinous horn at either side. Fl. August, Fr. Nov.-December.

Distribution

Free floating aquatic.

Parts Used

Fruit

Medicinal Properties and Uses

Fruit is sweetish, aphrodisiac, appetizer, antipyretic. Useful in chronic fevers, lumbago pain, sore throat and bronchitis. They are given in powder form with milk in nervous and general debility, leucorrhoea and seminal weakness.

Trema orientalis (L.) Bl.

Family

Ulmaceae

Vernacular Names

Oriya : Jivani, Kharkas; **Hindi :** Gio; **Sans :** Jeevanti.

The Plant

Small tree, trunck ringed with stipular scale branches with dense silky pubescence, bark smooth. White or pale. Leaves oblong, ovate, lanceolate. serrulate, acuminate, more or less white or silvery beneath with fine silky hairs. Flowers green. Drupe yellow. Fl. & Fr. most part of the year.

Distribution

Common in forests near streams

Parts Used

Root, bark.

Medicinal Properties and Uses

Decoction of root is given in diarrhoea and presence of blood in urine. Root bark and leaves are used in epilepsy.

Trewia nudiflora L.

Family

Euphorbiaceae

Vernacular Names

Oriya : Panigamhari, Munda, Tobu; **San** : Pindora; **Ko:** Goralo; **Hindi** : Bhillaura, Tumri.

The Plant

Deciduous tree, bark smooth, grey, Leaves large, broadly ovate, acuminate, glabros above, Flowers yellow, solitary. Drupe globose. Fl. Jan.-March, Fr. Oct.-December, Leafless Dec.-January.

Distribution

Occasional near stream.

Parts Used

Root.

Medicinal Properties and Uses

The poultice of roots applied in gout and rheumatism.

Ethnomedicinal Uses

Pounded bark is given in snakebite.

Tridax procumbens L.

Family

Asteraceae

Vernacular Names

Oriya : Bisalya karani, Bhumi poksunga; **Ko :** Bisal gacha.

The Plant

Procumbent hairy herb. Leaves rather distant, petiolate, ovate or lanceolocte, coarsely toothed. Capitula pale yellow. Fl. & Fr. all the year round.

Distribution

Common, waste places.

Parts Used

Leaves

Medicinal Properties and Uses

Leaves used in bronchial catarrh, dysentery and diarrhoea. Leaf juice insecticidal and piscidal, also used to check hemorrhage of wounds.

Ethnomedicinal Uses

Fresh leaf juice is applied as antiseptic cream for healing of cut wounds.

Triumfetta rhomboidea Jacq.

Family

Tiliaceae

Vernacular Names

Oriya : Bojormuli, Jotojuti; **Hindi :** Jhinjhira, Chikti; **Sans:** Jhinjhirita

The Plant

A stouty herb, 3-4 ft under shrub with more or less pubescent branches. Leaves broadly ovate or rhomboids, coarsely serrate or dentate, hairy, tomentose beneath. Flowers yellow. Capsule ellipsoid or sub globose. Fl. & Fr. July-January.

Distribution

Fairly common weed.

Parts Used

Bark, leaves, root, flowers, fruits.

Medicinal Properties and Uses

Root is bitter and diuretic. Root is used in dysentery. Bark and leaves used for diarrhoea and roots for dysentery. Pounded roots are given for intestinal ulcers and their hot infusion hasten parturition. Leaves and flowers are used against leprosy. Flowers, fruits and leaves are mucilaginous, demulcent, astringent, used with sugar during gonorrhoea.

Urena lobata L.

Family

Malvaceae

Vernacular Names

Oriya : Chikimiamanji, Rakta pheni, Bilokapasira; **Sans. :** Vana bhenda, Nagabala; Hindi : Bachita, Unga, Pithia.

The Plant

Annual or perennial erect undershrub. Leaves ovate to orbicular, angular, deeply palmilobed, cordate, rounded. Epicalyx copular in fruit dpressed to mericarp. Flower pink with purple centre. Seeds reniformed. Fl. & Fr. Aug.-December.

Distribution

Common weed in way sides and in open forests.

Parts Used

Root.

Medicinal Properties and Uses

Roots diuretic. Decoction of stem and roots used for flatulent colic. Flowers expectorant, there infusion used in aphthae and sore throat.

Urginea indica (Roxb.) Kunth.

Family

Liliaceae

Vernacular Names

Oriya : Bana-piyaza, Bana-ulli; Hindi: Jungli-piyaz; **Sans:** Vanapalandu.

The Plant

A glabrous herb. Bulb dull white or pale, 2.5-5 cm diameter or more. Leaves radicla, flat, narrow pointed. Flowers appearing before the leaves, drooping or spreading, distant in a terminal raceme, 15-50 cm long. Perianth long, bell shaped. 6-parting; segments white, with 3 green ribs in the center, tapering downwards; ovules several valved; seeds many, flat, blank. Fl. June-August.

Distribution

Occasional in open grassy places.

Parts Used

Bulbs.

Medicinal Properties and Uses

The bulb in action is anthelmintic, cardiac, stimulant, deobstruent, digestive, diuretic, emmenagogue, and expectorant.

Useful in asthma, aliments of hearts, calculous affections. Cough and bronchitis, paralytic affection, promotes urination, in reheumatism and skin diseases. Bulbs are source of raticide, and is used as an expectorant, stimulant, and cardio-tonic in small doses. Squill is used chiefly in chronic bronchitis and asthma. Alcoholic extracts of the bulbs possess anticancer activity against human epidermoid carcinoma. Also employed in dropsy, reheumatism and skin troubles. Externally used for removing corns and warts.

Ethnomedicinal Uses

The paste of bulb is externally used to remove warts and corns.

Vanda tessellata (Roxb.) G. Don

Family

Orchidaceae

Vernacular Names

Oriya : Kankata, Amdahaka, Bani; **Sans. :** Rasna; **Hindi:** Nai Rasna, Banda, Rasna; **Ko :** Gaccho Janaya.

The Plant

A small epiphytic herb, roots white, shiny, silvery grey coloured. The plant develops two kind of roots, the clinging roots and aerial roots. Leaves coriaceous in two rows, oblique at apex. Flowers axillary racemose or solitary. Fl & Fr. May-June.

Distribution

Common epiphyte on mango trees.

Parts Used

Whole plant.

Medicinal Properties and Uses

The plant is rheumatic disorders, local swellings, indigestion. The root of the plant is useful in inflammations, rheumatic disorders, osteoarthritis and allied disorder. It has been used for indigestion. It is also used as a laxative and stimulant to liver. The medicated oil is used for external application in rheumatic pains.

Ethnomedicinal Uses

Leaf-juice is heated and poured warm in the ears to check ear-ache.

Ventilago denticulata Willd.

Family

Rhamnaceae

Vernacular Names

Oriya : Pitchuli, Rainjhai, Kantamali; **Sant :** Bongasarjom; **Hindi :** Pitti-raidhani; **Sans :** Pittoli.

The Plant

A large, much branched, woody climber with branches hanging down and dark grey bark having vertical cracks exposing the inner vermilion surface. Leaves simple, alternate, oblong-lanceolate or elliptic-ovate, base rounded or acute, main nerves 4-8 pairs. Flowers greenish with an offensive odour in drooping pubescent terminal panicles. Fruits yellowish globular nuts, supported by the persistent calyx. Fl. Sept.-November, Fr. Feb.-April.

Distribution

Common in mixed forests.

Parts Used

Bark.

Medicinal Properties and Uses

Root bark is carminative, stomachic, stimulant and tonic. In the form of powder it is prescribed as a tonic to cure the dyspepsia, mild fever and debility. Stem bark is powdered mixed with gingelly oil and used as application for skin diseases and itch.

Ethnomedicinal Uses

The bark grounded into a paste and applied locally in bone fracture. The decoction of root bark about 15ml is taken 3 times a day for a fortnight in case of debility.

Vernonia anthelmintica (L.) Willd.

Family

Asteraceae

Vernacular Names

Oriya : Saoraj, Somraj; **Hindi** : Kalijira, Baksi; **Sans:** Somaraji.

The Plant

A tall robust, stout, erect annual with pubescent branches. Leaves long, lanceolate, denate or serrate, acute. Flowers purplish in subcorymbose head, outer involucral bracts linear and hairy, green with purplish obtuse tips, innermost bracts longest. Fruits achenes, oblong, cylindric, 10-ribbed, pubescent, pappus reddish, inner pappus long, outer short. Fl. Sept.-December, Fr. Nov.-January.

Distribution

Common, roadside and waste places.

Parts Used

Fruits

Medicinal Properties and Uses

The fruits are bitter, acrid, thermogenic, astringent, anti – inflammatory, anodyne, expectorant, depurative, demulcent, purgative, diuretic, stomachic, febrifuge and tonic. They are useful in inflammations, cough, asthma, leprosy, skin diseases, dyspepsia, colic, fever, vitiated conditions of *vata* and are very specific for round worm and threadworm.

Ethnomedicinal Uses

Fruits are pounded and taken to remove intestinal worms. Seeds are used as anthelmintic, especially for children, 2-5 g with water in empty stomach twice a day for 3 days.

Vernonia aspera Buch.-Ham.

Family

Asteraceae

Vernacular Names

Sant : Dorabohok.

The Plant

Erect stout herb, stems more or less striate, hairy. Leaves shortly petioled, elliptic, spinulose serrate. Heads purple. Fl. & Fr. Nov.-February.

Distribution

Frequent in forests.

Parts Used

Roots.

Medicinal Properties and Uses

Medicinal properties more or less similar to those of *V. cinerea*. Leaves are eaten as vegetable. Pulverized roots are used in articular rheumatism.

Vernonia cinerea (L.) Less.

Family

Asteraceae

Vernacular Names

Oriya : Badi poksunga, Poksunga; **Sant :** Birlopung-arak, Jhurjhuri; **Hindi :** Dautotpala, Sahadeyi, Sadodi; **Sans:** Sahadevi, Devasahra.

The Plant

An erect or somewhat decumbent annual herb with cylindric, striate, more or less pubescent branched stem. Leaves simple, alternate, variable in shape, ovate or lanceolate, shortly mucronate, irregularly toothed or shallowly crenate-serrate. Flowers many, pinkish violet, in small heads, involucral bracts oblong, lanceolate, acuminate, awned, silky on the back. Fruits oblong achenes, slightly narrowed at the base. Clothed with appressed white hairs. Fl. & Fr. most of the year.

Distribution

Fairly common weed.

Parts Used

Whole plant.

Medicinal Properties and Uses

The plants are bitter, acrid, thermogenic, anthelmintic, depurative, diuretic, anodyne, anti-inflammatory, stomachic, antibacterial, antifugal, antivitral and antiperiodic. The roots are useful in diarrhoea, stomachalgia, inflammations, skin diseases, leprosy, renal and versical calculi, chronic and intermittent fevers and vitiated conditions of *vata*. The leaves are useful in humid herpes, eczema, ringworm and elephantiasis. The flowers are useful in conjunctivitis, vitiated conditions of *vata* and fever. The seeds are useful in roundworms, thread-worms, cough, flatulence, leucoderma, skin diseases, colic and dysuria.

Vigna radiata (L.) Wilczek

Family

Fabaceae

Vernacular Names

Oriya : Mungo; **Hindi :** Mung; **Sans :** Masa.

The Plant

An erect pubescent herb. Leaflets ovate, oblong, lanceolate or rhomboid, Flowers yellow. Pods turgid, minutely appressedly hairy. Seeds green or yellow, smooth, long. Fl. & Fr. July-November.

Distribution

Found in moist area. Extensively cultivated.

Parts Used

Whole plant, root.

Medicinal Properties and Uses

Plant is considered hot and tonic. Root is narcotic and is a remedy for aching bones. Seeds are sweet, oily, tonic, laxative, aphrodisiac, appetizer. Cures piles, asthma, good for the heart and in fatigue. Seeds are used both internally and externally. Internally, a clear decoction is useful in dyspepsia, dysentery, diarrhoea, cough, piles, rheumatism, affection of liver and of the nervous system and in fever.

Vitex negundo L.

Family

Verbenaceae

Vernacular Names

Oriya : Begunia, Nirgundi; **Hindi :** Nishinda; **Ko :** Sant: Sinduari; **Sans :** Nirgundi

The Plant

Shrub or small tree, bark thin, grey finely hoary tomentose. Leaves 3-5 foliolate petiole long, leaflets lanceolate, entire or crenate, finely white tomentose beneath. Flowers bluish purple or white, in oblong panicles. Drupe globose. Fl. & Fr. most of the year.

Distribution

Frequent in waste ground, hedges and sometimes near thc banks.

Parts Used

Leaves, flower.

Medicinal Properties and Uses

Leaves are used as tonic and vermifuge. Leaves are smoked for relief in catarrh and headache. Their decoction is employed in medicinal baths for catarrhal and rheumatic affections. Leaves and roots possess tranquillizing effect and form a constituent of *Vishagarbha thaila,* an ayurvedic preparation. Leaves yield an essential oil. Extract of leaves showed anticancer activity against *Ehrlich ascites* tumour cells. Roots are used as tonic, febrifuge, diuretic, used in rheumatism and dyspepsia and as an anthelmintic. It is also employed as a demulcent in dysentery and piles. Flowers are astringent and used in diarrhoea, fever, and liver complaints.

Ethnomedicinal Uses

Decoction of root bark (about 15ml) with paste of 21 black peppers (*Piper nigrum)* is taken twice a day after food continuously seven days for the treatment of typhoid fever. Leaves are used as insect repellent in storing the food grains. Leaf powder is used in inflammation. Young leaves are heated with mustard oil and applied in ear to cure earache. Leaves are used to treat headache. Poisonous snake change their resting place keeping the peduncle on their hole. The root of the plant made into a fine paste is applied on the fore head during the labour pains for easy delivery. Leaves fried in ghee is used to check the blood vomiting.

Walsura trifoliata (A. Juss.) Harms

Family

Meliaceae

Vernacular Names

Oriya : Mundikabakam, Kuruwan.

The Plant

Bushy tree or shrub, bark grey, slightly cracked. Leaves pinnately 3-foliolate, leaflets oblong, rounded, both ends, very shining above. Flowers yellow, berry globous. Fl. & Fr. Feb.-June.

Distribution

Occasional in forests.

Parts Used

Bark.

Medicinal Properties and Uses

Bark stimulent, expectorant, emmenagogue, and emetic. An oily liquid obtained by heating the wood is used for itch.

Wendlandia tinctoria (Roxb.) DC.

Family

Rubiaceae

Vernacular Names

Oriya : Tilai, Icha, Dhulda; **Ko :** Tilai.

The Plant

Small tree or large shrub, bark brown stringy, branchlets pubescent. Leaves elliptic, obovate, acuminate, shining above. Flowers white. Capsule globose. Fl. Jan.-March, Fr. Mar.-April.

Distribution

Commonly found in forests.

Parts Used

Bark

Medicinal Properties and Uses

Bark used as a mordant in dyeing. An application prepared from the bark is used for cramps in cholera patients.

Withania somnifera (L.) Dunal

Family

Solanaceae

Vernacular Names

Oriya : Ashwagandha; **Hindi :** Asgandha, Punir; **Sans:** Asvagandha.

The Plant

An erect branching undershrub reaching about 150 cm in height usually clothed minutely stellate tomentum. Leaves ovate up to 10 cm long. Flowers greenish or lurid yellow in axillary fascicles. Fruits globose berries which are orange coloured when mature enclosed in persistent calyx. Fl. April-June, Fr. Aug.-October.

Distribution

Common in dry waste places and also cultivated.

Parts Used

Roots, leaves.

Medicinal Properties and Uses

The tuberous roots are astringent, bitter, acrid, somniferous, thermogenic, stimulant, aphrodisiac, diuretic and tonic. They are useful in vitiated conditions of *vata*, leucoderma, constipation, insomnia, tissue-building, and nervous breakdown. The leaves are bitter and are recommended in fever, painful swelling s and ophthalmitis. A paste of the root and bruished leaves are applied to carbuncles, ulcers and painful swellings.

Ethnomedicinal Uses

Decoction of flower with honey is taken in the ratio of 5:1 frequently for one month against seminal weakness. Root powder is given to improve general health. One teaspoonful of root powder with warm milk is given everyday for sexual vitality and to improve the sperm count.

Woodfordia fruticosa (L.) Kurz

Family

Lythraceae

Vernacular Names

Oriya : Dhatki, Dhai, Jalico, Harwari; **Hindi :** Dhatuki; Ko, **Sant :** Icha; **Sans :** Dhataki.

The Plant

Large spreading shrub, bark reddish brown, peeling off in thin strips, young parts hairy. Leaves and branches covered with black dots. Leaves sessile, lanceolate, and ovate. Flowers scarlet in fasciled cymes, axillary and from the old wood. Fruits ellipsoid, irregualarly dehiscent, capsules about 1 cm long. Seeds obovoid, smooth, brown. Fl. Nov.-April, Fr. Apr.-May.

Distribution

Common in open forests and on hill sides.

Parts Used

Flowers, bark, leaves.

Medicinal Properties and Uses

The flowers are astringent, acrid, refrigerant, stimulant, uterine sedative, constipating, and antibacterial. They are useful in vitiated conditions of *kapha* and *pitta*, leprosy, skin diseases, burning sensation, haemorrhages, menorrhagia, diarrhoea and dysentery. Bark is pungent, acrid, cooling, anthelmintic, toxic, uterine sedative. Leaves are used in bilious sickness.

Ethnomedicinal Uses

Paste of the flowers (5gm) and 'champa' (*Michelia champaca* L.) bark (10gm) is given twice a day for seven days to treat excess bleeding during menstruation. Dried flower powder (5gm) with honey (1ml) is given to women once a day continuously one month for the treatment of leucorrhoea. Flowers pasted and given to check nausea during pregnancy. Root paste is applied at the face of the anus for few minutes to expel intestinal worm.

Xanthium idicum Koenig

Family

Asteraceae

Vernacular Names

Oriya : Gokhru; **Hindi :** Shankeshwara; **Sans :** Sankesvara

The Plant

Herbs. Leaves long petioled, ovate-triangular, coarsely lobed and toothed. Male heads at the top of the inflorescence or stem. Fl. & Fr. through out the year.

Distribution

Common weed along road sides, waste places.

Parts Used

Root, leaves, fruit.

Medicinal Properties and Uses

Plant is diaphoretic, sedative. Useful in long-standing cases of malaria. Root is bitter, tonic and is useful in strumous diseases and cancer. Fruit is cooling, demulcent, given in small pox and for eye ailments as ointment.

Ethnomedicinal Uses

Seed oil used for resolving inflammatory swellings, herps and erysipelas.

Xantolis tomentosa (Roxb.) Rafin.

Family

Sapotaceae.

Vernacular Names

Oriya : Jyastha madhu, Jastimadhu, Kantabobhula; **Ko:** Garadhola.

The Plant

Small or medium sized tree, usually thorny, bark grey or light brown, blaze bright red, exuding drops of milky juice. Leaves obovate, margins wavy, obtuse or suddenly acute. Flowers white, small solitary. Berry yellowish, subglobose or broadly ovoid. Seeds usually 1 developed, deep brown. Fl. Apr.-

June, Fr. Nov.-February.

Distribution

Frequent in forests, especially in valleys.

Parts Used

Bark, fruits.

Medicinal Properties and Uses

Tonic prepared from boiling the bark, which is used to cure the cough and cold. Fruits contain a thermostable anti-choleric principles, which completely inhibits the growth of *Vibria comma,* fruit pulp given to patients of cholera.

Xylia xylocarpa (Roxb.) Taub.

Family

Mimosaceae

Vernacular Names

Oriya : Kongora, Boja, Dhamoni; **Sans :** Scimsapa, Kanakakuli; **Hindi :** Jambu, Suria, Tangan; **Ko :** Tingan.

The Plant

Small tree, branchlets brown-tomentose, thick, leaves long with a gland at the tip. Leaflets 5-6 pairs, ovate, oblong, acute, glabrous. Heads yellowish-white. Pods flat, woody, shoe shaped, rusty tomentose, seeds brown and long. Fl. Apr.-May, Fr. Nov.-April.

Distribution

Frequent in forests and commonly associated with sal.

Parts Used

Bark

Medicinal Properties and Uses

Decoction of bark given in gonorrhoea and diarrhoea and also used to stop vomiting and as a vermifuge.

Ziziphus mauritiana Lam.

Family

Rhamnaceae

Vernacular Names : Oriya: Barakoli, Boyer

Ko : Janumjan; **Sant** : Dedaori janum; **Hindi** : Ber, Beri; **Sans** : Badari

The Plant

A low, much branched, thorny, deciduous tree with spreading crown, dark greyish black bark having irregular cracks and strong reddish hardwood. Leaves oblong-elliptic, ovate or suborbicular, minutely serrulate or apex distinctly toothed, prominently 3-nerved. Flowers greenish yellow in axillary dense fascicles or sessile or short peduncled cyme. Fruits oblong, globose or ovoid drupes, turning from yellow to orange and finally red. Fl. Mar.-October, Fr. Jan.-March.

Distribution

Common in forest.

Parts Used

Leaves, fruits.

Medicinal Properties and Uses

The roots are bitter, cooling, anodyne and tonic and are useful in fever, wounds and ulcers. The bark is astringent, constipating and tonic and is useful in dysentery, diarrhoea and boils. The leaves are bitter, cooling, anthelmintic, antipyretic and are useful in stomatitis, ulorrhea, wounds, ulcers, asthma, typhoid fever and obesity. The fruits are sweet, cooling, anodyne, purgative, mucilaginous, pectoral, styptic, aphrodisiac, appetizer and tonic. They are useful in vitiated conditions of pitta, burning sensation, hyperdipsia, consumption, vomiting, constipation, leprosy, skin diseases, wound and ulcers. The seeds are acrid, sweet, astringent, soporific and tonic. They are useful in encephalopathy, ophthalmopathy, dipsia, cough, asthma, wounds and insomnia.

Ethnomedicinal Uses

Stem bark paste is taken twice a day after food as a cure for abdominal pain during pregnancy. The leaves mixed with turmeric are applied externally in skin diseases.

Ziziphus rugosa Lam.

Family

Rhamnaceae

Vernacular Names

Oriya : Chunkoli, Kotaikoli, Simukoli; **Hindi** : Suran Churna; **Sant** : Sekra; **Sans** : Tinkoli.

The Plant

Large armed shrub or small tree with long pendant scandent branches, young parts tomentose. Leaves elliptic, orbicular ovate, apex rounded 3-5 nerved, base cordate. Flowers greenish yellow. Seed obovoid, turgid. Fl. Mar.-April, Fr. May-July.

Distribution

Common in open forest near ravines.

Parts Used

Bark, flowers.

Medicinal Properties and Uses

Bark is given in diarrhoea. The powdered bark is mixed with ghee and applied to the swollen cheek in toothache and for ulcers in mouth. Flowers are used into medicines for menorrhagia.

Ethnomedicinal Uses

Pasty mass of leaves mixed with sugar (5 gm) and is taken as a preventive measure for pox. The dislocated joints are set right in one week time by applying hot root-paste and giving some support with the help of sticks.

Zornia gibbosa Span.

Family

Fabaceae.

Vernacular Names

Sant : Tandi japani.

The Plant

Prostrate herb. Leaves 2-foliolate, stipules peltate, lanceolate or ovate, apex acute, obtuse, Flowers yellow, sessile. Joints of pods very reticulately venose with retrosely scabrid prickles. Fr. & Fr. Aug.-December.

Distribution

Common in open grassy places.

Parts Used

Root.

Medicinal Properties and Uses

Plant is used for dysentery and root given to children as a soporific.

2

BIOTECHNOLOGICAL POTENTIALS OF MEDICINAL PLANTS

The medicinal plants are in great demand in traditional system of medicine *i.e.* Ayurveda, Siddha Unani, and Tibetan systems as well as preparation of modern medicine. Nearly 80% of people worldwide rely chiefly on traditional medicines to meet their primary health care needs. The Indian system of medicine is fascinating people all over the world for its crude drug use with the least side effects and effective cure. Various technologies have been adopted for enhancing bioactive molecules in medicinal plants. Biotechnological tools are important for the multiplication and genetic enhancement of the medicinal plants by adopting techniques such as *in vitro* regeneration and genetic transformation. Modern method of tissue culture, combined with improvement in genetic engineering techniques specifically transformation technology, have opened up new avenues for high volume production of pharmaceuticals, nutraceuticals and other beneficial substances. The modern pharmaceutical industry also requires a large quantity of authentic plants for manufacture of drugs. Extraction of active principles and manufacture of drug formulations is a sophisticated technology and capital intensive. Medicinal plants thus constitute an important component of the plant resource of our country.

When we speak about medicinal plants we have to consider three important sectors *i.e.*

(1) Modern medicines which utilize some 30 to 35 medicinal plants,

(2) The traditional medicine which are organized, codified with written treatise texts like Ayurveda, Siddha, Unani, Amchi and Tibetan systems of medicine which use about 1200-2000 medicinal plant species, and

(3) The Local Health Traditions which based on the oral traditions practiced by villagers folk healers, vaidyas and tribal people who use over 8000 species of medicinal plants for primary healthcare purposes.

Modern pharmacopoeia still contains at least 25% drugs derived from plants and many others which are synthetic analogues built on prototype compounds isolated from plants. Interest in medicinal plants as a re-emerging health aid has been fuelled by the rising costs of prescription drugs in the maintenance of personal health and well being. There is an increasing reliance on the use of medicinal plants in the industrialized societies attributed to the extraction and development of several drugs and chemotherapeutics from these plants as well as from traditionally used herbal remedies. The medicinal properties of these plants could be based on the antioxidant, antimicrobial antipyretic effects of the phytochemicals in them.

Survey and Documentation on Medicinal Plants of India

India is one among the 12-mega biodiversity countries of the world. It is estimated that out of 17,500 species of flowering plants, 140 genera and 5285 species are endemic to the country. The endemic flora is concentrated mainly in three major hot spot centers of flora viz. the Eastern Himalayas (3500 species), the Western Ghats (1600) and Andaman & Nicobar Islands (185). The East Himalayas and the Western Ghats are the two identified 'global hot spots' of biodiversity. In India species richness is complemented by enormous genetic diversity found within individual species. The occurrence of several ecotypes, chemotypes and cytotypes even within a single plant species offer ample opportunities to systematically survey, study, characterize and evaluate the economic uses and potentials of the plant resources of India, particularly the medicinal plants.

A number of organizations in the country are engaged in survey, inventory and documentation on medicinal plants of India. The important among them are Botanical Survey of India (BSI), Kolkata and its regional circles (IO) located in different parts of the country; laboratories under Council of Scientific & Industrial Research (CSIR) like Regional Research Laboratory

(RRL), Jammu, Central Institute of Medicinal & Aromatic Plants (CIMAP), Lucknow, National Botanical Research Institute (NBRI), Lucknow, RRL- Jorhat and IMMT, Bhubaneshwar; Indian Council of Agricultural Research (ICAR) centers, Agricultural Universities, Botany Departments of various Universities, Ayurvedic University of Gujarat; Govt. Ayurvedic Colleges, and State Government R&D institutions like Tropical Botanic Garden and Research Institute (TBGRI), Trivandrum; Kerala Forest Research Institute (KFRI), Peechi (Kerala). Apart from these the Foundation for Revitalization of Local Health Traditions (FRLHT) was established with the Headquarters at Bangalore as an autonomous voluntary organization by an initiative of Ministry of Environment & Forests, Government of India. FRLHT has been generously funded by Danida for inventory, documentation and conservation of medicinal plants used in Traditional systems of Medicines in the country.

Ministry of Environment & Forests, Department of Science & Technology (DST) and Department of Biotechnology (DBT) have launched many project programmes for inventory, documentation, conservation, cultivation and sustainable utilization of medicinal plant wealth of India. Important among them is a massive All India multi-institutional (27 centres) and multidisciplinary All India Coordinated Research Project on Ethnobiology (AICRPE), originally launched by DST in 1982 and then transferred to Ministry of Environment & Forests, Govt. of India which was concluded in 1998. It has documented over 8000 plant species used by the tribal communities for medicinal purpose. A Digitized Data Base of the vast information generated from AICRPE about the wild plants used by the tribal communities of India has been taken up at NBRI, Lucknow. Dept of Biotechnology had launched a gene bank programme in 1993 and established 4 major Gene *Banks* for Medicinal & Aromatic Plants at TBGRI, Trivandrum; CIMAP, Lucknow and National Bureiu of Plant Genetic Resources (NBPGR), Delhi and RRL, Jammu which focus on *ex situ* conservation of medicinal and aromatic plant wealth of India. Another major effort for establishing a comprehensive national database *on* medicinal plants was launched under the National Bioresource Development Board (NBDB) constituted by Ministry of Science

& Technology, Govt. of India. An expert group on medicinal plant bioresources has reviewed the scenario of medicinal plant research in India and identified the gaps in knowledge. The expert group has reported that out of the 8000 plants used by different traditional communities only 1800 are well studied and documented. Also many drugs mentioned in the classical medical texts of Ayurveda, Unani, Siddha and Amchi are not correctly identified. The expert group also observed that a complete inventory of medicinal plants with quantified details with respect to their intraspecific variability, distribution and extent of their extraction etc. from wild sources is lacking. Therefore, it was decided to initiate an All India Coordinated Project on Inventorying the Medicinal Plant Resources of India with the participation of 6 major organizations in the country namely, Botanical Survey of India (BSI), Kolkata; NBRI, Lucknow; CIMAP, Lucknow; NBPGR, New Delhi; Central Council for Research in Ayurveda and Siddha, Pune and J.N. Centre for Advanced Scientific Research, Bangalore.

COLLECTION, PREPARATION AND EVALUATION OF HERBAL MEDICINES

According to World Health Organization nearly 80 per cent of people still rely mainly on traditional remedies such as herbs for their medicines. It has been reported that a number of preparations/application of medicinal plants are being made by traditional communities. So far about 3000 wild plant species are used in the codified systems of Indian medicine like Ayurveda (900 species), Siddha (800), Unani (700) and Amchi (300), modern medicine (30). It is estimated that approximately one quarter of prescribed drugs contain plant extracts or active ingredients obtained from or modelled on plant substances. Aspirin, atropine, artimesinin, colchicine, digoxin, ephedrine, morphine, physostigmine, pilocarpine, quinine, quinidine, reserpine, taxol, tubocurarine, vincristine and vinblastine are a few important examples of what medicinal plants have given us in the past. Most of these plant-derived drugs were originally discovered through the study of traditional cures and folk knowledge of indigenous people and some of these could not be substituted despite the enormous advancement in synthetic chemistry.

The most common method of preparing medicines was cutting the particular bark, roots or leaves in pieces and boiling them in water. The *decoction* was then drunk as tea, sometimes mixed with milk and sugar to camouflage its unpleasant taste. Decoctions were also used as steam baths or to bathe the body. Few infusions (solutions of plant material in cold water) were used. When the undiluted sap from herbs was needed to disinfect cuts or sores, leaves were briefly heated over a fire until they became soft, and then rolled firmly between the hand palms and squeezed. Amerindians used most plants singly. Complicated mixtures of several different species were prescribed only occasionally. Most herbal treatments included leaves (34%), followed by bark (15%), the whole plant (12%, mostly in the case of smaller herbs), roots (10%, including tuberous rhizomes and bulbs), and exudate (8%, including latex, resin, or gum).

The herbal drugs are inconsistent in quality. Even the active principles involved in exerting the therapeutic efficacy (and toxicity if any) are not known in herbal medicines. One of the drawbacks in traditional medicine is that the spectrum of biological activities and the requirement of each ingredient to combat specific diseases are not clear. Even, in traditional medicine numerous therapeutic values are attributed to one single herb (without pinpointing the major therapeutic effect from the minor therapeutic effect). Herbal drugs in traditional use should be validated using experimental animal models rather than isolated organ or cell studies. Such studies can give some indications of efficacy and safety. However, animal experiments may not be totally reflection of human beings as minor metablic diversity between animal and human and role of psyche unique to human exists. Even ecotype (including seasonal) and genotype variations could interfere with the overall phytochemical picture and pharmacological profile of the herbal medicines.

Different ecotypes differ in the efficacy of medicinal plants in some cases. This is more important when medicinal plants are collected from wild and used as a phytomedicine. Some of the medicinal plants used in traditional medicine exhibit variations in their habitats from sea coast to hills. Depending ecological conditions medicinal plants exhibit variations in pharmacological properties and phytochemical profile. Knowledge in ecotype variations in efficacy and safety can help in determining cultivation condition for maximum efficacy and minimum toxicity (if any). Further, the pharmacological and toxicological properties of medicinal plants could be altered by soil conditions including nutritional as well as by their association with other organisms such as bacteria, fungi, and other plants. In many cases genotype variations could be confused with variations arising from differences in ecological conditions. Man-made interference in the ecosystem such as use of pesticides and contamination of the ecosystem with heavy metals, industrial toxins influence the efficacy and safety of medicinal plants. The major task in herbal drug development is ensuring uniform quality raw materials in sufficient amounts as per requirement.

Pharmacological studies have to be carried out to determine the most suitable ecotype and genotype for phytomedicine preparation. Lack of standards of safety and efficacy of the traditional herbal drugs is the main reason for not accepting them by the drug controlling system of most of the scientifically advanced counties. Under this context the therapeutic agents used in traditional medicines for various diseases can form the basis for the development of standardized herbal drugs for various diseases. During the past decade West Germany developed many phytopharmaceuticals for on wide variety of medical problems. China has scientifically validated and upgraded the quality of a large numbers of traditional herbal drugs. However, in India herbal drug research is not integrated and focused to develop phytomedicines (or allopathic medicine) with modern standards of safety and efficacy.

BIOTECHNOLOGICAL TOOLS IN MEDICINAL PLANT RESEARCH

Biotechnological tools are important for multiplication and genetic enhancement of the medicinal plants by adopting techniques such as *in-vitro* regeneration (Plant tissue culture) and genetic transformations. Apart from this, several other biotechnological tools are also available for regeneration, and genetic transformation leading to enhancement of *in-vitro* secondary metabolite production from medicinal plants. It can also be harnessed for production of secondary metabolites using plants as bioreactors.

PLANT TISSUE CULTURE

Biotechnological tools such as plant tissue culture techniques are important in order to select, multiply and conserve the critical genotypes of medicinal plants.

Tissue culture refers to growing and multiplication of cells, tissues and organs of plants on defined solid or liquid media under aseptic and controlled environment. The commercial technology is primarily based on micropropagation, in which rapid proliferation is achieved from tiny stem cuttings, axillary buds and to a limited extent from somatic embryos, cell clumps in suspension cultures and bioreactors. The cultured cells and tissues can take several pathways. The pathways that lead to the production of true-to-type plants in large numbers are the preferred ones for commercial multiplication. The process of micropropagation is usually divided into several stages such as pre-propagation, initiation of explants, subculture of explants for proliferation, shooting and rooting and hardening. These stages are universally applicable in large-scale multiplication of plants. Micropropagation (*in vitro* propagation of axillary and/ or adventitious buds as well as somatic embryos) is presently used as an advanced biotechnological system for the production of identical pathogen-free plants for agriculture and forestry. Protocols for cloning of some medicinal plants such as *Catharanthus roseus* (Apocynaceae), *Chlorophytum borivilianum* (Liliaceae), *Datura metel* (Solanaceae) and *Bacopa monnieri* (Scrophulariaceae) have been developed. Similarly micro-propagation protocols have been achieved for several medicinal plants such as *Withania somnifera, Hoslundia opposita, Cinchona ledgeriana, Digitalis* spp. and *Rauvolfia serpentina* etc.

PLANT BIOREACTORS

Micropropagation by conventional techniques is typically a labour-intensive means of clonal propagation. Bioreactors containing liquid media are used for large-scale growth of various tissues. The use of bioreactor for the micropropagation was first reported in 1981 for Begonia. Since then it has proved applicable to many species including shoot, bulbs, microtubers, corms and somatic embryos. Bioreactors are vessels designed for large-scale cell, tissue or organ culture in liquid media. Functionally, plant culture bioreactors can be divided into two broad types: those in which the cultures are immersed partially or temporarily in the medium and those in which the cultures are continuously submerged. Bioreactors provide more precise control of the medicinal plant growth, gaseous exchange, illumination, medium agitation, temperature and pH than the conventional culture vessels. Bioreactor-based propagation of plants can increase the rate of multiplication and growth of cultures and reduce the space, energy and labour requirements in commercial micropropagation. Three main classes of culture systems in bioreactors can be distinguished: (1) those producing biomass (cells or organogenic or embryogenic propagules, shoots or roots as the final product); (2) those producing metabolites and enzymes; and (3) biotransformation of exogenously added metabolites (which may be precursors in the pathway).

COMBINATORIAL BIOSYNTHESIS

The basic concept of combinatorial biosynthesis is to combine metabolic pathways in different organisms at the genetic level, where genes from different microorganisms are combined for the production of new and interesting plant secondary metabolites. From pharmaceutical point of view, hydroxylations and glycosylations are considered to be particularly useful bioconversions. They can yield new drugs and existing drugs can be improved as to increased activity and decreased toxicity. An increasing number of natural products are being biosynthesized in low quantities. Some of the examples are *artemisinin*, paclitaxel, podophyllotoxin, and *Vinca*-alkaloids. The use of genetically modified plant cell cultures, such as hairy root cultures for Solanaceae or for artemisinin offers a rational approach to allow the overexpression of genes encoding biosynthetic enzymes, and to overcome the rate-limiting steps of the biosynthesis. Combinatorial biosynthesis is a new tool in the generation of novel natural products, as well as for the production of rare and expensive natural products. Combinatorial biosynthesis is carried out for important classes of natural products, including alkaloids (vinblastine, vincristine), terpenoids (artemisinin, paclitaxel), and flavonoids.

GENETIC TRANSFORMATION TECHNOLOGY & PRODUCTION OF TRANSGENIC PLANTS

The use of biotechnological tools in medicinal plant science is very limited as compared to other crops. However, in recent years the engineering of agronomic traits in medicinal plants led to interesting developments for genetic transformation, both *in vivo* and *in vitro*. Genetic transformation with bacterial vector systems has been widely used for several medicinal plants, including *Artemisia annua*, *Taxus* sp., *Papaver somniferum*, *Ginkgo biloba* and *Camptotheca acuminata* and species from the Solanaceae. Plant transformation mediated by *Agrobacterium tumefaciens*, a soil plant pathogenic bacterium, has become the most commonly used method for the introduction of foreign genes into plant cells and the subsequent regeneration of transgenic plants. The rapid progress in the area of crop biotechnology is mainly because of the development of efficient regeneration and suitable *Agrobacterium* mediated transformation protocols for different crop species. *Agrobacterium* mediated genetic transformations has been reported for various medicinal plants. Sucessfull regeneration of transgenic neem plants (*Azadirachta indica*), *Atropa belladona* and *Echinacea purpurea* using *Agrobacterium tumefaciens* has been reported with improved medicinal properties.

ENGINEERING AGRONOMIC TRAITS IN MEDICINAL PLANTS

There has been relatively few reports of biotechnology applied to abiotic stresses and other aspects of agronomic performance of medicinal plants although the approach is considered to have great potential. Just as resistance to herbicides, pests and diseases are the characters that have led the way in the introduction of transgenic crop species so too have these characters been among the first targets for medicinal plant biotechnology.

GENOMIC PROFILING OF MEDICINAL PLANTS BY DNA MICROARRAY TECHNIQUE

DNA microarray was developed in response to the need for a high throughput efficient and comprehensive strategy that can simultaneously measure all the genes or a large defined subset encoded by a genome. Several methodologies including differential display PCR, northern blots, quantitatives PCR, serial analysis of gene expression (SAGE) and TIGR Orthologous Gene Alignments (TOGA) are used along side microarrays as research tools. DNA microarray is an orderly arrangement of thousands of oligo nucleotides or identified sequenced genes printed on an impermeable solid support, usually glass, silicon chips or nylon membrane. Novel technologies such as SAGE and DNA microarray allow rapid and detailed analysis of thousands of transcripts providing revolutionary approach to the investigation of gene expression. Recently microarray have been applied for the DNA sequence based identification of medicinal plants. DNA microarray can also be used for studying herbal drug interactions and the mechanisms underlying these interactions.

MARKER ASSISTED BREEDING

Marker assisted breeding invloves the use of DNA markers linked with DNA sequences of interest. Inheritance pattern of sequences/traits can be confirmed even prior to expression using RFLP, RAPD, AFLP and minisatellite markers. A high content artimisinin producing plant variety "CIM Arogya" was developed at CIMAP, Lucknow through marker assisted breeding. Marker assisted breeding could also be used in developing high secondary metabolite yielding plants.

BIOANALYTICS AND METABOLOMICS

Metabolomics is an important biotechnological tool in functional genomics. It concerns with the analysis of all metabolites in an organism. *Metabolic profiling* aims at measuring a selected group of metabolites in an organism where as *Metabolic fingerprinting* aims at measuring a "fingerprint" of the metabolite(s) in an organism, but without identifying all of the compounds present. In addition to this basic scientific approach, metabolomics has been applied to a wide array of other fields. For example, it is an important tool for the chemotaxonomy of botanicals, or for studying the equivalence of genetically modified and wild-type organisms, especially in the case of plants. Metabolomics also represents a major diagnostic tool, for example in the analysis of urinary metabolites using nuclear magnetic resonance (NMR) spectrometry in order to diagnose disease. Today, in drug development, metabonomics is used as a major means of detecting the toxicity of novel compounds on the kidney and liver, and more recently has attracted much attention from systems biology approaches to drug development.

DRUG DEVELOPMENT

Since bioactive phytochemical compounds are used directly as theurapeutic agents and also used as starting material for the synthesis of drugs or as models for pharmacologically active compounds they are very useful for drug development. Exploiting traditional herbal medicines in the context of modern science is the need for optimum and proper utilization of traditional plant drugs.

It is true that a lot of scientific studies has been done on a large number of medicinal plants in India. In spite of this, we have not developed a considerable number of marketable drugs as plant derived chemical entities or traditional herbal preparations with modern standards of safety and efficacy. This is due to the fact that in India, to a large extent, integrated research focusing the development of commercially viable and useful phytomedicines (or even plant derived allopathic drugs) is not carried out.

PHARMACEUTICAL EVALUATION

There are two main approaches to develop successful drugs from medicinal plants. One is a **phytochemical approach** and the other is **phytotherapeutic approach**. In the former approach, the plant materials are subjected to chemical analysis and individual chemical compounds are isolated and characterized. Then the defined chemical entities are tested for their pharmacological activity and therapeutic value. The pharmacological properties are very often predicted based on their chemical structure.Then structure and activity relationship are studied. If it can control, prevent and/or cure a disease then detailed studies are carried out in experimental animals. If it successfully passes animal experiments, detailed clinical trials of chemical entity may be approved as a medicine for human use.

Although there are success stories of ancient insights on medicinal plants leading to the discovery of chemical entities as drugs, this type of drug discovery, in general, is expensive and time consuming. In India, The Central Drug Research Institute, Lucknow, studied approximately 2500 plants over a period of more than two decades. This did not result in the development of even a single marketable drug (chemical entity), though many leads were uncovered. It has been estimated that development of a chemical entity from plant as drug may cost as much as US$ 1-20 crore in developed countries.

The second approach to drug development is a phytotherapeutic approach wherein crude plant preparations, (extracts, active fractions or mixtures of them) or ayurvedic types of formulations can be used as drugs with modern standards of safety and efficacy. It is cost-effective and more relevant to our conditions. Even standardised phytomedicines are increasingly accepted in Europe.

Although opportunities for developing ayurvedic and other traditional herbal drugs with international acceptance are vast, at present, there is hardly any concerted effort in this direction in our country. Many research publications on medicinal plants show marginal or insufficient pharmacological activities, which are not satisfactory to develop into a herbal drug or phytomedicine. Further, in some cases, a medicinal plant is credited with innumerable pharmacological activities without focusing practical therapeutic benefits. Details of the both the approaches are discussed below :

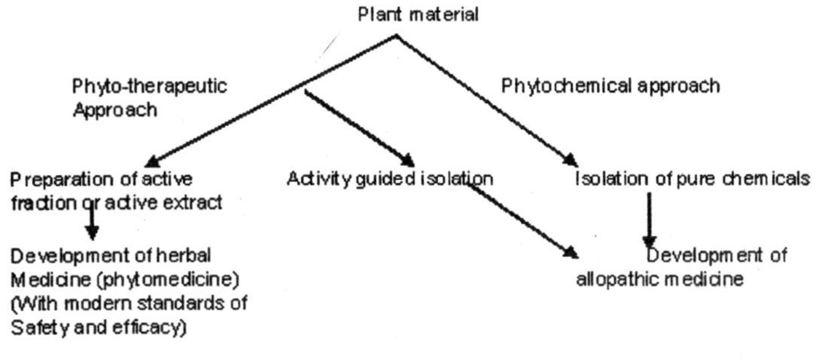

Fig. 1 : Flow chart showing the development of allopathic type of medicines and phytomedicines.

PHYTOCHEMICAL APPROACH

Medicinal plants are plants containing inherent active ingredients used to cure disease or relieve. Modern pharmacopoeia still contains at least 25% drugs derived from plants and many others which are synthetic analogues built on prototype compounds isolated from plants. Medicinal plants contain physiologically active principles that over the years have been exploited in traditional medicine for the treatment of various ailments. The drugs contained in medicinal plants are known as active principles. Plants usually contain a wide variety of active principles. There is a reasonable likelihood that medicinal plants with a long history of human use will ultimately yield novel drug prototypes. There are several standard methods used for the phytochemical screening of medicinal plants. The phytochemicals includes alkaloids, steroids and phlobatannins, phenolics and flavonoids, saponins and cardiac glycosides, tannins etc. Methods are available for quantitative and qualitative analysis of phytochemicals in medicinal plants.

Phytochemicals are the chemicals extracted from plants. These chemicals are classified as primary or secondary constituents, depending on their role in plant metabolism. Primary constituents include the common sugars, aminoacids, proteins, purines and pyrimidines of nucleic acids, chlorophylls etc. They are essential for growth of metabolites of plants. Secondary constituents are the remaining plant chemicals such as alkaloids (derived from amino acids), terpenes (a group of lipids) and phenolics (derived from carbohydrates). Unlike primary metabolites, absence of secondary metabolities does not result in immediate death, but rather in long-term impairment of the organism's survivability, or perhaps in no significant change at all. Secondary metabolites are often restricted to a narrow set of species within a phylogenetic group. The most commonly encountered secondary metabolites of plants (phytochemicals) are saponins, tannins, flavornoids, alkaloids, anthraquinones, cardiac glycosides and cyanogenic glycosides. The presence of these secondary metabolites in plants probably explains the various uses of plants for traditional medicine.

Saponins are glycosides of both triterpenes and steroids having hypotensive and cardiac depressant properties. Saponins bind to cholesterol to form insoluble complexes. Dietary saponins in the gut of monogastric combine with endogenous cholesterol excreted via the bile. This prevents cholesterol reabsorption and results in a reduction of serum cholesterol. Saponins have been found to be potentially useful for the treatment of hypercholesterolaemia which suggests that saponins might be acting by interfering with intestinal absorption of cholesterol.

Tannins is a general descriptive name for a group of polymeric phenolic substances capable of tanning leather or precipitating gelatin from solution, a property known as astringency. These are complex phenolic polymers which can bind to proteins and carbohydrates resulting in reduction in digestibility of these macromolecules and thus inhibition of microbial growth. They are found in almost every plant part: bark, wood, leaves, fruits and roots.

Flavonoids are phenolic structures containing one carbonyl group (as opposed to the two carbonyls in quinones). The addition of a 3-hydroxyl group yields a flavonol. Flavonoids are also hydroxylated phenolic substances but occur as a C6-C3 unit linked to an aromatic ring. These are a group of phyto-chemicals found in varying amounts in foods and medicinal plants which have been shown to exert potent anti-oxidant activity against the superoxide radical. It's consumption has been documented not to be associated with mortality due to coronary heart disease. This may be as a result of its antioxidant activity and subsequent inhibitions of low density lipoproteins (LDL) oxidation known to have been attributed to the dietary and supplemental intake of flavonoids and other micronutrients. Epidemiologic studies indicate an inverse relationship between intake of dietary flavonoids and coronary artherosclerotic.

Alkaloids are heterocyclic nitrogen compounds. These are basic natural products occurring primarily in many plants. They are generally found in the form of salts with organic acids and they are haemolytically active and are also toxic to micro-organisms. Alkaloids, comprising a large group of nitrogenous compounds are widely used as therapeutic agents in the management of cancer. Alkaloids also interfere with cell division. The first medically useful alkaloid was morphine isolated in 1805 from the opium poppy *Papaver somniferum*. Diterpenoid alkaloids, commonly isolated from the plants of the Ranunculaceae or buttercup family are commonly found to have antimicrobial properties. Solamargine, a glycoalkaliods from the berries of *Solanum khasianum* and other alkaloids are useful against HIV infections as well as intestinal infections associated with AIDS.

Cardiac glycosides are cardioactive compounds belonging to triterpenoids class of compounds. Their inherent activity resides in the aglycone portions of their sugar attachment. Their clinical effects in cases of congestive heart failure are to increase the force of myocardiac contraction. They exert their hypotensive effect by inhibiting Na^+–K^+ ATPase. They also act directly on the smooth muscle.

PHYTOTHERAPEUTIC APPROACH (Pharmacological Approach)

The second approach is a phytotherapeutic approach. In this approach the extraction, fractionation, isolation and separation of chemical entities from plant materials are guided by pharmacological activity (bioactivity). In the activity guided step-wise isolation procedure, if activity is not detected in one step, the next step will not be carried out. This phytotherapeutic approach is also employed to discover new compounds as medicine (Fig. 2). The phytotherapeutic approach will enable the development of crude plant materials as standardized medicines. Development of standardized phytomedicines following traditional leads is relatively inexpensive and less time consuming. Pharmacological evaluation is an essential component in the development of herbal drugs (phytomedicine). In traditional medicine, generally whole plants or plant parts (leaves, roots flowers, seeds, bark, stem etc.) fresh or dried, are used as crude homogenates, extracts, decoctions and tinctures. These herbal drugs are mixture of numerous phytochemicals. Out of these a few chemicals or one may be involved in exhibiting the said pharmacological property in a given herbal medicine. The active principle(s) are not identified in most of the herbal drug preparations and in the traditional medicinal plants. The phytochemicals of certain medicinal plants may exhibit toxicity which needs to be evaluated.

Standardized pharmacological methods are available to evaluate most of the pharmacological parameters. Demonstrating activity in an *in-vivo* bio-assay should be the first step in the verification or validation of herbal drugs. Animal experimental models simulating human diseases are used, to a large extent, to determine efficacy. Efficacy and toxicity determinations of many potential herbal drugs consist of orally administering the crude drugs into experimental animals and watching changes in key physiological, biochemical and behavioural parameters.

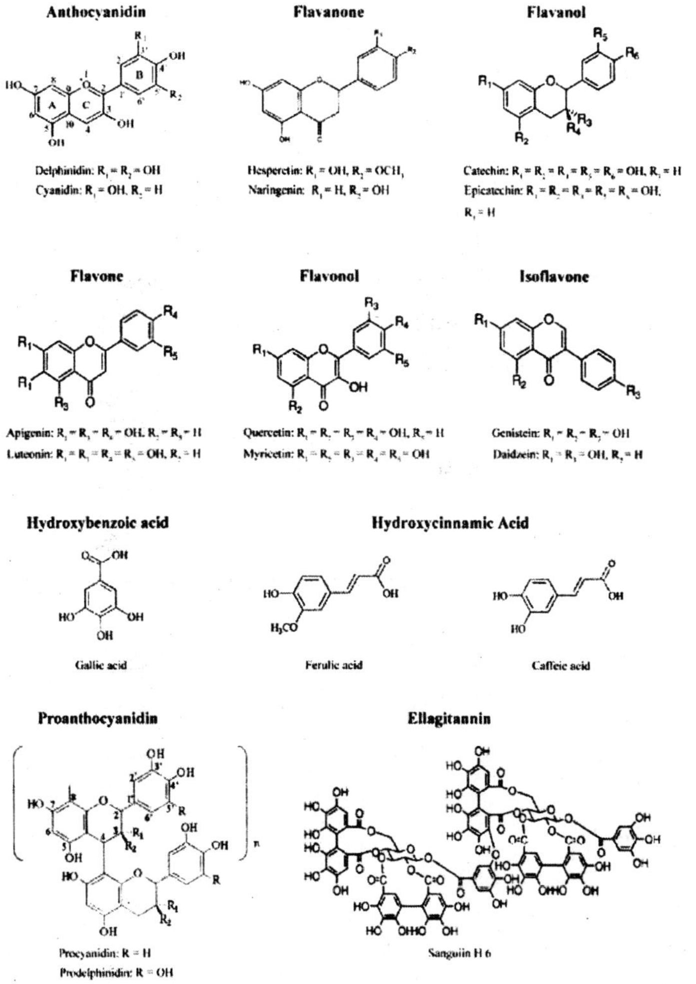

Fig. 2 : Structures of flavonoids, phenolic acids and tannins

After establishing *in vitro* effects, attempts can be made to set up simple *in vitro* assays to reflect *in vivo* effects. These *in vitro* assays can be used for setting up pharmacological standards for efficacy. Isolated organs such as smooth muscle, pieces of intestine, heart, lung etc. can be used to test plant extracts for muscle contraction, heartbeat, secretion and other function. Unraveling the mechanism of action of herbal drugs could help to devise simple test–system to assess efficacy. Many diseases are caused by defect in important functional protein such as G– proteins, receptor ligands and key enzymes. Many assays are used to assess the effect of the drugs on the function of a single protein involved in the biochemical interactions that underlie a disease. Fully automated *in vitro* tests for many enzymes are now available for example, if the mechanism of action of an anti-inflammatory drug is inhibition of phosphokipase A2 activity, this enzyme assay under cell free assay condition can serve as a tool to determine efficacy. Similarly, inhibition of histamine action or mast cell stabilization is useful as anti-allergic drug. Thus many *in vitro* simple tests could reflect the therapeutic efficacy and these assays can also be used to set efficacy standards of herbal extracts/active fraction. Anti-microbial and anti–helminthes effects are tested under *in vitro* conditions when the drug acts directory of the organism without significant involvement of host immune system. Further, simple and effective tests have to be developed in some cases in light of the advancement in physiology pathology, biochemistry, pharmacology etc.

DEVELOPMENT OF PHYTO-MEDICINE

Current research in drug discovery from medicinal plants involves a multifaceted approach combining botanical, phyto-chemical, biological, and molecular techniques. Medicinal plant drug discovery continues to provide new and important leads against various pharmacological targets including cancer, HIV/AIDS, Alzheimer's, malaria, and pain. Although drug discovery from medicinal plants continues to provide an important source of new drug leads, numerous challenges are encountered including the procurement of plant materials, the selection and implementation of appropriate high-throughput screening bioassays, and the scale-up of active compounds.

The first major step in the development of a phytomedicine is to prepare a therapeutically valuable extract or active fraction (in rare cases crude homogenate may prove better than extract or active fraction regarding therapeutic value). As given in flow chart (Fig. 3) the process of medicine development has to begin with identification of promising plants for combating a particular disease. The plants may be selected based on ethnomedical leads. The identified plant has to be evaluated for its likely efficacy in suitable experimental animal models. To start with, the part of the plant used in ethnomedical practices has to be tested. The crude homogenate or preparation used in ethnomedical practice may be evaluated in 2 or 3 doses including 1 reasonably high dose. If there is any signs of bioactivity (therapeutic action) three different extracts may be tried (e.g. n-hexane (nonpolar), alcohol and water (polar). We prefer to do each of this extraction separately from the original plant material (dry powder). Some investigators prefer sequential extraction. These extractions may be done at room temperature because biological activity of some of the compounds could be destroyed by heat. The yield of the extract has to be determined in each case. One or two doses of each of these extracts may be tested for pharmacological activity. (The dose selection could be guided by the activity in the original homogenate and the yield of each extract). Based on the bioactivity one out of the three extracts may be selected for further studies. The appropriate extract (active extract) prepared from different parts of the plant has to be tested to determine the most suitable plant part.

After identification of the promising extract, it has to be subjected to detailed studies (Fig. 3). Then the active extract may be fractionated by sequential solvent extraction, column chromatography, etc. to obtain an active fraction (Fig. 4). In rare cases the fraction or even the extract can develop toxic side effect. Therefore, therapeutic does of crude homogenate extract and active fraction may be compared for their possible toxicity in general toxicity evaluation in experimental animals.

Development of toxicity indicates that the extract contain one or more compounds (which is removed during fraction), which attenuates or abrogates the toxicity of therapeutically valuable compounds (active principles) or other compounds present in the extract.

Selection of plants based on ethono-medicinal leads

↓

Screening (crude suspension of plant parts)
for anticipated therapeutic efficacy using animal models

↓

Selection of therapeutically valuable plants

↓

Pharmacological evaluation

↓

Identification of the following

↓

-the best plant part

-the best ecotype

-the best genotype

-the best extract/active fraction

Fig. 3 : Identification of promising plants

The bioactivity screening of the plant parts for antimicrobial activity, antioxidant activity, anticancer activity, antihelminthes activity, immunomodulatory activity, antitumour screening, cytotoxic screening etc. are done to evaluate the pharmaceutical importance of the medicinal plants. The presence of bioactive compounds in the various organic solvent extracts are determined by using different separation techniques such as extraction of active principles, isolation of bioactive compounds using Thin Layer Chromatography, HPLC, HPTLC, Gas chromatography, Mass Spectroscopy etc. Prediction of the structure and chemical nature of the isolated compound is done using Nuclear Magnetic Resonance (NMR) techniques etc.

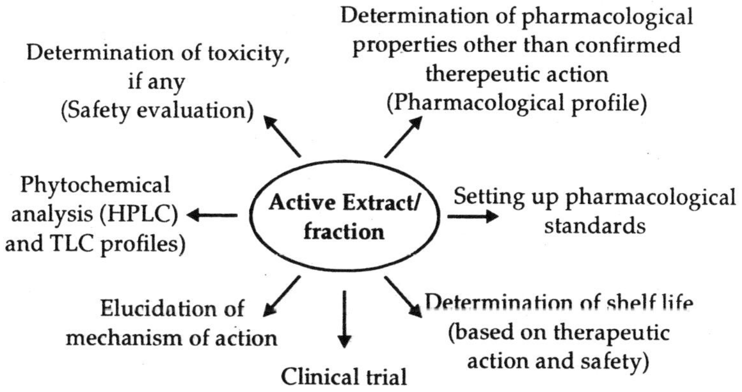

Fig. 4 : Isolation, identification of bioactive compound in medicinal plant

Plants can be considered as chemical factories that have their biosynthetic pathways to synthesise an array of compounds whose structural diversity is often beyond the imagination of even the most imaginative organic chemists. The isolation and characterization of the bioactive chemicals from plants have become possible with the advent of modern sophisticated techniques such as chromatographic methods, multidimensional NMR and mass spectrometry. The ability to screen natural product sources for biological activities has resulted in *uncovering* of many novel structures-activity relationship producing both new product drugs as well as new leads from rational drug design.

Structural Elucidation

The elucidation of the chemical structure is critical to avoid the re-discovery of a chemical agent that is already known for its structure and chemical activity. Mass spectrometry, often used to determine structure, is a method in which individual compounds are identified based on their mass/charge ratio, after ionization. Chemical compounds exist in nature as mixtures, so the combination of liquid chromatography and mass spectrometry (LC-MS) is often used to separate the individual chemicals. Databases of mass spectras for known compounds are available. Nuclear magnetic resonance spectroscopy is another important technique for determining chemical structures of natural products. NMR yields information about individual hydrogen and carbon atoms in the structure, allowing detailed reconstruction of the molecule's architecture

Elucidation of mechanisms of action is an important aspect of modern drug development. The mechanisms of action of an extract or active fraction can be studied with the same methods and tools, which are used to study the mechanisms of action of pure isolated chemical entity. The effect of an extract can be studied in cell free biochemical systems, cell culture systems as well as *in vivo* systems. If there are more than one chemical involved in therapeutic efficacy expression, there could be more than one mechanism of action. These different mechanisms of action have to be elucidated step by step using present state of knowledge in cell function regulation, physiology, biochemical processes, etc. If the extract or active fraction is found suitable based on the above mentioned efficacy and safety study, shelf-life determination, mechanism of action etc., the phytomedicine may be subjected to direct clinical trials according to WHO guidelines (WHO 1993).

EVALUATION OF BIOACTIVITY

Antimicrobial Activity of Medicinal Plants

Infectious diseases represent an important cause of morbidity and mortality among the general population, particularly in developing countries. Therefore, pharmaceutical companies have been motivated to develop new antimicrobial drugs in recent years, especially due to the constant emergence of microorganisms resistant to conventional antimicrobials. Owing to their popular use as remedies for many infectious diseases, searches for substances with antimicrobial activity in plants are frequent. Plants are rich in a wide variety of secondary metabolites, such as tannins, terpenoids, alkaloids, and flavonoids, which have been found *in vitro* to have antimicrobial properties. A number of literature is available on antimicrobial compounds that have been isolated from a variety of medicinal plants. Despite the abundant literature on the antimicrobial properties of plant extracts, none of the plant derived chemicals have successfully been exploited for clinical use as antibiotics. A significant part of the chemical diversity produced by plants is thought to protect plants against microbial pathogens. A number of plant compounds often classified as antimicrobial produce MIC ranges greater than 1,000 microgram/ml which are of no relevance from a clinical perspective. A vast majority of plant compounds showing little *in vitro* antibacterial activity are not antimicrobial but are regulatory compounds playing an indirect role in the plant defence against microbial infections. It is generally observed that plant derived compounds are generally weak compared to bacterial or fungal produced antibiotics and these compounds often show considerable activity against gram-positive bacteria than but no activity against gram-negative species. Plants produced compounds can be considered as an effective antimicrobials if they find their way into the cell of the pathogen especially across the double membrane barrier of Gram negative bacteria.

A number of plants have been documented for their antimicrobial properties. For example, *Anethum graveolens* (Dill), *Foeniculum vulgare* (Fennel), *Trachyspermum ammi* (Omum) and *Elettaria cardamomum*—queen of spices (Chotti elaichi)—have been commonly used to treat gastrointestinal disorders; *Viola odorata* has been in use to treat respiratory diseases and as an anti-inflammatory agent, while *Syzygium aromaticum* (clove) is used for toothache due to its local anaesthetic activity. *Anethum graveolens, Elettaria cardamomum, Foeniculum vulgare, Trachyspermum ammi* and *Viola odorata* were found to be better/equally effective compared to standard antibiotics. Apart from these, the acetone and alcoholic extracts of the leaves of *Cassia alata* showed significant *in vitro* antibacterial activity against *Staphylococcus aureus, Bacillus subtilis, Bacillus stearothermophillus, Escherichia coli, Salmonella typhi* and *Salmonella dysentriae*. Further, the alcoholic extracts of this plant also inhibited the growth of

Klebsiella pneumoniae where as the acetone extract inhibited the growth of *Vibrio cholerae*. The alcoholic extract of dry nuts of *Semecarpus anacardium* showed bactericidal activity *in vitro* against 3 gram negative strains (*Escherichia coli, Salmonella typhi* and *Proteus vulgaris*) and 2 gram positive strains (*Staphylococcus aureus* and *Corynebacterium diphtheriae*). Subsequent studies have shown that the alcoholic extracts of different parts of the plant (leaves, twigs, green fruits) also possess antibacterial properties especially the leaf extracts. Substantial antibacterial, and anti-fungal activities were observed with the hexane extract of the stem bark of *Amona glabra*. Volatile components of the hexane extracts of certain medicinal plants like *Eugenia caryophyllus, Thymus vulgaris, Cinnamonum zeylanium and Cuminum cyminum* were tested against standard gram positive and gram negative bacteria grown on agar slants showed antibacterial properties. The aqueous and ethanolic extracts of *Azadirachta indica* leaves have been shown to have anti-dermatophytic activity when tested *in vitro* against 88 clinical isolates of dermatophytes using the agar dilution technique. Similarly anti-mycotic activity was observed by certain plants like *Eucalyptus globules, Catharanthus roseus, Ocimum sanctum, Azadirachta indica, Ricinus communis, Lawsonia inermis* and *Jatropha curcas* against the test pathogen *Pestalotiopsis mangiferae*. Essential oil obtained from the herb of *Santolina chamaecyparissus* showed significant antifungal activity both *in vitro* and *in vivo* experiments. The essential oil isolated from the leaves of *Aegle marmelos* exhibited significant antifungal activity against different fungal isolates.

Scientists have realized an immense potential in natural products from medicinal plants to serve as alternate source of combating infections in human beings which may also be of lower cost and lesser toxicity. Clinical microbiologists have two reasons to be interested in the topic of antimicrobial plant extracts. First it is very likely that these phytochemicals will find their way into the arsenal of antimicrobial drugs prescribed by the physicians; several are already being tested in humans. Second the public is becoming increasingly aware of the problems with the over prescription and misuse of traditional antibiotics.

Antimicrobial Activity Mechanisms of Natural Products

Most plants contain several compounds with antimicrobial properties for protection against aggressor agents, especially microorganisms. The chemical structures of some antimicrobial compounds, obtained from plants are shown in Fig. 6. Active compounds found in some plants have antiseptic action; for example, thyme has thymol and carvacrol, clove has eugenol and isoeugenol, and oregano has carvacrol and terpinenol-4. In some cases, terpenes from essences that are soluble in water have higher antibacterial power than others.

The sites or structures of the bacterial cell that are considered targets for action by the components of natural products are shown in Fig. 5. The action mechanisms of natural compounds are related to disintegration of cytoplasmic membrane, destabilization of the proton motive force (PMF), electron flow, active transport and coagulation of the cell content. Not all action mechanisms work on specific targets and some sites may be affected due to other mechanisms.

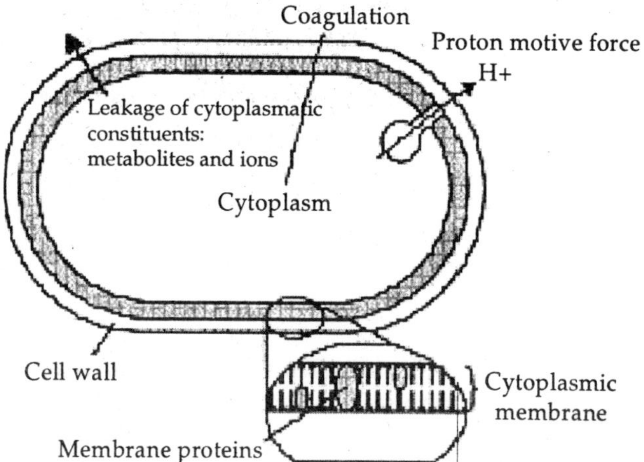

Fig. 5 : Sites in a bacterium where natural compounds are active

Important characteristics responsible for the antimicrobial action of essential oils include hydrophobic components that allow the participation of lipids from the bacterial cell membrane, which disturbs cell structures and make them more permeable.

Several compounds and their mechanisms of action on microorganisms are listed below.

Carvacrol and Thymol

The structure of thymol is similar to that of carvacrol; however, they differ as to the location of the hydroxyl group in the phenolic ring. Both substances seem to make the membrane permeable. Their structure disintegrates the external membrane of gram-negative bacteria, releasing lipopolysaccharides (LPS) and increasing the permeability of the cytoplasmic membrane to ATP. The presence of magnesium chloride does not influence this action, suggesting a chelating mechanism of different cations on the external membrane.

Eugenol

Different concentrations of eugenol may inhibit the production of amylase and protease by *B. cereus*. Furthermore, cell wall degradation and cell lysis were also reported.

p-Cymene

A precursor of carvacrol, this hydrophobic compound provokes greater swelling of the cytoplasmic membrane compared to carvacrol.

Carvone

When tested at concentrations higher than its minimum inhibitory concentration, carvone dissipates gradient pH and cell membrane potential. The growth of *E. coli, Streptococcus thermophilus* and *Lactococcus lactis* may decrease according to the concentrations of carvone, suggesting that it acts by disturbing the general metabolic status of the cell.

Cinnamaldehyde

Cinnamaldehyde is known to inhibit *E. coli* and *Salmonella* typhimurium growth at concentrations similar to those of carvacrol and thymol. However, it neither disintegrates the outer membrane nor weakens the intracellular ATP. Its carbonyl group has affinity for proteins, prèventing the action of decarboxylase amino acids on *E. aerogene*.

METHOD TO EVALUATE ANTIMICROBIAL ACTIVITIES

Antimicrobial Susceptibility Testing

Successful discovery of novel natural antimicrobials has necessitated the development of new bioassay techniques which are sensitive enough to detect small amounts of biologically active chemicals. In ethnopharmacology research the antimicrobial susceptibility test (AST) is used to determine the efficacy of potential antimicrobials from biological extracts against a number of different microbial species. AST methods are used to screen plant extracts for antimicrobial activity but are largely used to determine the usefulness of an antimicrobial in combating infections by determining its minimum inhibitory concentration (MIC). In clinical research *in vitro* susceptibility tests are particularly important if an organism is suspected to belong to a species that has shown resistance to frequently used antimicrobial agents. They are also important in epidemiological studies of susceptibility and in comparisons of new and existing microbial agents. AST standard tests can be conveniently divided into diffusion and dilution methods. Common diffusion tests include agar well diffusion, agar disk diffusion and bioautography, while dilution methods include agar dilution and broth micro/macrodilution. The broth and agar based methods are the conventional reference methods for AST. There are other commercial custom-prepared methods like the agar screen plate, Epsilometer test and the Vitek system which could be used in place of the standard reference methods but these are not common in routine AST and are not common for testing activity of plant extracts. The major problem in the diffusion and dilution based AST is one of availability of the active principles which is a function of the solubility of the test compound.

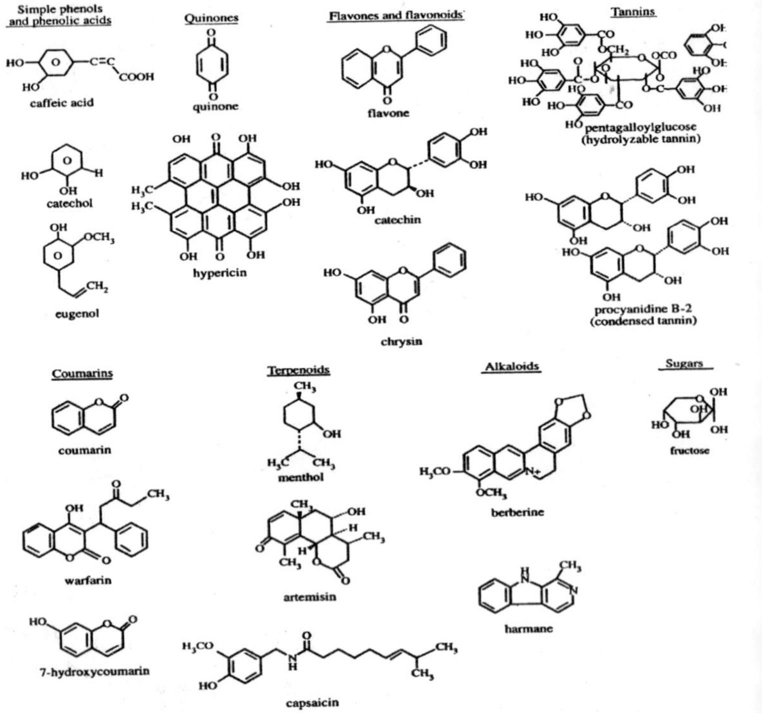

Fig. 6 : Chemical structures of antimicrobial compounds

AGAR DISK DIFFUSION ASSAY

Agar diffusion techniques have been widely used to assay plant extracts for antimicrobial activity, although there are limitations with the technique. Disk diffusion is suitable for identification of leads but not effective for quantification of bioactivity. These diffusion techniques generally do not distinguish bactericidal and bacteriostatic effects. The MIC can not be determined and these are usually used for preliminary screening that is, as qualitative tests, since the amount of extract that adheres to the disk is not quantitatively determined. Some researchers however have reported MIC values obtained by the agar diffusion method although high activity in the disk diffusion assay does not necessarily correlate to low MIC values in the microtitre plate method. The agar disk diffusion technique can only be used for AST of pure substances because when it

Table 1 : Main groups of plant compounds with antimicrobial activity

Class	Subclass	Examples	Mechanism
Phenolics	Simple phenols	Catechol	Substrate deprivation
		Epicatechin	Membrane disruption
	Phenolic acid	Cinnamic acid	?
	Quinones	Hypericin	Adhesin binding, complex with cell wall, enzyme inactivation
	Flavonoids	Chrysin	Adhesin binding
	Flavones	–	Complex with cell wall
		Abyssinone	Enzyme inactivation
			HIV reverse transcriptase inhibition
	Flavonols	Totarol	?
	Tannins	Ellagitannin	Protein binding
			Adhesin binding
			Enzyme inhibition
			Substrate deprivation
			Complex with cell wall
			Membrane disruption
			Metal-ion complexation
	Coumarins	Warfarin	Interaction with eucaryotic DNA (antiviral activity)
Terpenoids, essential oils	–	Capsaicin	Membrane disruption
Alkaloids	–	Berberine	Intercalation into cell wall and/or DNA
		Piperine	
Lectins and polypeptides	–	Mannose-specific agglutinin	Block of viral fusion or adsorption
		Falxatin	Disulfide bridge formation
Polyacetylenes	–	8s-heptadeca-2(Z),9(Z)-diene-4,6-diyne-1,8-diol	?

is applied to mixtures containing constituents, which exhibit different diffusion rates, results may be unreliable. In the method, 6 mm paper disks, saturated with filter sterilized plant extract at the desired concentration, are placed onto the surface of a suitable solid agar medium. Muller Hinton is usually the medium of choice, although Tryptone soy agar or Nutrient agar have sometimes been used by other researchers. The media is preinoculated with the test organism and authors have reported inoculum sizes of 1 × 10^8 cfu/ml of bacteria for inoculating diffusion plates. There have been some variations noted on whether the disks are impregnated with antimicrobial substances after or before placing on the inoculated plate. Some impregnate before placing on the agar while others place the disk on the plate and then impregnate with antimicrobial substance. According to some the paper disks were soaked in the leaf extract for about 2 h and the disks was left to dry under a laminar flow cabinet overnight. Others refrigerate the plates for an hour or two at 4°C to allow pre-diffusion of the extracts from the disk into the seeded agar layer before incubation. The plates are then incubated at 37°C for 24 h for bacteria and 48 h for fungi. Some incubate for 18 h at 37°C for the same bacteria. Zones of inhibition are then measured from the circumference of the disks to the circumference of the inhibition zone or recorded as the difference in diameter between the disks and the growth free zones around the disks.

AGAR WELL DIFFUSION

The principle of the agar well diffusion is the same as that of the agar disk diffusion method. A standardized inoculum culture is spread evenly on the surface of agar plates. Wells of between 6 and 8 mm are aseptically punched on the agar using a sterile cork borer allowing at least 30 mm between adjacent wells and the Petri dish. Fixed volumes of the plant extract are then introduced into the wells. The plates are then incubated at 37°C for 24 h for bacteria.

BIOAUTOGRAPHY

This is a variation of the agar diffusion method where the analyte is adsorbed onto a Thin Layer Chromatography (TLC) plate. Bioautography is also employed as a preliminary phytochemical screening technique, by bioassay guided fractionation, to detect active components. Bioautography overcomes the challenge of isolating antimicrobial compounds from crude extracts with complex chemical components by simplifying the process of their isolation and identification. It relatively uses very little amount of sample which is ideal for plant extracts and also allows the determination of the polarity of the active compounds. Compared to different methods of AST, bioautography is a practical, reproducible test which is easy to perform. In the bioautography agar overlay procedure, a determined amount of the extract is applied to silica 60 gel plates and developed with an appropriate solvent system. A suspension of the test bacteria is sprayed onto the TLC plate. Some authors reported using an inoculum of 0.84 absorbance at 560 nm, while others report using a suspension of 106 CFU/ml. The bioautograms are then incubated at 25°C for 48 h in humid conditions. Microbial indicators (usually tetrazolium salts) are used as a growth detector. These are sprayed onto the plates after which the plates are reincubated at 25°C for 24 h or at 37°C for 3-4 h. Clear (white) zones on the TLC plate indicate antimicrobial activity of the extracts. However some authors' state that direct bioassay on TLC plates is not an ideal method for the quantification of bioactivity of plant extracts. They suggest that TLC causes disruption of synergism between active constituents in an extract thereby reducing its activity.

BROTH MICRODILUTION

The micro-titre plate or broth microdilution method has provided a potentially useful technique for determining MICs of large numbers of test samples. Its advantages over diffusion techniques include increased sensitivity for small quantities of extract which is important if the antimicrobial is scarce as is the case for many natural products; ability to distinguish between bacteriostatic and bactericidal effects; and quantitative determination of the MIC. This method can also be used for a wide variety of microorganisms, it is not expensive and it presents reproducible results. In the micro-titre plate method, a stock solution of the extract is first obtained in solvent, usually the solvent used for extraction DMSO. Methanol and acetone are sometimes chosen as solvents because, in addition to dissolving the extracts completely they show no inhibition of the microorganisms even at 2% final concentration. Most authors report on filter sterilizing with a 0.22 or 0.45 μm membrane filter before the procedure. When membrane filtration is used the samples, before and after sterilization, should be compared by assay to ensure that adsorption has not occurred. Mueller Hinton Broth or water are often used as diluents in the wells of the microtitre plate before transferring an equal volume of stock solution to the plate. Cation-supplemented Muller-Hinton broth is some times recommended for non-fastidious microorganisms. Two fold serial dilutions are then made from the first well to obtain a concentration range. For full range MIC, 5–8 concentrations representing achievable concentrations for the antimicrobial are usually tested, although some authors have reported from even 3 concentrations. An equal volume of a fixed bacterial culture is added to the wells and incubated at 37°C for 24 h, the recommended temperature is 35–37°C in air for 16–20 h for nonfastidious organisms. The inoculum size for the microtitre plate procedure is usually 1×10^6 cfu/ml. Others have used a microbial culture with an optical density of 0.4 (log-phase) at 620 nm or a 12 h broth culture adjusted to a turbidity standard. This recommends that plates be inoculated within 30 min of standardization of inoculum, to avoid changes in inoculum density. Plates are then examined for changes in turbidity as an indicator of growth. The first well that appears clear is taken to be the MIC of the extract. Some researchers use indicators or spectrophotometry to determine presence of growth in microtitre plates. Indicators (usually tetrazolium salts or resazurin dye) are added after the incubation period and left for about 6 h and changes in color or absence of color, depending on the indicator, is used to detect the MIC breakpoint. The use of calorimetric indicators eliminates the need for a spectrophotometric plate reader and avoids the ambiguity associated with visual comparison or measurement of growth inhibition rings on agar plates. When the spectrophotometric method is used the absorbance, usually at 620 nm with the negative control as a blank, is used to detect the breakpoint. The concentration at which there is a sharp decline in the absorbance value, or the lowest concentration which gives a zero absorbance reading is deemed to be the MIC. The minimum bactericidal concentration (MBC) is determined by subculturing the preparations that would have shown no evidence of growth in the MIC determination assay. These subcultures are made either in broth or in agar plates. In broth, the MBC is regarded as the lowest concentration of extract which does not produce an absorbance reading at 620 nm relative to the negative control. On agar the lowest concentration showing lack of growth represents the MBC.

AGAR DILUTION ASSAY

The agar dilution test is more versatile than the broth dilution assay and does not present problems encountered with the latter that is, sample solution, contamination and determination of MIC breakpoints. In this method a stock solution of the extract is prepared in its extracting solvent, filter-sterilized (0.22 ìm) and then incorporated in molten agar, cooled to 50°C in a water bath, to obtain different concentrations of the extract in the agar. Usually Muller-Hinton is used although some authors have used nutrient agar. Inoculum preparation also differs between authors and others have used overnight culture dilutions of 1:100 or 1:10 in broth. The inoculum density of about 1×10^7 cfu/ml is usually recommended and using replicator pins, micropipette or standard loop about 1 µl (1×10^4 cfu/ml) of the inoculum is transfered. Some publications have reported leaving the plates overnight, before streaking, to allow the solvent to evaporate. The organisms are streaked in radial patterns on the agar plates and incubated at 37°C for 24 to 48 h. The MIC is defined as the lowest concentration of the extract inhibiting the visible growth of each microorganism on the agar plate.

GUIDELINES FROM STANDARDIZATION BODIES

Given the diversity of the methods used in the study of the antimicrobial potential of plant compounds, the comparison of results by different laboratories is very difficult. Breakpoints for MIC and MBC are defined differently by researchers and standardization bodies. MIC can 'be defined as the lowest concentration of antimicrobial that will inhibit the visible growth of a microorganism after overnight incubation and MBC as the lowest concentration of antimicrobial that will prevent the growth of an organism after subculture on antimicrobial free media. The EUCAST (2000) defines MIC as the lowest concentration, expressed in mg/L, that under defined *in vitro* conditions, prevents the growth of bacteria within a defined period of time and the MBC as the lowest concentration of an antimicrobial agent, expressed in mg/L, that under defined *in vitro* conditions reduces by 99.9% (3 logarithms) the number of organisms in a medium containing defined inoculum, within a defined period of time.

The ethnomedicinal study of plants is important for modern day medicine but its usefulness cannot be over-emphasized if methods are not standardized to obtain comparable and reproducible results. Other pharmacological studies like time kill assays; potentials for combination antimicrobial chemotherapy and mechanisms of action are important ingredients as additional tests to fully assess anti-microbial activity of plant extracts. Some of the medicinal plants with strong antimicrobial properties are summerized in Table-2.

ANTIVIRAL ACTIVITY OF MEDICINAL PLANTS

Many traditional medicinal plants have been reported to have strong antiviral activity and some of them have already been used to treat animals and people who suffer from viral diseases. Research interests for antiviral agent development was started after the Second World War in Europe and in 1952 the Boots drug company at Nottingham, England, examined the action of 288 plants against influenza a virus in embryonated eggs. They found that 12 of them suppressed virus amplification. During the last 25 years, there have been numerous broad-based screening programmes initiated in different parts of the globe to evaluate the antiviral activity of medicinal plants for *in vitro* and *in vivo* assays. Canadian researchers in the 1970s reported antiviral activities against herpes simplex virus (HSV), poliovirus type 1, coxsackievirus B5 and echovirus 7 from grape, apple, strawberry and other fruit juices. The extracts of *Rosa nutkana* and *Amelanchier alnifolia* were very active against an enteric corona virus. A root extract of *Potentilla arguta* and a branch tip extract of *Sambucus racemosa* completely inhibited respiratory syncytial virus (RSV). An extract of *Ipomopsis aggregata* demonstrated good activity against parainfluenza virus type 3. A *Lomatium dissectum* root extract completely inhibited the cytopathic effects of rotavirus. In addition to these, extracts prepared from *Cardamine angulata, Conocephalum conicum, Lysichiton americanum, Polypodium glycyrrhiza* and *Verbascum thapsus* exhibited antiviral activity against herpes virus type 1. The extracts of 40 different plant species have been used in traditional medicine and were investigated for antiviral activity against a DNA virus, human cytomegalovirus (HCMV), and two RNA viruses, Ross River virus (RRV) and poliovirus type 1, at noncytotoxic concentrations. The most active extracts were the aerial parts of *Pterocaulon sphacelatum* (Asteraceae) and roots of *Dianella longifolia* var. grandis (Liliaceae), which inhibited poliovirus type 1 at concentration of 52 and 250 μg/ml respectively.

METHODS FOR EVALUATION OF ANTIVIRAL ACTIVITY

Use of animal models

The earliest method for the study of viruses had been the use of animal host systems. Louis Pasteur for instance, began to study rabies in animals in 1881 and over a number of years he developed methods of producing attenuated virus preparations by progressively drying spinal cord of rabbits experimentally infected with the agent. Also through experimental transmission to mice, in 1900, Walter Reed demonstrated that yellow fever was caused by a virus and spread by mosquitoes. This discovery eventually enabled Max Thailler in (1937) to propagate the virus in chick embryo and to produce an attenuated vaccine – the 17

D strain that is still in use today. The success of this approach had led to increased use of animal systems to identify and propagate pathogenic viruses even with the adoption/ perfection of tissue culture technique.

Animal Protection Studies

As already indicated, the earliest method of virus study had been the use of animal hosts. In the area of antiviral chemotherapeutic research, animal models have been used either primarily as screening tools or applied in testing the efficacy of the test compound when it had been identified as effective/potent using any other method.

Egg Inoculation Studies

Inoculation of fertilized hen eggs with the virus strain under study has been a powerful virological tool especially in the area of virus identification, vaccine production and in the evaluation of compounds for antiviral activities. In the later event, after obtaining the virus titre and the cytotoxicity of the extract under study, different time course studies are carried out using varying concentrations of the extracts. The use of egg inoculation in virological studies especially in developed countries is waning with the advent of faster and cheaper biotechnological tools.

Cell Culture Methods

Cell culture began in the 20th century with whole organ cultures, then progressed to methods involving individual cells, either primary cell cultures or immortalized cell lines which when given appropriate conditions, continue to grow in culture indefinitely. In 1949, Enders and his colleagues were able to propagate poliovirus in primary human cell cultures. This opened what many regard as the 'golden age of virology', the identification and isolation during the 1950s and 1960s of many viruses and their association with human disease. Among the cell culture techniques are the plaque reduction techniques, viral cytopathic effect assay and haemagglutination inhibition techniques.

ANTIOXIDANT PROPERTY OF MEDICINAL PLANTS

Oxidants or reactive oxygen species are produced in our body during aerobic metabolism. Generation of free radicals or reactive oxygen species (ROS) during metabolism and other activities beyond the antioxidant capacity of a biological system gives rise to oxidative stress. Oxidative stress plays a role in heart diseases, malaria, neurodegenerative diseases, AIDS, cancer and in the aging process. This concept is supported by increasing evidence that oxidative damage plays a role in the development of chronic, age-related degenerative diseases, and that dietary antioxidants oppose this and lowers the risk of disease, thus there arises a necessity to extract these antioxidants from the plant matrices. Antioxidants are the chemicals that neutralize these oxidants. Natural antioxidants are the secondary metabolites of phytochemicals found naturally in the body and in plants such as fruits and vegetables and are preferred over synthetic antioxidants, which are found to impose side effects. An antioxidant can be defined in simple terms as anything that inhibits or prevents oxidation of a susceptible substrate. Plants produce a very impressive array of antioxidant compounds that includes carotenoids, flavonoids, cinnamic acids, benzoic acids, folic acid, ascorbic acid, tocopherols and tocotrienols to prevent oxidation of the susceptible substrate. These plant-based dietary antioxidants are believed to have an important role in the maintenance of human health because our endogenous antioxidants provide insufficient protection against the constant and unavoidable challenge of reactive oxygen species (ROS; oxidants).

Enzymes

Superoxide dismutase (SOD), Catalase (CAT), Glutathion peroxidase (GP), etc. are the well known enzymes present in plasma which act as antioxidants by transforming reactive oxygen species and reactive nitrogen species into the stable compounds.

High Molecular Weight Compounds

These include proteins like albumin, transferin, ceruplasmin. They restrict the production of metal catalysed free radicals.

Low Molecular Weight Compounds

These can be further divided into two categories *i.e.* lipid soluble antioxidants and water soluble antioxidants.Tocopherol, quinines, bilirubin antioxidants; and ascorbic acid, uric acid and some polyphenols come under water soluble antioxidants.

Minerals

Minerals like selenium, copper, manganese, zinc, etc. are well-known antioxidants.

Vitamins

Vitamin A, C, E and certain compounds called carotenoids (like lutein and beta-carotene) are the popular antioxidants, which play a crucial role in preventing peroxidation damage in the biological system.

Antioxidant Assays

Screening of plants is done by measuring the antioxidant activity through various *in vitro* models like DPPH method, Nitric oxide method, DMPD method, ABTS method, ORAC method, TBARS assay. Total antioxidant capacity, reducing assay etc. and via various *in vivo* models using rats or mice.

ANTIULCEROGENIC ACTIVITY

Several indigenous medicinal plants heve been indicated in the Ayurvedic system of medicine to possess anti-ulcerogenic activity and effectively employed in the treatment of gastric ulceration. *Withania somnifera* possesses antiulcerogenic activity. The antiulcerogenic activity of *W. somnifera* is tested on albion rats by first inducing gastric ulcers by injecting asprin suspended in 1 % carboxymethyl cellulose to the rats and the root powder of the plant suspended in 1% gum acacia was injected to test the antiulcer activity of the plant extract.

ANTICANCER ACTIVITY OF MEDICINAL PLANTS

Cancer is one of the most dreaded disease of the 21st century and spreading further with continuance and increasing incidence. Recently a greater emphasis has been given towards the researches on complementary and alternative medicine that deals with cancer management. Plants have a long history of use in the treatment of cancer. Plant-derived compounds have played an important role in the development of several clinically

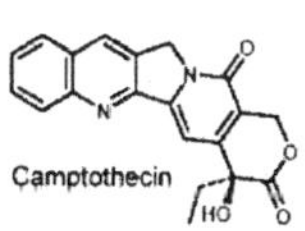

Camptothecin

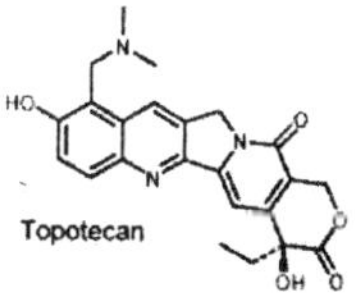

Topotecan

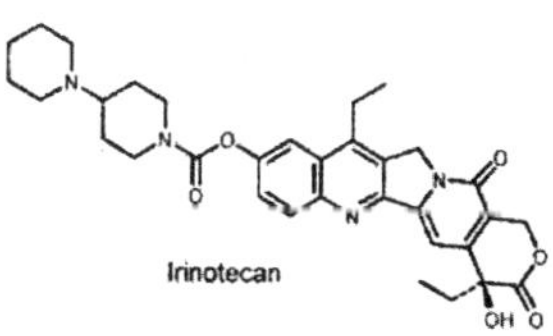

Irinotecan

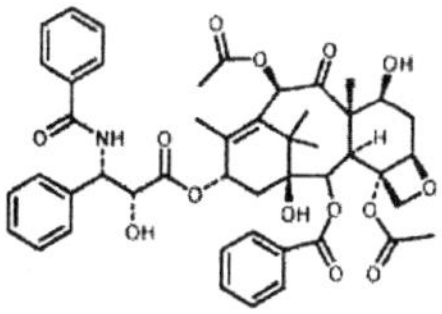

Taxol

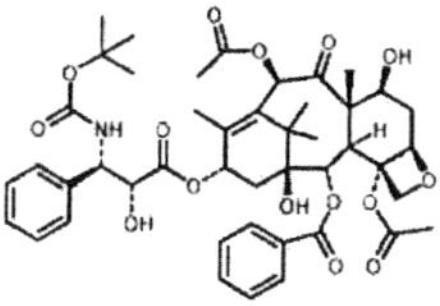

Docetaxel

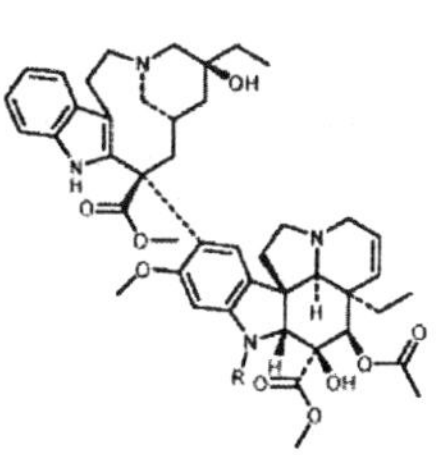

Vinblastine; R = CH_3
Vincristine; R = CHO

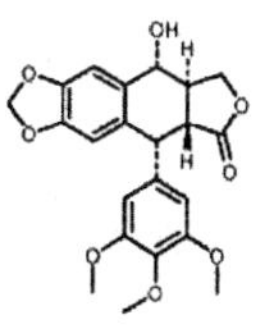

Podophyllotoxin

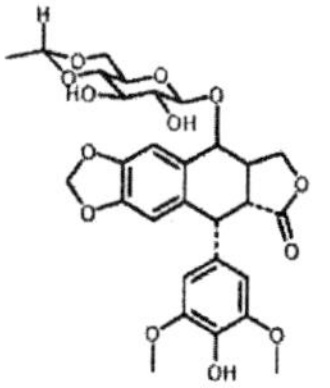

Etoposide

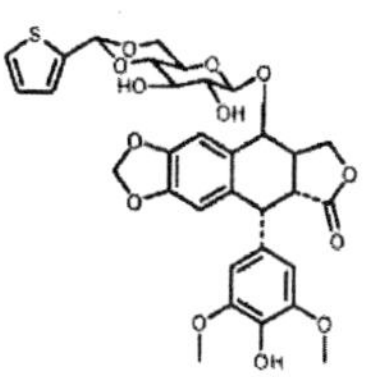

Teniposide

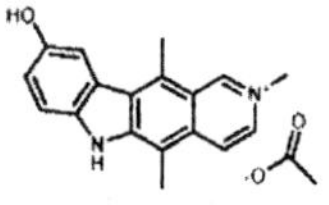

Elliptinium

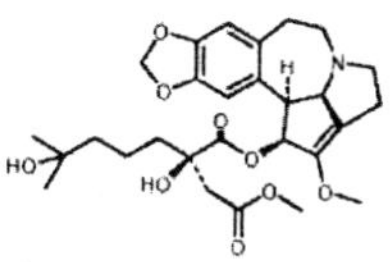

Homoharringtonine

Fig. 1 : Plant-derived anti-cancer agents in clinical use

useful anti-cancer agents. These include vinblastine, vincristine, the camptothecin derivatives, topotecan and irinotecan, etoposide, derived from epipodophyllotoxin, and paclitaxel (taxol). Several promising new agents are in clinical development based on selective activity against cancer-related molecular targets, including flavopiridol and combretastin A4 phosphate, and some agents which failed in earlier clinical studies are stimulating renewed interest. A number of tests on medicinal plants is going on throughout the world to find out an alternative medicine to cure this dreadful disease. Some of the assays are discussed above.

ANTI TUMOR ASSAY

MTT Assay

Cytotoxic activity or anticancer properties of medicinal plant extracts can be done using the microtitration colorimentic method of MTT reduction against human tumor cell lines like HT-29 (colorectal cancer), MCF-7 (breast cancer), HEp-2 (Larynx cancer) and MKN-45 (gastric cancer), HCT-8 (human colon carcinoma), CEM and HL-60 (leukemia) tumor cell lines, MCF 7 (breast carcinoma), T 24 (bladder carcinoma) etc. These cells can be obtained from the cell bank. The list of some important medicinal plants with anticancer properties is shown in Table 2. Growth of tumoral cells was quantitated by the ability of living cells to reduce the yellow dye 3-(4,5-dimethyl-2-thiazolyl)-2,5-diphenyl-2*H*-tetrazolium bromide (MTT) to a blue formazan product (Mosmann, 1983).

Brine Shrimp Assay

Brine shrimp (*Artemia salina* Leach) assay as per Meyer *et. al.*, 1982. Brine shrimp (*Artemia salina* Leach) eggs are hatched in a beaker filled with seawater under constant aeration. After 48 h the nauplii are collected by pipette and counted macroscopically in the stem of the pipette against a lighted background. Ten nauplii are transferred to each well of 24-multiwell plates containing the samples. The extract concentration ranged from 10 to 1000μg/ml. The plates are maintained under illumination. Survivors counted after 24 h of incubation and the percentage of deaths at each dose and control (seawater plus vehicle) were determined (Meyer *et. al.*, 1982).

Hemolytic assay

The test was performed in 96-well plates following the method described by Costa-Lotufo *et al.* (2002). Each well received 100 μl of 0.85% NaCl solution containing 10mM $CaCl_2$. The first well was the negative control that contained only the vehicle (distilled water or DMSO 10%), and, in the second well, 100 μl of test substance that was diluted in half was added. The extracts are tested at concentrations ranging from 10 to 2500 μl/ml. The serial dilution continued until the 11th well. The last well received 20 μl of 0.1% Triton X-100 (in 0.85% saline) to obtain 100% hemolysis (positive control). Then, each well received 100 μl of a 2% suspension of mouse erythrocytes in 0.85% saline containing 10mM $CaCl_2$. After incubation at room temperature for 30 min and centrifugation, the supernatant was removed and the liberated hemoglobin was measured spectroscopically as absorbance at 540 nM.

Potato Disc Assay

Antitumor activity can be assessed by potato disc method using *Agrobacterium tumefaciens*. This assay is used to determine the antitumor property of the plant extract against tumor induced by *Agrobacterium tumefaciens* on potato tuber. This method is commonly known as potato disc assay. In this process first of all tumor is induced on disc made up of potato and the effect of antineoplastic activity was tested for the plant extracts.

Alamar Blue Method

In order to estimate the amount of viable cells after treating them with plant extracts, the Alamar Blue method can be used. Alamar Blue (Promega, Biofellows, Finland) is a redox indicator which contains blue non-fluorescent resazurin which is reduced to pink fluorescent resorufin by the metabolic activity of living cells. The cytotoxicity can be assessed using the resazurin reduction test as described by O'Brien (2000).

Hoechst Staining

Hoechst staining was used to investigate if the antiproliferatively most effective extract caused fragmentation of the nucleus in the cancer cell lines.

The list of some important medicinal plants from Similipal Biosphere Reserve, Orissa with anticancer properties is shown in Table 2.

ANNEXURE-I

Table 2 : Checklist of Medicinal Plants found in Similipal Biosphere Reserve evluated for phytochemicals, antimicrobial and anticancer properties based on the literature surveys.

Medicinal Plants	*Phyto-chemicals*	*Antimicro-bial Properties*	*Anti-canceros Properties*
Acacia leucophloea (Roxb.)Willd	✔		-
Achyranthes aspera L.	✔	✔	✔
Achyranthes bidentata Blume	✔	✔	✔
Acorus calamus L. -	✔		
Acronychia pedunculata (L.) Miq.	✔	✔	-
Adenostemma lavenia (L.) Kuntz	✔	-	
Adhatoda zeylanica Medik	-	-	
Adiantum philippense L.	✔	✔	-
Aegle marmelos (L.) Correa	✔	✔	✔
Ageratum conyzoides L.	✔	-	✔
Alangium salvifolium (L.f.) Wang	✔	✔	-
Alstonia scholaris (L.) R.Br.	✔	✔	✔
Alternanthera sessilis (L.) R.Br. ex DC.	✔	✔	-
Ammannia baccifera L.	-	-	-
Ampellocissus latifolia Planch	-	-	-
Anacardium occidentale L.	✔	-	✔
Anaphalis adnata DC.	✔	-	-
Andrographis paniculata Nees	✔	✔	-
Annona reticulata L.	✔	-	✔
Annona squamosa L.	a	a	a
Anogeissus latifolia (Roxb.) Wall. ex Bedd	a	a	-
Anthocephalus chinensis (Lam.) Rich. Ex. Walp	a	a	-
Ardisia solanacea Roxb.	a	a	-
Argemone mexicana L.	a	a	a
Argyreia nervosa (Burm.f.)Boj.	a	-	-

Medicinal Plants	*Phyto-chemicals*	*Antimicro-bial Properties*	*Anti-canceros Properties*
Argyreia speciosa Sweet	a	a	-
Aristolochia indica L.	-	a	a
Asparagus racemosus Willd	-	a	-
Atylosia scarbaeoides (L.) Benth.	a	a	-
Azadirachta indica A. Juss.	a	a	
Bacopa monnieri (L.)Pennell	a	a	-
Baliospermum montanum (Willd.) Muell-Arg	-	-	
Barleria cristata L. a	a	-	
Barleria strigosa. Wild.	a	a	-
Barringtonia acutangula (L.)Gaertn	✔	✔	✔
Bauhinia variegata L	✔	✔	✔
Bauhinia purpurea L.	a	-	a
Bauhinia vahlii Wight & Arn	-	-	
Bidens pilosa L.	✔	✔	✔
Bischofia javanica Blume	a	-	
Bixa orellana L.	✔	✔	✔
Blumea lacera (Burm.f.) DC.	a	-	a
Boerhavia diffusa L.	a	-	
Buchanania lanzan Spreng.	a	a	-
Butea monosperma (Lam.) Taub	✔	✔	✔
Butea superba Roxb	✔	✔	✔
Callicarpa macrophylla Vahl	a	a	-
Callicarpa tomentosa (L.) Murr.	-	-	-
Calotropis gigantea R.Br.	a	a	
Calycopteris floribunda Lam.	a	-	a
Camellia sinensis (L.) Kuntze	✔	✔	✔
Canscora decussata (Roxb.) Schult.	a	-	-
Canscora diffusa (Vahl.) R.Br.	✔	✔	✔
Canthium dicoccum (Gaertn.) Teijsm. & Binnend	a	a	-
Carica papaya L.	a	-	a
Cassia fistula L.	a	a	-
Cassia occidentalis L.	a	a	-
Cassia tora L.	a	a	-

Medicinal Plants	*Phyto-chemicals*	*Antimicro-bial Properties*	*Anti-cancerous Properties*
Catharanthus roseus (L.) G. Don	✓	✓	✓
Catunaregam spinosa (Thunb.)Tirveng	-	-	
Celastrus paniculatus Willd.	a	a	
Celosia argentea L.	✓	✓	✓
Centella asiatica (L.) Urb	-	a	-
Centipeda minima (L.) A. Braun & Asch.	-	a	a
Chlorophytum arundinaceum Baker	a	a	-
Chrysanthemum indicum L.	a	a	-
Cissus quadrangularis L.	a	a	-
Citrus aurantium La	a	-	
Citrus medica L	-	-	-
Clausena excavata Burm	a	a	-
Cleome viscosa L.	a	a	-
Clerodendrum indicum (L.) Kuntze	-	a	-
Clerodendrum serratum (L.) Moon	-	a	-
Clerodendrum viscosum Vent. Jard. Malm.	-	a	-
Clitoria ternatea L. a	a	-	
Coccinia grandis (L.) Voigt	a	-	-
Cochlospermum religiosum (L.) Alston	a	a	-
Combretum roxburghii Spreng	a	a	-
Commelina benghalensis L.	a	a	-
Costus speciosus (Koenig) Sm.	a	a	-
Crinum defixum Ker-Gawl.	a	-	-
Croton roxburghii Balak	✓	✓	✓
Curcuma amada Roxb.	-	a	-
Curcuma aromatica Salisb	a	-	a
Cyathocline purpurea (Buch-Ham. ex Don Kuntze)	a	a	-
Cymbopogon martinii (Roxb. Wats.)	-	a	-
Cyperus rotundus L.	a	a	
Dalbergia lanceolaria L.f.	a	a	
Dalbergia latifolia Roxb.	a	-	-
Datura metel L.	✓	✓	✓

Medicinal Plants	*Phyto-chemicals*	*Antimicro-bial Properties*	*Anti-canceros Properties*
Dendrophthoe falcata (L.f.) Etting.	a	a	-
Desmodium gangeticum (L.) DC.	✔	✔	✔
Desmodium oojeinensis (Roxb.) Ohashi	-	a	-
Desmodium triflorum (L.)DC.	a	-	-
Dioscorea pentaphylla L.	a	-	-
Diospyros malabarica (Desr.) Kostel.	-	a	-
Diospyros melanoxylon Roxb.	-	a	-
Drosera indica L.	a	a	-
Eclipta prostrata Roxb.	a	a	-
Elephantopus scaber L.	✔	✔	✔
Embelia tsjeriam-cottam A. DC	-	-	
Enydra fluctuans Lour.	a	a	-
Erioglossum rubiginosum Blume-	a	-	-
Erycibe paniculata Roxb.	-	-	-
Euphorbia hirta L.	a	a	-
Euphorbia nivulia Buch.-Ham.	a	-	-
Exacum bicolor Roxb	-	-	-
Flacourtia indica (Burm.f.) Merr	a	a	-
Flacourtia jangomas (Lour.)Raeusch	a	a	-
Flemingia strobilifera R.Br.	-	-	-
Floscopa scandens Lour.	-	-	-
Gardenia gummifera L. f.	a	-	-
Glochidion lanceolarium (Roxb.) Dalz	a	a	-
Gloriosa superba L.	-	-	-
Gmelina arborea Roxb	a	a	-
Grewia hirsuta Vahl	-	-	-
Grewia tilifolia Vahl	-	-	-
Haldinia cordifolia (Roxb.) Ridsd.	a	-	
Hedychium coronarium Koenig	a	-	a
Heliotropium indicum L.	✔	✔	✔
Hemidesmus indicus R. Br.	-	a	-
Heteropogon contortus (L.) Beauv. ex R. & S.	-	-	-
Hiptage benghalensis (L.) Kurz.	-	-	-

Medicinal Plants	*Phyto-chemicals*	*Antimicro-bial Properties*	*Anti-canceros Properties*
Holarrhena pubescens (Buch. Ham.) Wall ex Don	a	-	
Holoptelea integrifolia(Roxb.) Planch	a	-	-
Homonoia riparia Lour	-	-	a
Hygrophila auriculata(Schum.) Heyne	-	-	a
Hypericum japonicum Thunb. ex Murr.	a	a	-
Hyptis suaveolens Poit	a	-	
Ichnocarpus frutescens (L.) R. Br.	a	-	-
Imperata cylindrica (L.) P. Beauv.	-	a	
Indigofera glabra L.	a	a	-
Iphigenia indica (L.) A. Gray	-	-	-
Ipomoea nil (L.) Roth.	a	-	-
Ixora pavetta Andr.	-	-	-
Jasminum arborescens Roxb.	-	-	-
Jasminum scandens Vahl.	-	-	-
Jatropha gossypifolia L.	✔	✔	-
Justicia adhatoda L.	-	-	-
Justicia betonica L.	✔	✔	-
Kaempferia rotunda L.	-	-	-
Kalanchoe pinnata (Lam.) Pers.	✔	✔	✔
Leea indica (Burm.f.) Merr.	-	-	-
Lannea coromandelica (Houtt.) Merr.	a	-	-
Lawsonia inermis L.	a	-	a
Lagerstroemia speciosa (L.) Pers.	✔	✔	✔
Ludwigia octovalvis (Jacq.)Raven	-	a	a
Litsea glutinosa (Lour.) Robins	✔	✔	-
Litsea monopetala (Roxb.) Pers.	a	-	-
Lantana camara L. var. aculeata (L.) Mold.	a	-	a
Leucas indica (L.) Druce	-	-	-
Leucas mollissima Wall. ex Benth	-	-	-
Leea asiatica (L.) Ridsdale	-	-	-
Litchi chinensis (Gaertn.) Sonn	-	a	
Lagerstroemia parviflora Roxb.	a	-	-

Medicinal Plants	*Phyto-chemicals*	*Antimicro-bial Properties*	*Anti-canceros Properties*
Lagerstroemia reginae Roxb	-	-	-
Lawsonia inermis L.	a	-	-
Linum usitatissimum L	a	-	a
Leea macrophylla Roxb.	-	-	-
Labalb purpureus L.	-	-	-
Laggera alata (D. Don) Sch.-Bip.ex Oliver	a	-	-
Limnophila indica (L) Druce	-	-	-
Lindernia crustacea (L.) F. Muell	-	-	-
Michelia champaca L.	✔	✔	✔
Mesua ferrea L.	a	-	-
Murraya koenigii (L.) Spreng.	a	a	
Mangifera indica L.	✔	✔	✔
Mimosa pudica L.	a	-	
Mucuna pruriens (L.) DC	a	-	-
Melaleuca leucadendron L.	a	-	-
Mitragyna parvifolia (Roxb.) Korth	a	-	-
Morinda pubescens J. E.Smith	-	-	-
Morinda citrifolia L	a	-	a
Mussaenda incana Wall.	-	-	-
Madhuca indica (Koenig) Macbride	-	-	
Merremia umbellata (L.) Hall. f.	-	-	-
Mosla dianthera (Buch. Ham. ex Roxb.)Maxim	-	-	-
Morus australis Poir.	✔	✔	✔
Mallotus philippensis (Lam.) Muell. Arg.	-	-	-
Mucuna nigricans (Lour.) Steud.	-	-	-
Macaranga peltata (Roxb.) Muell. Ar	-	-	-
Nyctanthes arbor-tristis L.	a	a	-
Oxalis corniculata L.	a	-	-
Oroxylum indicum (L.) Kurz	a	-	-
Ocimum gratissimum L.	-	-	-
Ocimum basilicum L.	-	a	a
Olax scandens Roxb.	-	-	-
Osyris wightiana Wall. ex Wight	-	-	-

Medicinal Plants	*Phyto-chemicals*	*Antimicro-bial Properties*	*Anti-canceros Properties*
Pongamia pinnata (L.) Pierre	-	a	
Pterocarpus marsupium Roxb.	a	-	-
Punica granatum L.	a	-	a
Paederia foetida L.	a	a	-
Plumbago zeylanica L.	✓	✓	✓
Phyllanthus fraternus Webster,	a	a	-
Prunus ceylanica (Wight) Miq.	-	-	-
Petalidium barlerioides (Roxb.)Nees	-	-	-
Premna coriacea C.B.Cl.	-	-	-
Polygonum hydropiper L.	a	a	-
Peperomia tetraphylla (Forster.f.) Hook. & Arn.	-	-	-
Piper trioicum Roxb.	-	-	-
Phyllanthus emblica L	a	a	-
Phoebe lanceolata Nees,	-	-	-
Pueraria tuberosa (Roxb. ex Willd.) DC	✓	✓	-
Pergularia daemia (Forsk.) Chiov.	✓	-	
Pogostemon benghalensis (Burm. f.) Kuntze	-	-	-
Plesmonium margaritiferum (Roxb.) Schott	-	-	-
Pothos scandens L.	-	-	-
Polyalthia longifolia (Sonn.) Thw.	✓	✓	✓
Panicum sumatrense Roth ex R & Schult.	-	-	-
Parthenium hysterophorus L.	a	a	-
Paspalum scrobiculatum L.	✓	-	-
Quisqualis indica L.	-	-	-
Rubia cordifolia L.	✓	✓	-
Rauvolfia serpentina (L.) Benth.ex Kurz	-	-	-
Rhus chinensis Miller	✓	✓	-
Ranunculus pensylvanicus L.f.	-	-	-
Rhinacanthus nasutus (L.) Kurz.	✓	-	-
Rungia pectinata (L.) Nees.	a	-	-
Rhynchostylis retusa (L.)Bl.	-	-	-
Shorea robusta Gaertn.f.	-	-	-
Sida acuta Burm. F	a	a	-

Medicinal Plants	*Phyto-chemicals*	*Antimicro-bial Properties*	*Anti-canceros Properties*
Sida cordata (Burm.f.)Borssum	-	-	-
Sida rhombifolia L.	a	-	-
Soymida febrifuga (Roxb.) A. Juss.	a	-	-
Semecarpus anacardium L.f	a	a	-
Schleichera oleosa (Lour) Oken	a	-	-
Spondias pinnata (L.f.) Kurz	a	-	-
Saraca asoca (Roxb.) de Willde.	a	-	
Syzygium cumini (L.) Skeels	a	a	-
Schrebera swietenioides Roxb.	-	-	-
Strychnos nux-vomica L.	-	-	-
Strychnos potatorum L.f.	a	a	-
Solanum erianthum D.Don,	a	a	-
Solanum torvum Sw	-	-	-
Solanum virginianum L.	-	-	-
Scoparia dulcis L.	a	a	-
Strobilanthes auriculatus Nees	a	-	-
Stachytarpheta jamaicensis (L.) Vahl,	✓	✓	-
Stephania japonia (Thuab.) Miers,	-	-	-
Streblus asper Lour. Fl.	✓	✓	-
Salix tetrasperma Roxb.	a	-	-
Sigesbeckia orientalis L.	a	-	-
Smilax perfoliata Lour	a	-	a
Setaria palmifolia (Koenig) Stapf	-	-	
Sesbania bispinosa (Jacq.) W.F. Wight	-	-	-
Strychnos potatorum L.f.	✓	✓	-
Symplocos racemosa Roxb.	-	-	-
Sterculia urens Roxb.	-	-	-
Solanum surattense Burm.f.	-	-	
Scindapsus officinalis (Roxb.)Schott.	-	-	-
Syzygium cerasoides (Roxb.) Raizad	a	-	-
Syzygium jambos (L.) Alston	-	a	-
Solena heterophylla Lour.	-	-	-
Spermacoce hispida L.	-	-	-
Sphaeranthus indicus L.	-	-	
Sesamum indicum L.	a	-	-

Medicinal Plants	*Phyto-chemicals*	*Antimicro-bial Properties*	*Anti-canceros Properties*
Sauropus quadrangularis (Willd.) Muell. Arg	-	-	-
Triumfetta rhomboidea Jacq.	a	-	-
Toddalia asiatica (L.) Lam	-	-	-
Toona ciliata Roem.	✓	✓	✓
Tamarindus indica L.	✓	✓	-
Tephrosia purpurea (L.) pers	✓	✓	-
Terminalia arjuna (Roxb.ex.DC.) Wight.& Arn	✓	✓	✓
Terminalia bellirica (Gaertn.) Roxb.	-	-	-
Terminalia chebula Retz.	-	-	-
Tridax procumbens L.	✓	✓	✓
Thevetia peruviana (Pers.) K. Schum.	a	-	
Terminalia alata Heyne ex Roth,	a	-	
Trema orientalis (L.) Bl. Mus.	a	-	-
Trapa natans L.	a	-	-
Teramnus labialis (L.f.) Spreng.	✓	-	-
Trewia nudiflora L	a	-	-
Urena lobata L.	a	-	
Vernonia anthelmintica Willd.	-	-	-
Vernonia cinerea (L.) Less.	-	-	-
Vernonia aspera Buch.-Ham.	-	-	-
Vitex negundo L.	✓	✓	-
Ventilago denticulata Willd.	-	-	-
Vigna radiata (L.) R. Wilezek var *radiat*	-	-	-
Walsura trifoliata (A. Juss) Harms	✓	✓	-
Woodfordia fructicosa (L.) Kurz	-	a	-
Wendlandia tinctoria (Roxb.) DC.	a	-	-
Xantolis tomentosa (Roxb.) Rafin.	-	-	-
Xanthium strumarium L.	a	-	-
Xylia xylocarpa (Roxb.) Taub.	-	-	-
Ziziphus mauritiana Lam.	a	-	-
Ziziphus rugosa Lam	-	-	-
Zornia gibbosa Span.	-	-	-

Keynote: "a"= present, "- " = absent

Annexure-II

GLOSSARY OF MEDICAL TERMS

abortifacient : An agent that induces abortion.

abscess : A localized collection of pus caused by suppuration in a tissue.

absorbent : Any agent which attracts and sucks up gases or secretions from a wound.

acne : A term denoting an inflammatory disease occurring in or around the sebaceous glands.

acrid : Biting, pungent.

acute : Short and severe, not long drawn out or chronic.

agalactia : Absence or failure or secretion of milk.

ague : Malaria fever with successive stages of fever and chills.

albuminuria : The presence of serum albumin and serum globulin in the urine.

alterative : Causing a favourable change in the disordered functions of the body or metabolism.

amenorrhoea : Failure of menstruation.

anaemia : Lack of enough blood causing paleness.

analgesic : A drug which relieves pain.

anaphrodisiac : Having the power to lessen or inhibit sexual feeling.

anasarca	:	Diffused dropsy in the skin and sub-cutaneous tissue.
anodyne	:	A medicine that allays pain.
anorexia	:	A condition of having lost the appetite for food.
anthelmintic	:	Destroying or expelling worms.
antidote	:	An agent which neutralizes or opposes the action of a poison.
antiematic	:	An agent that relieves vomiting.
antiperiodic	:	Preventing the regular recurrence of a disease.
antiphlogistic	:	Acting against heat or inflammation.
antipruntic	:	Preventing or relieving itching.
antipyretic	:	Counteracting fever.
antiscorbutic	:	Acting against scurvy.
antiseptic	:	A chemical sterilizing substance to kill or control pathogenic microbes.
antispasmodic	:	Opposing spasms or convulsions.
anuria	:	Complete cessation of the secretion and excretion of urine.
aperient	:	A laxative or mild cathartic.
aphrodisiac	:	A drug which stimulates sexual desire.
apthae	:	Ulcer on the surface of a mucous membrane.
apoplexy	:	A sudden loss of consciousness.
arthralgia	:	Pain in a joint.
arthritis	:	Inflammation of a joint.
ascites	:	Abnormal accumulation of fluid in the peritoneal cavity.

asphyxia	:	Inability to breath.
atrophy	:	Wasting of a tissue or organ.
beriberi	:	A deficiency disease caused by imbalance of carbohydrate and Vitamin B.
blennorrhagia	:	Free discharge of mucus.
bronchopathy	:	Any disease of the bronchi.
cachexia	:	Depressed habit of mind.
calculus	:	A concretion formed in any part of the body usually compounds of salts of organic or inorganic acids.
calmative	:	Sedative.
carbuncle	:	An infection of the skin and subcutaneous tissue by *Staphylococcus aureus*.
cardiodynia	:	Pain in the region of the heart.
cardiopathy	:	A morbid condition of the heart.
carminative	:	Drug curing flatulence.
cataract	:	Opacity in the crystalline lens of the eye which may be partial complete.
catarrh	:	Inflammation of a mucous membrane, usually associated with an increase in the amount of normal secretion of mucus.
cathartic	:	Having the power of cleaning the bowels-purgative cephalagia headache.
cephalic	:	A remedy for disorders of the head.
cerebropathy	:	Any disorder of the brain.
cholera	:	A severe infectious epidemic disease due to *Vibrio cholerae*.
colic	:	A severe spasmodic griping pain.
conjunctivitis	:	Inflammation of the conjunctiva.

consumption	:	Pulmonary tuberculosis.
contraceptive	:	Any agent or device used to prevent conception.
convulsion	:	A violent involuntary contraction of the skeletal musculature.
coxalgia	:	Pain in the hip.
cystalgia	:	Pain in the urinary bladder.
cystitis	:	Inflammation of a bladder, especially the urinary bladder.
dandruff	:	Dead scarf-skin separating in small scales and entangled in the hair.
demulcent	:	Soothing.
dentalgia	:	Soothache.
deobstruent	:	Relieving or removing obstruction.
deodorant	:	Removing the odour.
depurative	:	An agent that purifies blood.
dermatopathy	:	Any skin disorder.
diaphoresis	:	Sweating.
diaphoretic	:	A drug which induces perspiration.
diptheria	:	A specific infectious disease caused by virulent strains of a bacillus.
disinfectant	:	Having a lethal effect upon germs.
diuretic	:	Promoting the flow of urine.
dizziness	:	Any sensation of imbalance of a stable relationship with the immediate environment.
dropsy	:	An excessive accumulation of clear or watery fluid in any of the tissues or cavities of the body.

dysmenorrhoea	:	Difficult or painful menstruation.
dyspepsia	:	Indigestion.
dysuria	:	Difficulty or pain while passing urine.
eczema	:	A noncontagious inflammatory disease of the skin with much itching and burning.
elephantiasis	:	Gross lymphatic oedema of the limbs leading to hypertrophy.
emetic	:	Causing vomiting.
emmenagogue	:	Medicine intended to restore the menses.
emollient	:	Softening.
epilepsy	:	An affection of the nervous system resulting from excessive or disordered discharge of cerebral neurons.
epistaxia	:	Bleeding from the nose.
expectorant	:	Aiding the secretion of the mucous membrane of the air passages and the removal of fluid by splitting.
febrifuge	:	Anything which reduces fever.
filariasis	:	Infection with filarial nematode worms.
fistula in ano	:	An open channel from the anus or rectum to the skin near the anus.
flatulence	:	Presence of excessive gas in the stomach or intestine.
galactagogue	:	Medicine that promotes secretion of milk.
galactorrhea	:	Excessive of spontaneous flow of milk.
gastralgia	:	Pain in stomach.
glaucoma	:	A term signifying increased intraocular pressure and its consequences.
glycosuria	:	Excretion of the sugar in the urine.

gonorrhoea : An inflammatory diseases of the genito-urinary passages characterized by pain and discharge.

gout : A disease of purine metabolism characterized by attacks of arthritis with an associated raised level of serum uric acid.

haematernesis : Vomiting of blood.

haematuria : The presence of blood in the urine.

haemoptysis : Spitting of blood.

haemostatic : Stypic.

helminthiasis : Morbid state due to infestation with worms.

hematorrhea : Copious haemorrhage.

hemicrania : Headache confined to one side.

hepatitis(viral) : Inflammation of the liver, jaundice.

hepatosis : Downward displacement of the liver.

hepatalgia : Pain in the liver.

hernia : The protrusion of an internal organ through a defect in the wall of the anatomical cavity in which it lies.

herps : Inflammation of the skin or mucous membrane with clusters of deep seated vesicles.

hydragogue : Promoting expulsion of water or serum.

hydrocele : A circumscribed collection of fluid in the tunica vaginalis testis.

hydrophobia : Exaggerated fear of water as in rabies.

hyperdipsia : Intense thirst of relatively brief duration.

hyperoxia : Excessive appetite.

hypertension : High arterial blood pressure.

hypotension	:	A fall in blood pressure below the normal level.
hysteria	:	A neurotic disorder with varying symptoms.
impotence	:	Inability to perform the sexual act due to failure of the reflex mechanism.
insecticides	:	Any agent which kills or destroys insects.
insanity	:	Mental disease of a grave kind.
insomnia	:	The condition of being unable to sleep.
laxative	:	Having the action of loosening the bowel.
leucoderma	:	Any white area on the skin.
leucorrhoea	:	An abnormal mucous discharge from the vagina.
lumbago	:	Pain in mid or lower back.
melalgia	:	Pain in the limbs.
menolipsis	:	Temporary cessation of menstruation.
menorrhagia	:	Excessive or prolonged menstruation.
migraine	:	A periodic condition with localized headaches, frequently associated with vomiting and sensory disturbances.
narcotic	:	A drug that induces sleep.
nephralgia	:	Pain in the kidney.
nephritis	:	Inflammation of the kidneys.
neuralgia	:	A painful affection of the nerves due to functional disturbances or neuritis.
obesity	:	An excessive accumulation of fat in the body.
opacity	:	An opaque or non-transparent area.
ophthalmia	:	A term usually applied to conjunctivitis.

ostalgia	:	Pain in the bones.
pneumonia	:	A general disease in which the essential lesion is an inflammation of the spongy tissue on the lung with consolidation of the alveolar exudates.
poultice	:	A soft mush prepared by various substances with oily or watery fluids.
pyorrhoea	:	A discharge of pus.
refrigerant	:	Cooling.
rheumarthritis	:	Rheumatoid arthritis.
rheumatalgia	:	Rheumatic pain.
rickets	:	A disturbance of the calcium/phosphorus metabolism which occurs in the growing child as a result of vitamin D deficiency.
scabies	:	Sarcoptic infestation of the human skin particularly a contagious skin disease caused by invasion of the epidermis.
scurvy	:	A deficiency disease due to lack of Vitamin C.
sinusitis	:	Inflammation affecting the mural epithelium of a sinus.
splenopathy	:	Any disease of the spleen.
stomatopathy	:	Any disorder of the mouth.
styptic	:	Having the power to arrest bleeding.
syphills	:	A contagious venereal disease.
tetanus	:	An infective diseases due to the toxins of *Clostridium tetani.*
tonsilitis	:	Inflammation of the tonsil.
trauma	:	A pathological alteration of the supporting tissues of a tooth due to abnormal occlusion.

urethrorrhoea	:	Abnormal discharge from the urethra.
urodynia	:	Pain on urination.
urorrhoea	:	Involuntary flow of urine.
vaginitis	:	Inflammation of the vagina.
vermifuge	:	A drug that expels worms.
vesical	:	Referring to the urinary bladder.
wart	:	A circumscribed cutaneous excrescence.

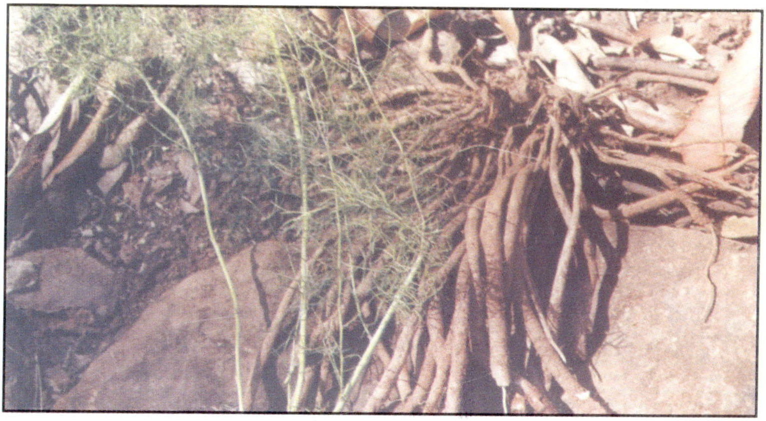

16 Asparagus

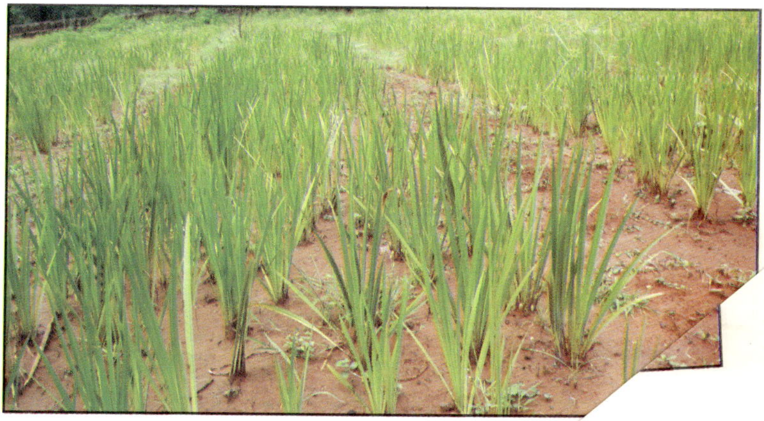

Acorus calamus

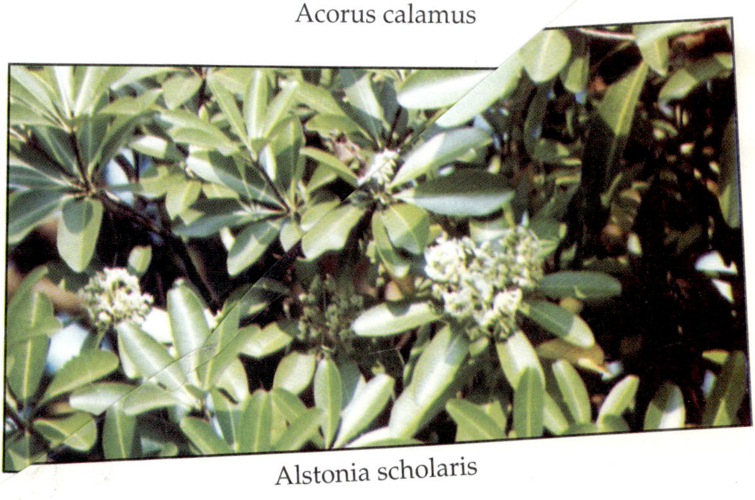

Alstonia scholaris

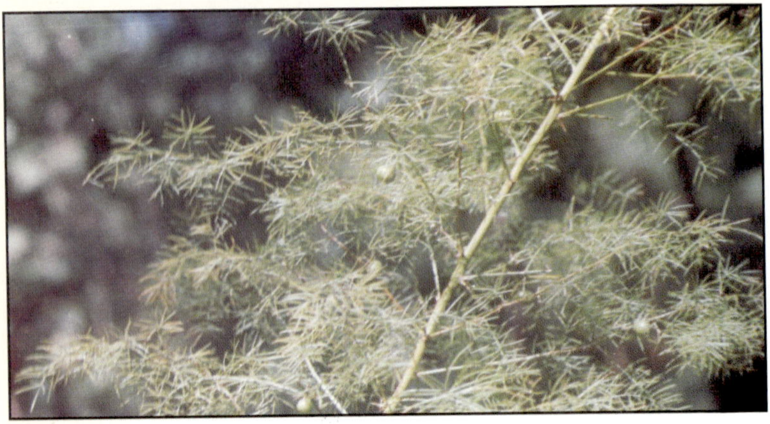

Asparagus racemosus

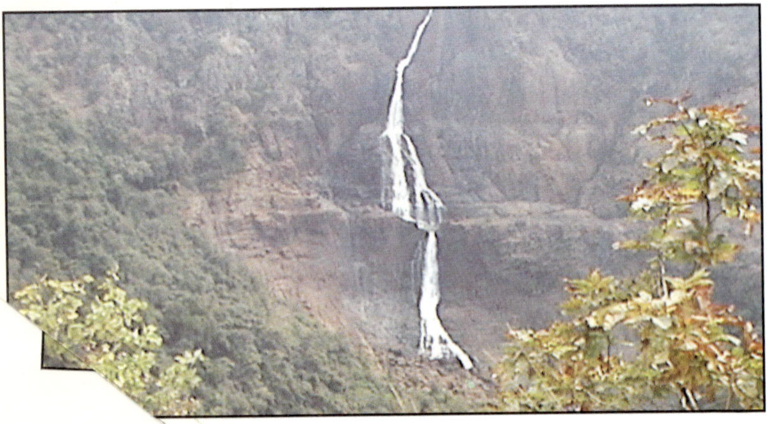

Barehipani 2

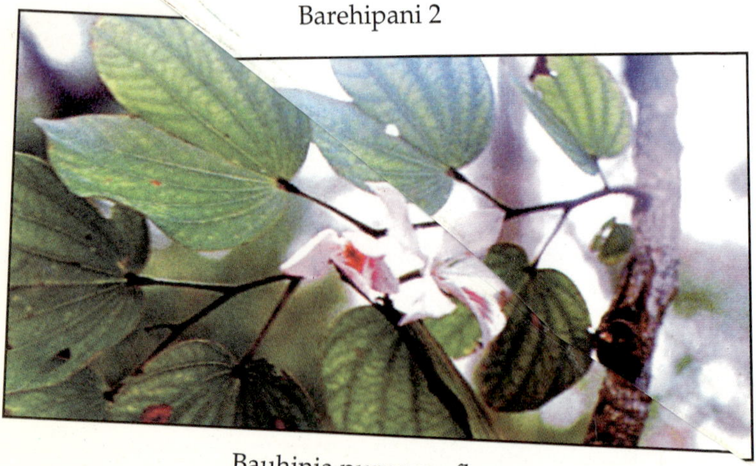

Bauhinia purpurea flower

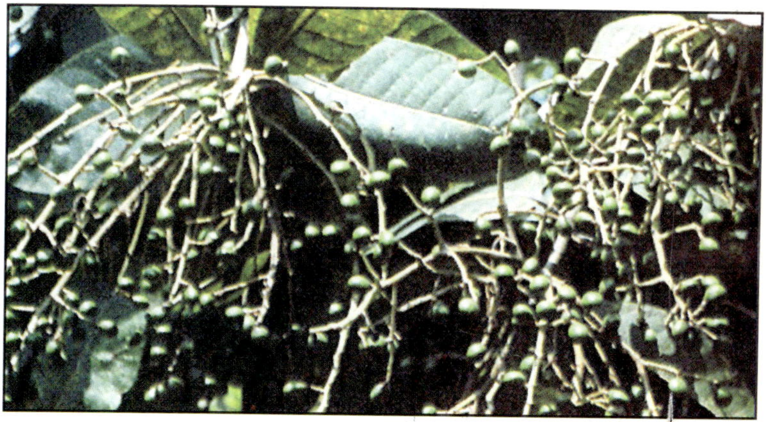

Buchanania lanzan

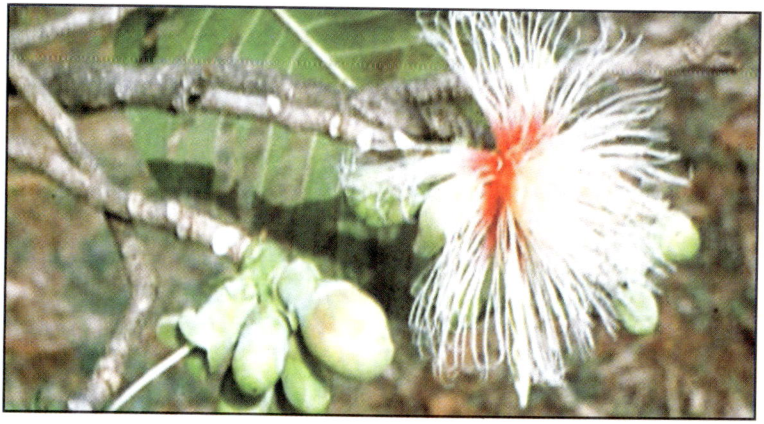

Careya arborea

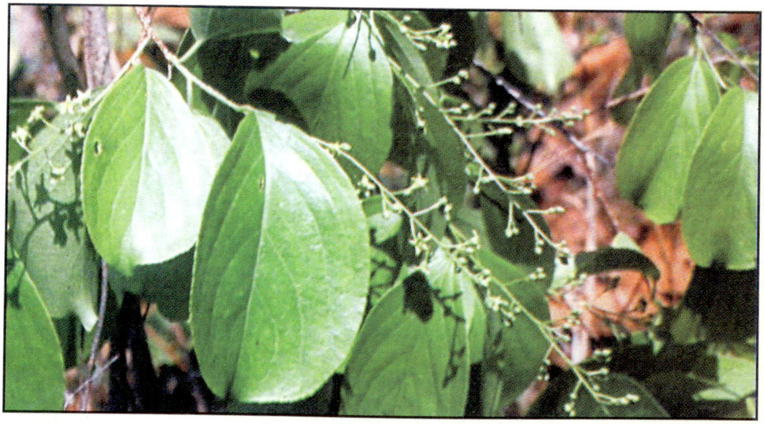

Celastrus paniculatus

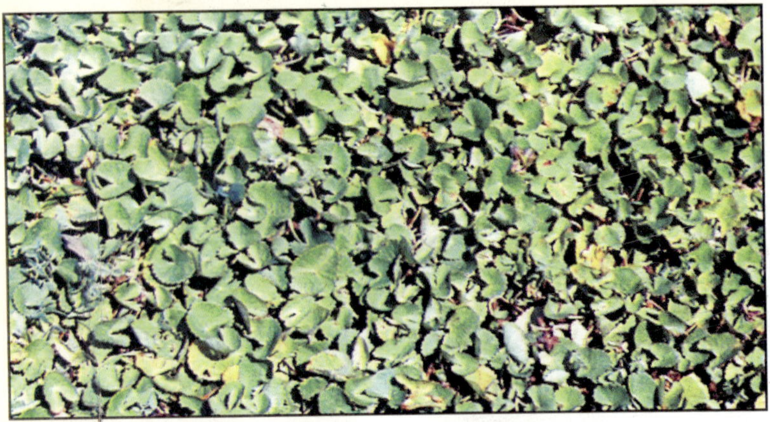

Centella assiatica

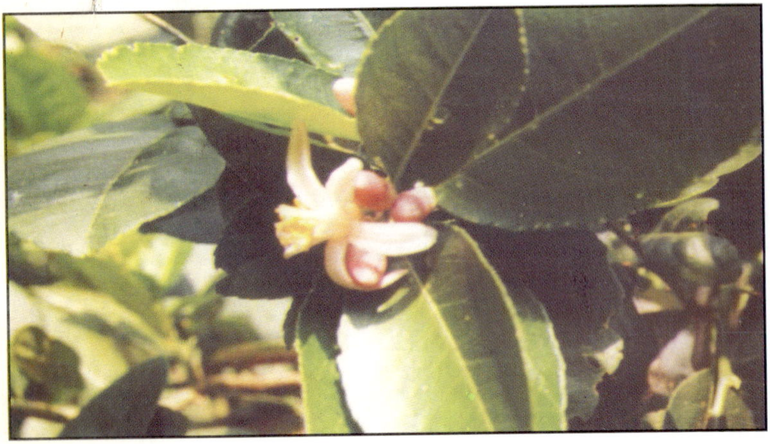

Citrus medica

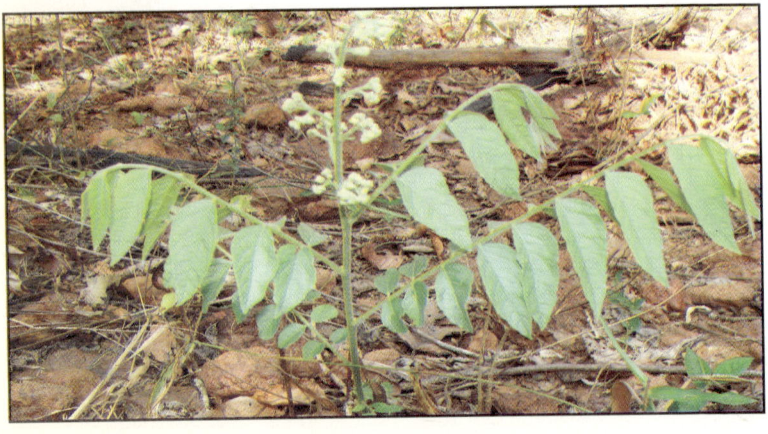

Clausena excavata

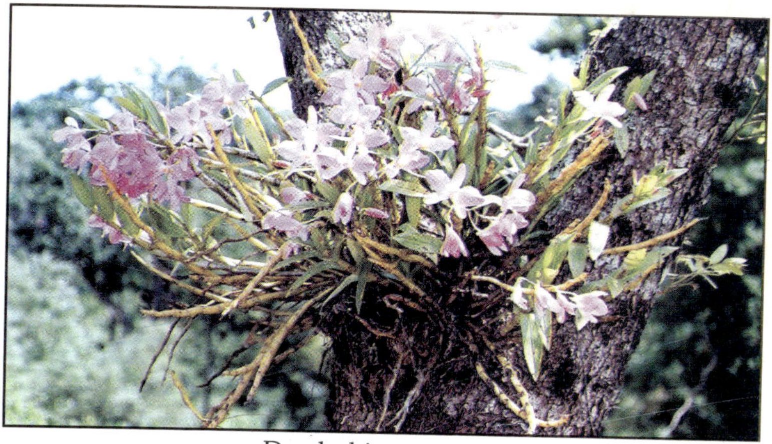

Dendrobium regium

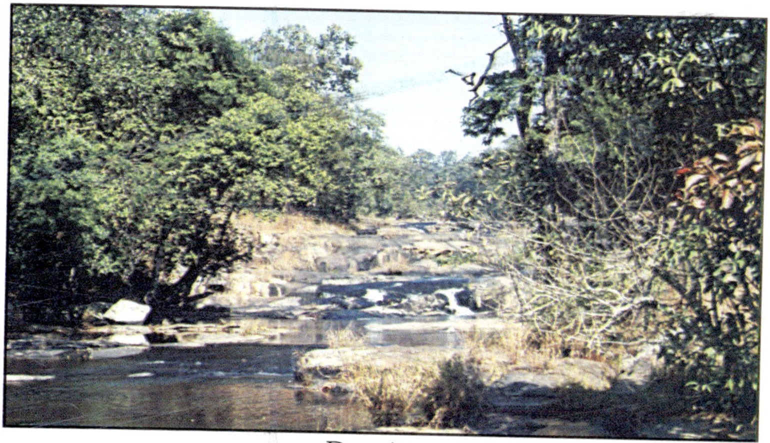

Deo river

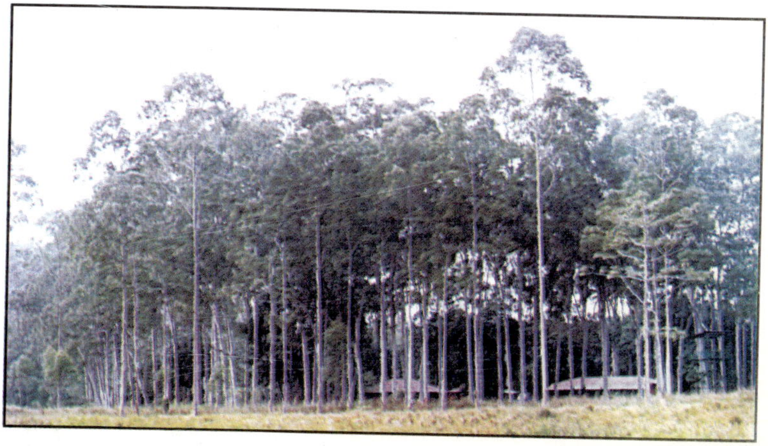

E. Villa Chahala

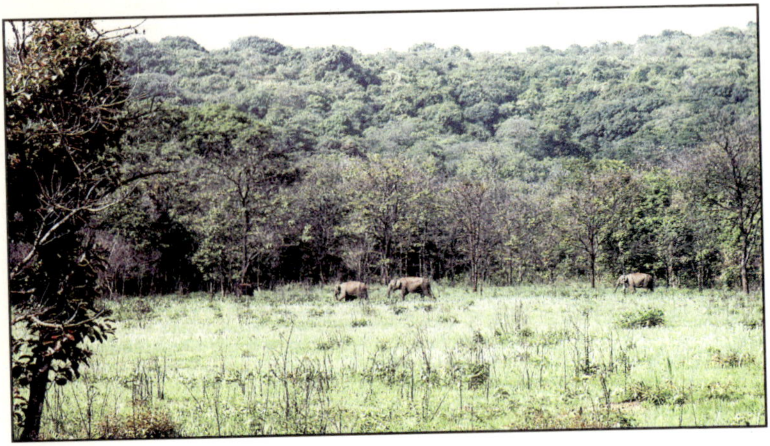

Elephant 6 matughar

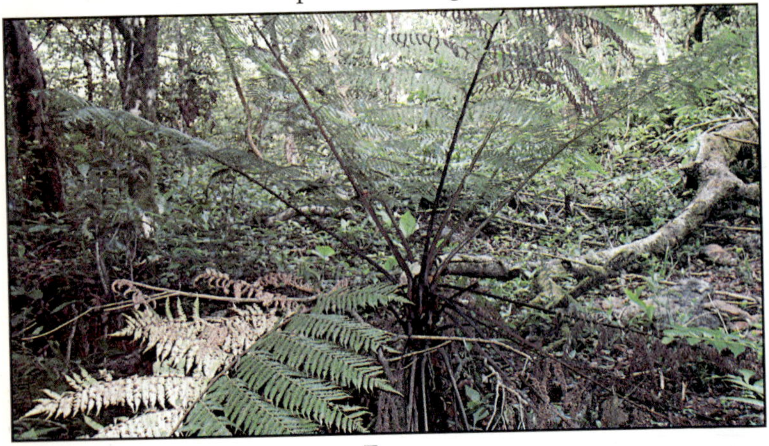

Fern

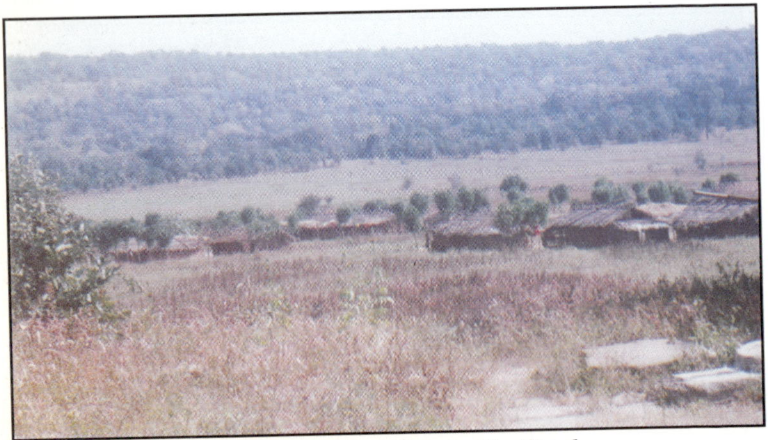

Huts of Khadia tribes in Similipal

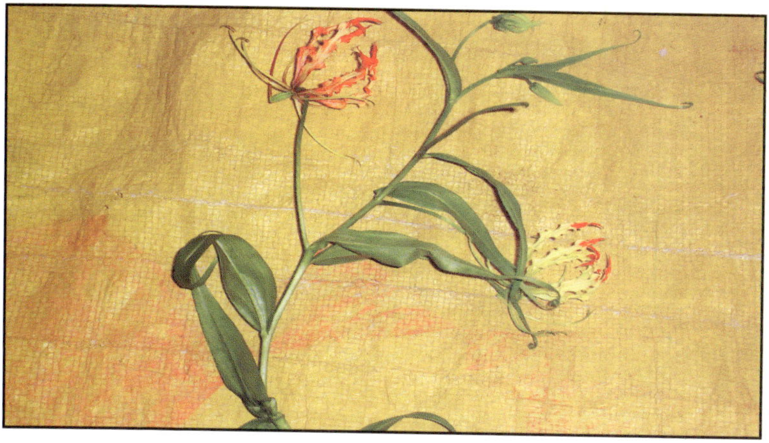

Gloriosa superba

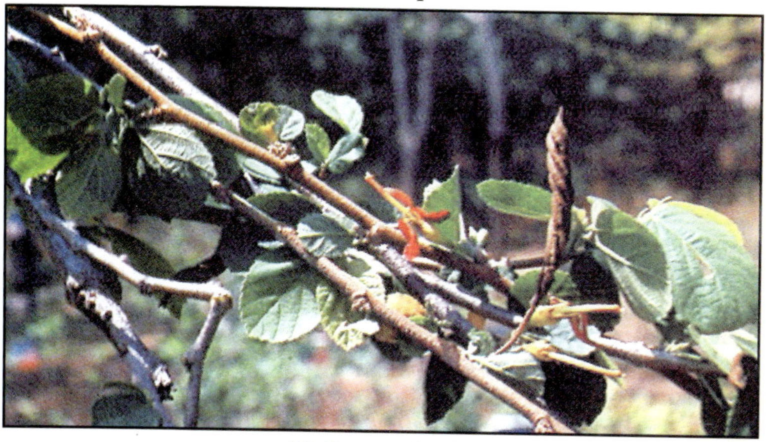

Helicteres isora

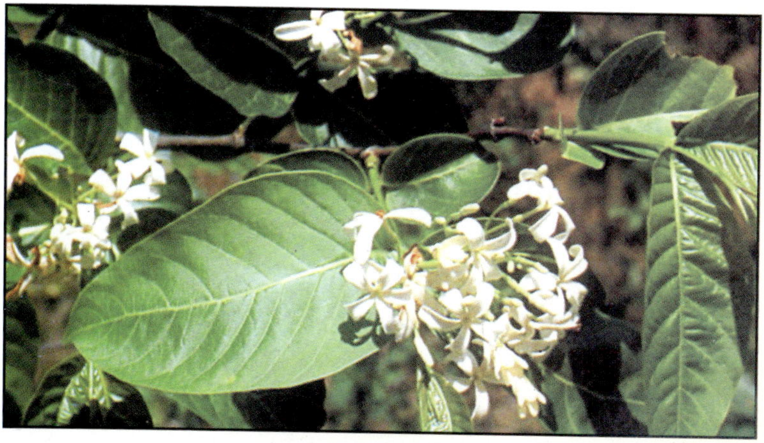

Holarrhena pubescens

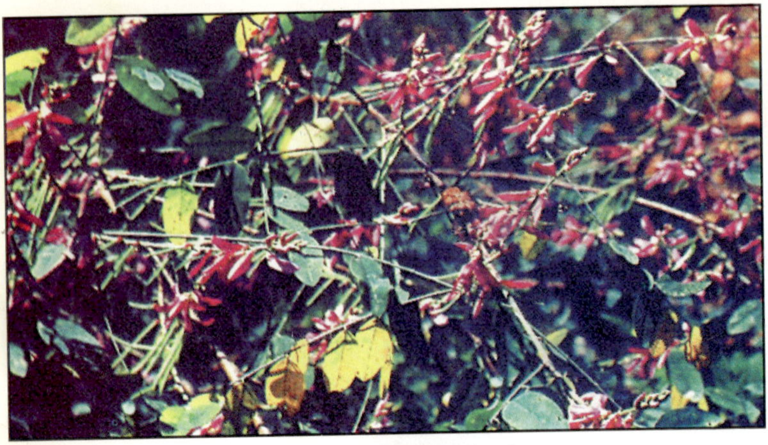

Indigofera cassioides-2

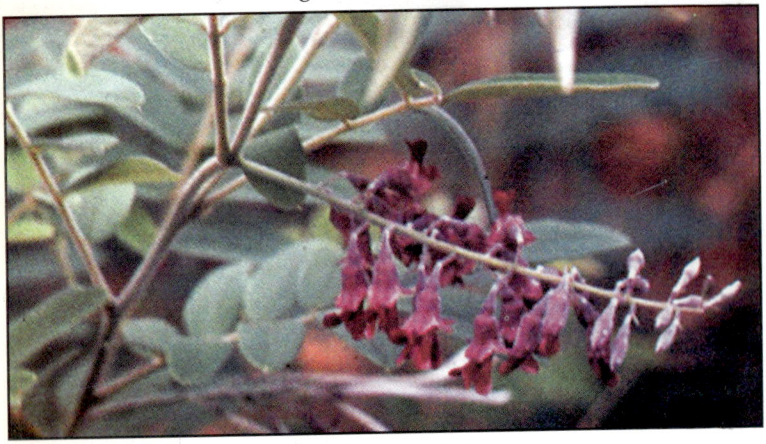

Indigofera cassioides

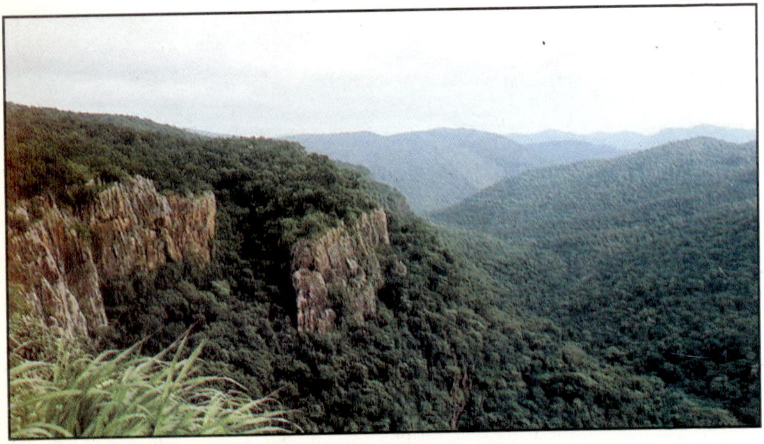

Joranda forest view 2

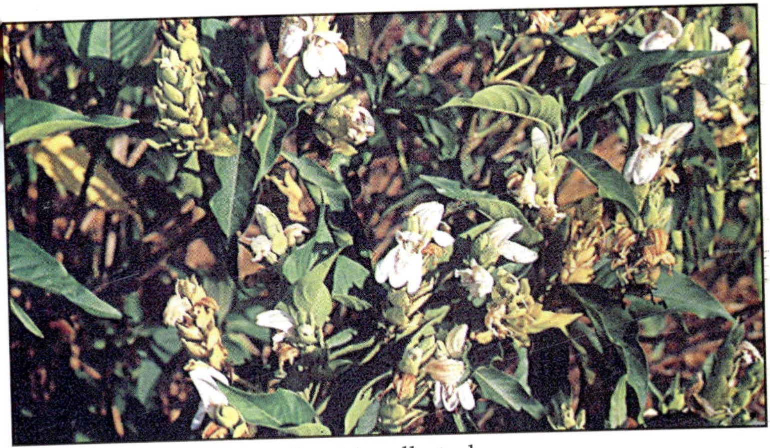

Justicia adhatoda

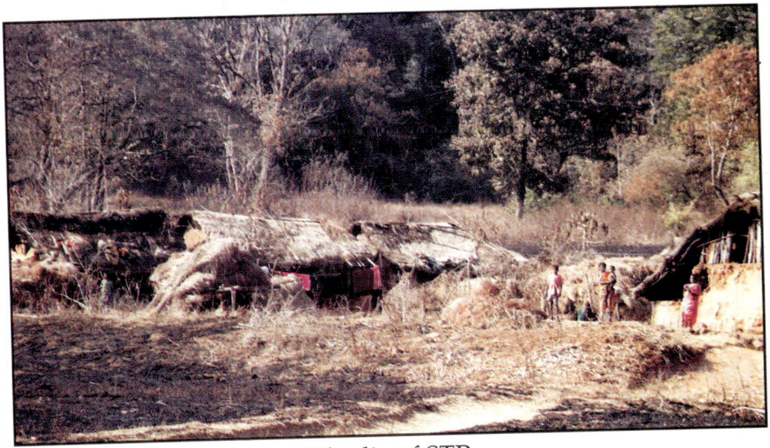

Khadia of STR

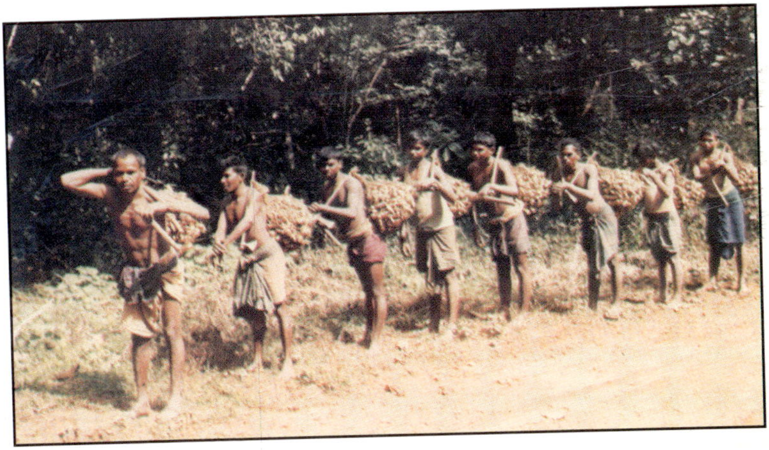

KHADIA 2

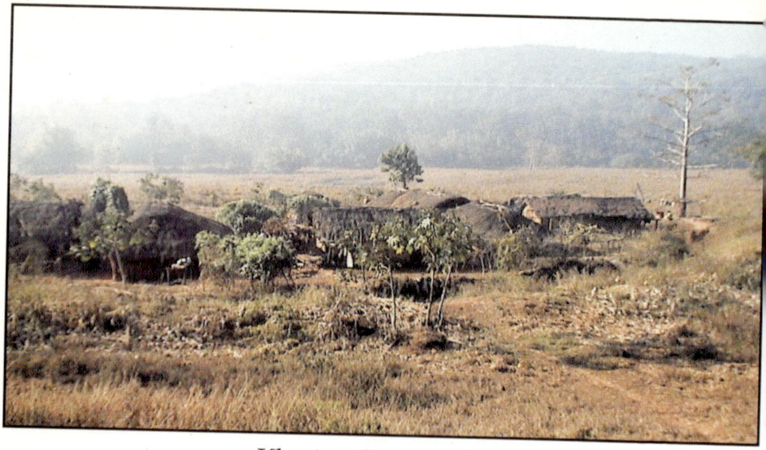

Kharia village at UBK

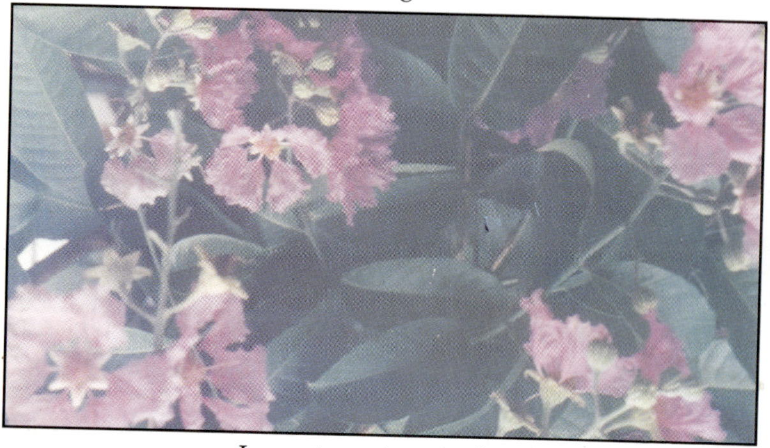

Lagerstroemia parviflora

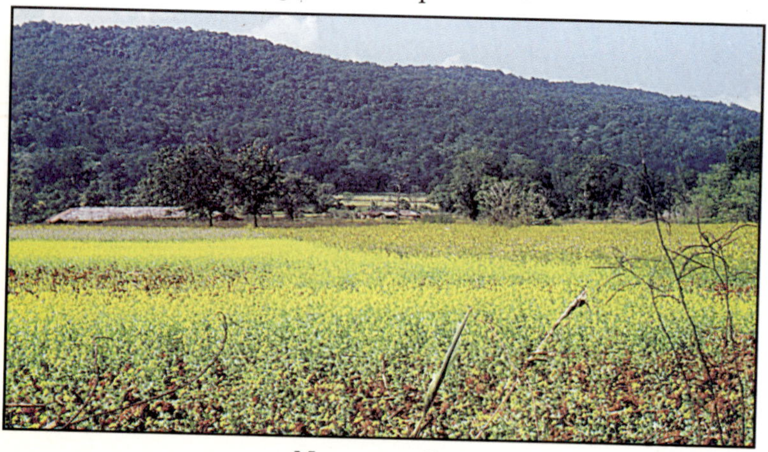

Nawana valley

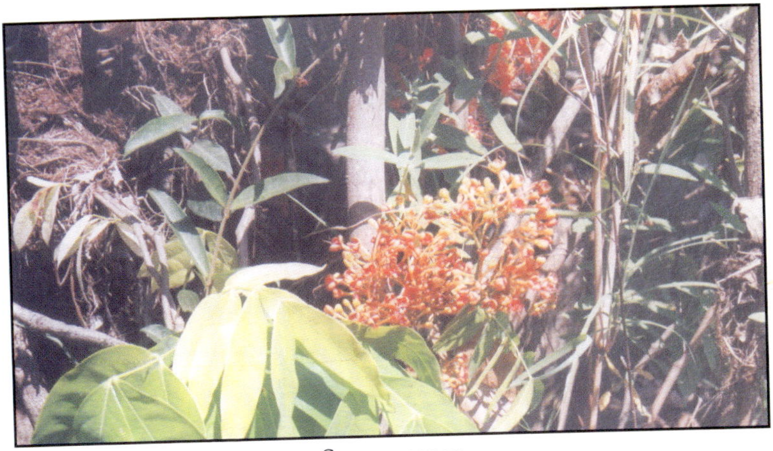

Saraca asoca

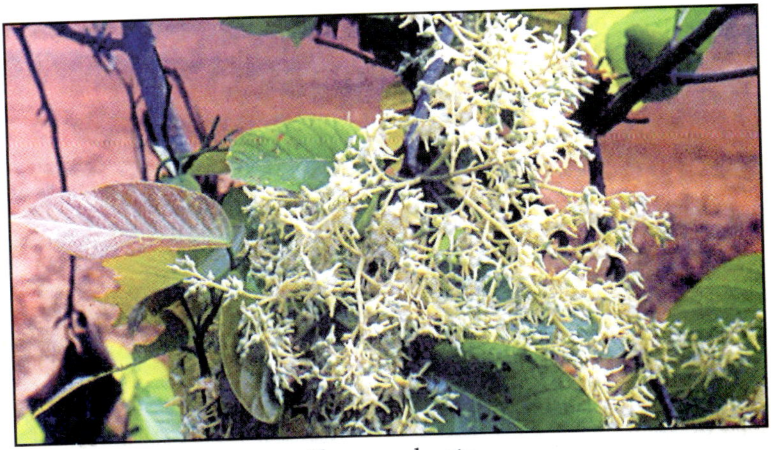

Shorea robusta

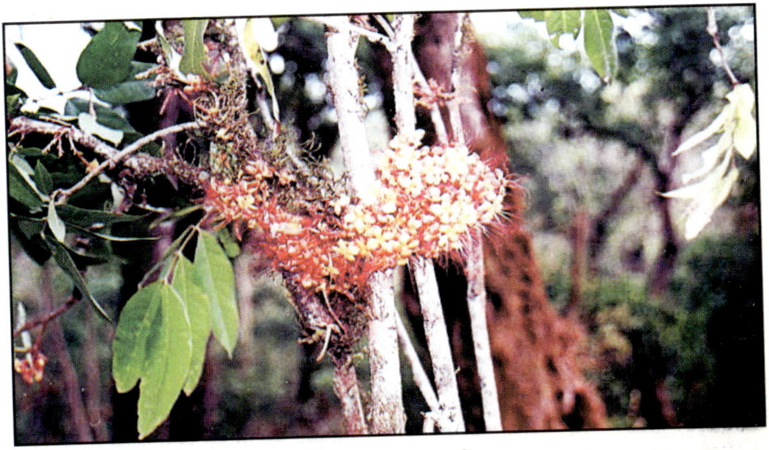

Saraca asoca-2

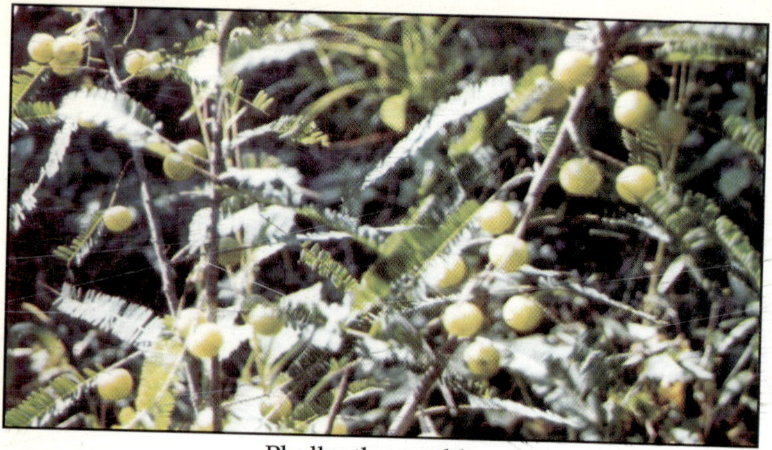

Phyllanthus emblica

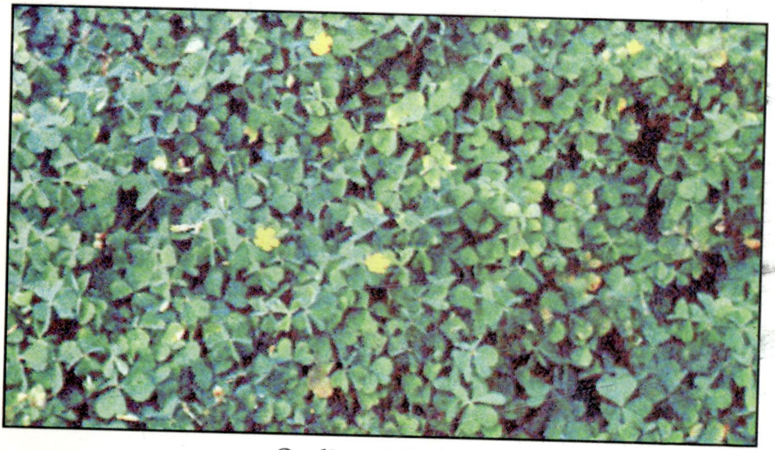

Oxalis corniculata

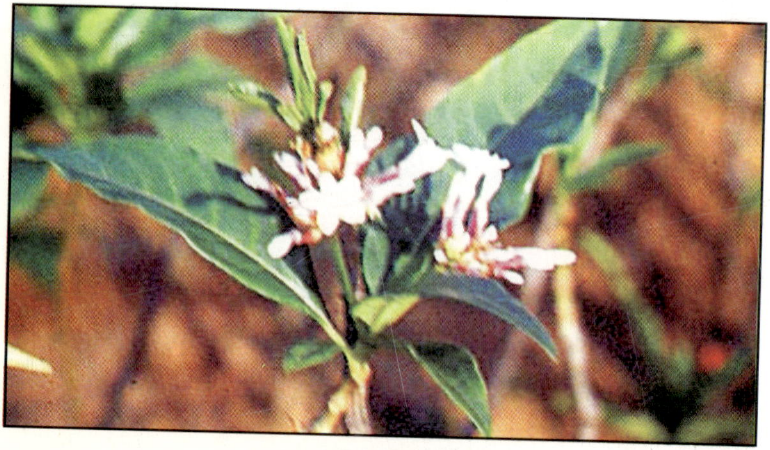

Rauvolfia serpentina

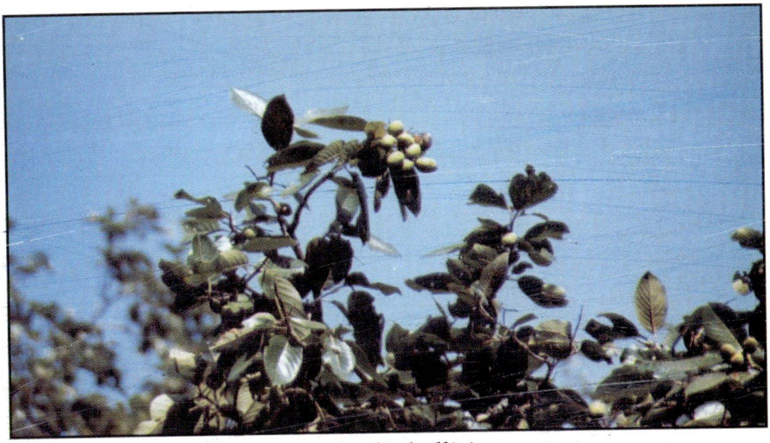

Terminalia bellirica

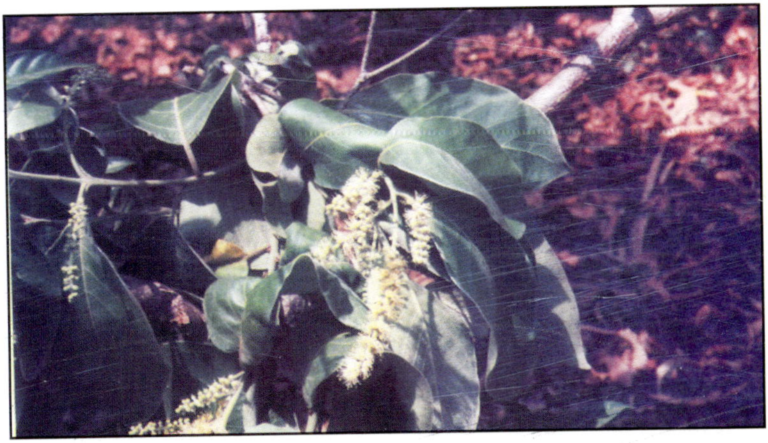

Terminalia chebula

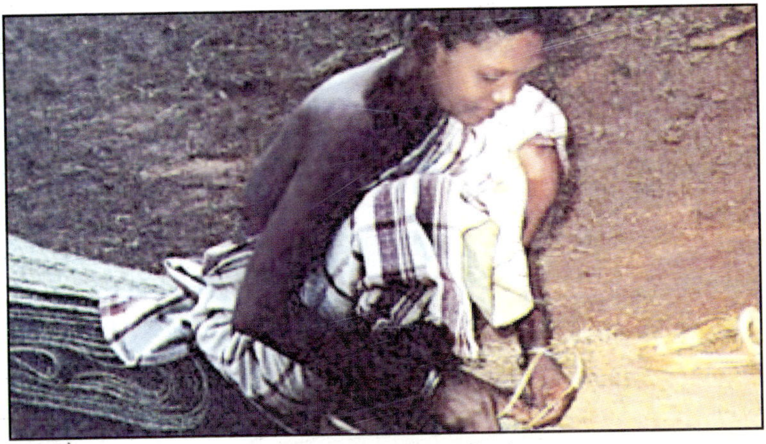

Tribal in preparing Patia

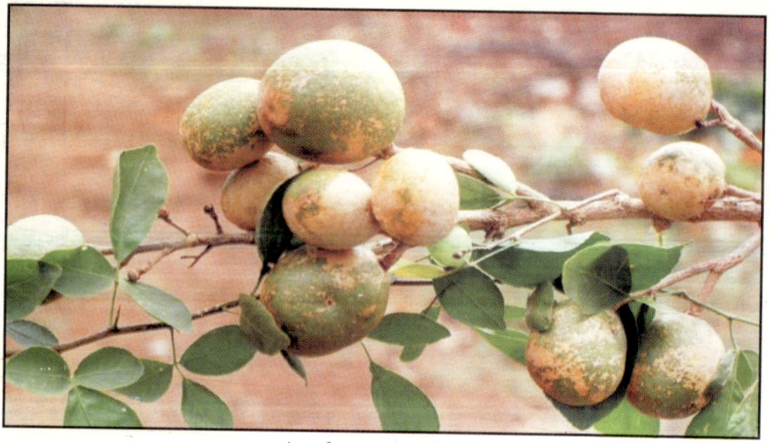
Aegle marmelos 2

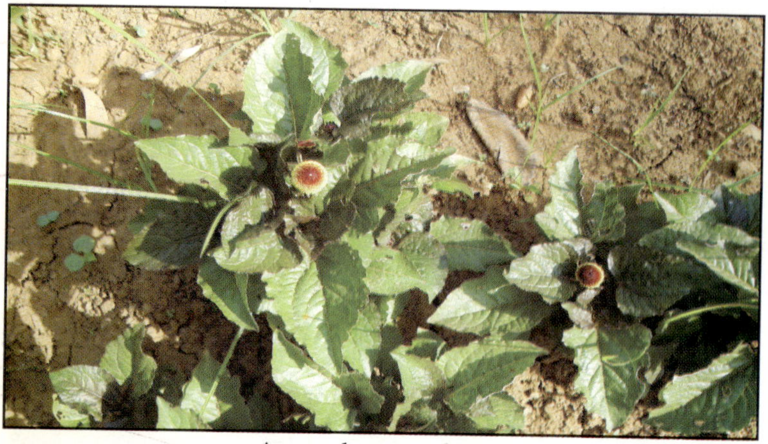
Anacyclus pyrethrum

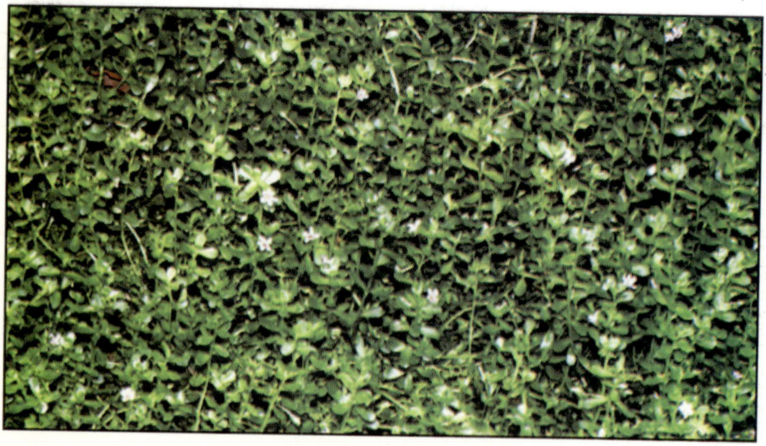
Bacopa monnieri 1

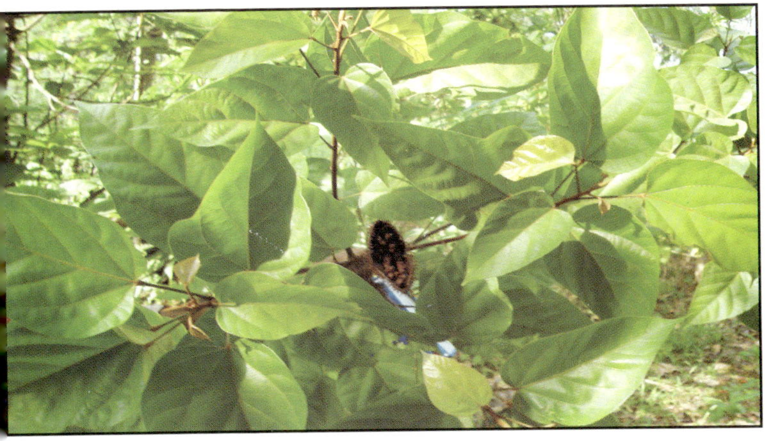

Bixa orellana

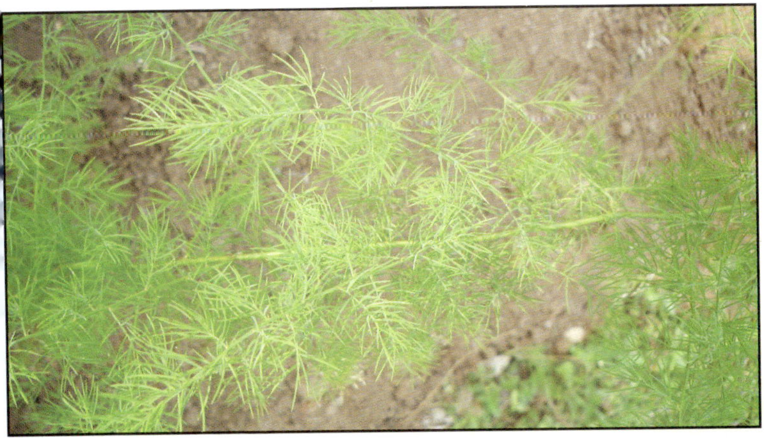

Asparagus racemosa

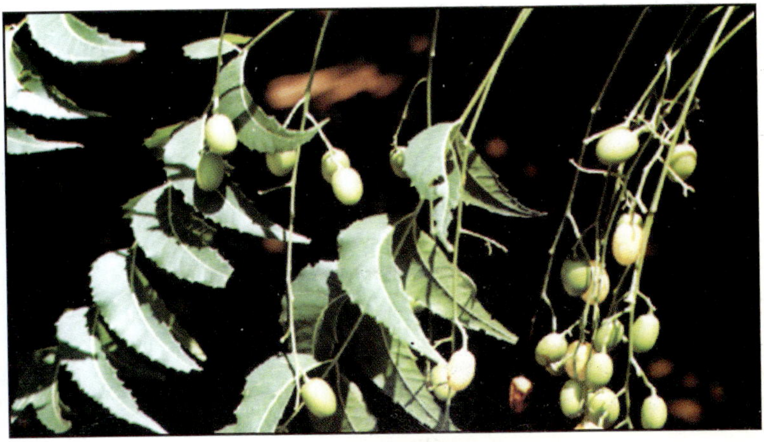

Azadirachta indica 1

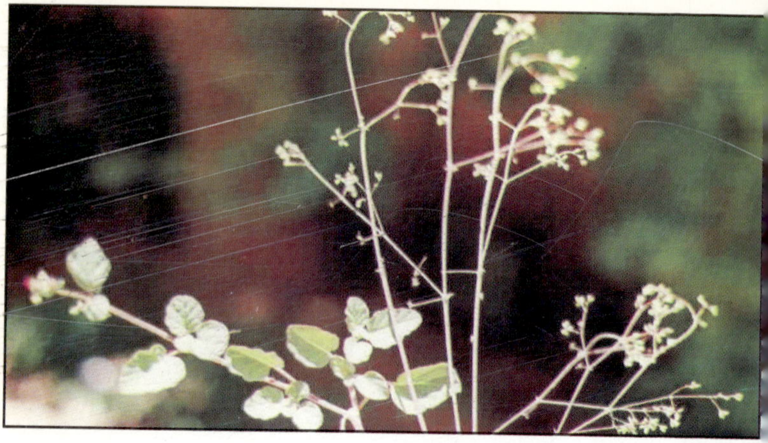

Boerhavia diffusa 1

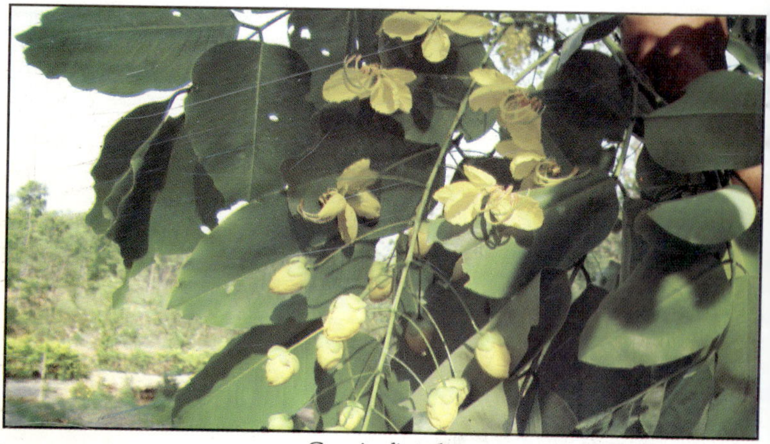

Cassia fistula

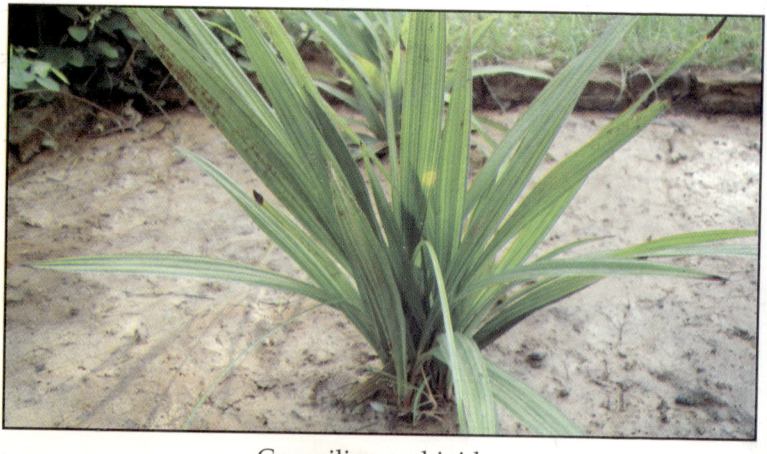

Curcuiligo orchioides

BIBLIOGRAPHY

Ambasta, S.P. (1986). The Useful Plants of India. Publication and Information Directorate, C.S.I.R. New Delhi.

Ahmmedullah, M. and M.P. Nayar (1986). Endemic Plants of the Indian Region Vol. I. Botanical Survey of India. Howrah.

Annonymous (1989). Botanical exploration of Puri district (Orissa), Central Council for Reserch in Ayurveda & Sidha (Ministry of Health and F.W Govt of India), New Delhi Publication.

Annonymous (1989). Medico-Botanical exploration of Puri District, of Orissa. Central Council for Research in Ayurveda and Siddha (Ministry of Health and Family Welfare, Govt. of India, New Delhi.

Babu, S.S. and Madhavi, M. (2001) Green Remedies, Pustak Mahal, Delhi.

Bal, S.N. (1942). Useful plants in Mayurbhanj State in Orissa. Rec. Bot. Surv. India, 61-119.

Choudhury, B.P., Biswal, A.K. and Subudhi, H.N. (1993). Enumeration of some potential medicinal plants in the district of Cuttack (Orissa). Bioscience Research Bulletin, 9(1-2) : 11-16.

Das, A.P. and Pandey A.K. (2007). Advances of in Ethnobotany. Bishen Singh Mahendra Pal Singh. Dehradun.

Girach, R.D., Singh, S., Brahmam, M. and Misra, M.K., (1999). Traditional treatment of skin diseases in Bhadrak District, Orissa. Eco & Tax. Bot. 23(2) : 499-504.

Haines, H.H. (1921-25). The Botany of Bihar and Orissa. 6 parts London. Reprint, Bot. Surv. India, Calcutta. 3 Vol. 1961.

Jain, S.K. and R.R. Rao (1983). "An Assessment of Threatened Plants of India" (Proc. of the Seminar held at Dehra Dun 14-17th Sept. 1981). Botanical Survey of India, Howrah.

Kayser O. and Quax W. (2007). Medicinal Biotechnology. From basic Research to Industrial Applications. WILEY-VCH Verlag GmbH & Co. KGaA, Weinheim. pp. 1-18.

Kirtikar, K.R. and B.D. Basu (1935). Indian Medicinal Plants. (2nd Ed. Revised by E. Blatter, J.F. Calus and K.S. Mhaskar, Allahabad, 4 Vols).

Khan M.Y., Aliabbas S., Kumar V. and Rajkumar S. (2009). Recent advances in medicinal plant biotechnology. Indian Journal of Biotechnology, 8: 9-22.

Kumar, J., S.D. Rout and M.K. Das, 2006. The Medicinal plants of Hatikote forests of district Mayurbhanj, Orissa–Need for Conservation. *Indian Forester,* 132(1): 43-53.

Kumar. J. Rout S.D., and Das, M.K. (2006). The medicinal plants of Hatikote Forests of District Mayurbhanj, Orissa-Need for Conservation. Indian Forester, 132(1):43-53.

Kumar, J. and S.D. Rout. 2005 Ethnomedicinal Study of Mayurbhanj district of North Orissa. Step towards participatory documentation of indigenous knowledge of Medicinal Plants. Revival of Local Health Traditions & Conservation of Medicinal Plants. pp. 51-60 (Ed. Bibhu Kalyan Mohanty). SAMBADH, Bhubaneswar, Orissa, India.

Mooney, H. (1950). Supplement to the Botany of Bihar and Orissa, Ranchi.

Mohanta, R.K. S.D. Rout and H.K. Sahu (2006). Ethnomedicinal plant resources of Similipal Biosphere Reserve, Orissa, India. *Zoos' Print Journal* 21(8) : 2372-2374.

Mandal, P. and Mukherjee, P.K. (1992). Notes on Ethnobotany of Keonjhar District, Orissa. J. Econ. Tax. Bot. Addl. Ser 10: 7-18.

Nayar, M.P. and A.R.K. Sastry (1987-88). "Red Data Book of Indian Plants". Vol. I & II. Botanical Survey of India. Howrah.

Nayar, M.P., M. Ahmed and D.C.S. Raju (1984). Endemic and Rare Plants of Easternghats. Indian Journal of Forestry, 7(1): 35-42.

Pradhan, J. (2001). Health Care, Satpathy Prakasan, Cuttack.

Prajapati, N.D., S.S. Purohit, A.K. Sharma and T.Kumar (2003). A handbook of Medicinal Plants–A Complete Source Book. Jodhpur, Agrobios (India).

Panda, Tribhuban and Padhy, Rabindra N. (2008). Ethnomedicinal Plants used by Tribes of Kalahandi District, Orissa; *Indian Journal of Traditional Knowledge.* 7(2), pp. 242-249.

Pandey, A.K., S.D. Rout (2006). Ethnobotanical uses of Plants by Tribals of Similipal Biosphere Reserve, Orissa. *Ethnobotany,* 18 : 102-106.

Pandey, A.K. and S.D. Rout and N. Pandit (2002). Medicinal Plants of Similipal Biosphere Reserve–Perspectives of Plant Biodiversity. pp. 681-696 (ed. A.P. Das); Bishen Singh Mahendra Pal Singh, Dehra Dun.

Pareek, S.K. and Gupta Rajendra (1993). Medicinal and Aromatic Plants Improved Profitability of Cropping Systems in India. Glimpses in Plant Research.

Park S.U., Park N.I., Kim Y.K., Suh S.Y., Eom S. H. and Lee S.Y. (2009). Application of plant biotechnology in the medicinal plant, *Rehmannia glutinosa* Liboschitz. Journal of Medicinal Plants Research, 3(13), 1258-1263.

Rout, S.D., J. Kumar and D. Swain (2005). Conservation Strategy for Medicinal Plants in Orissa, India. *The International Journal of Biodiversity Science & Management,* Vol. 1 (4): 205-211.

Rout, S. D. (2007) Ethnobotany of Diversified Wild Edible Fruit Plants in Similipal Biosphere Reserve, Orissa. *Ethnobotany,* 19: 137-139.

Rout, S.D. (2007). Observations on the use of ethno veterinary herbal practices in Similipal Tiger Reserve, Orissa, Souvenir, ADRI, Cuttack pp. 41-43.

Rout, S.D., A.K. Pandey and H.N. Thatoi 2007. Medicinal Plants used by Tribals of Similipal Biosphere Reserve. *Similipal Biosphere Reserve,* 2 (1&2): 14-17.

Rout S.D., Kumar J. and Swain, D. (2005) Conservation Strategy for Medicinal Plants in Orissa, India. *International Journal of Biodiversity Science and Management.* (4) : 205-211.

Rout, S.D. 2004. *Medicinal plants of Similipal Biosphere Reserve.* Ph.D. Thesis, T.M. Bhagalpur University, Bhagalpur.

Rout, S.D.J. Kumar and D. Swain (2005). Medicinal Plants Biodiversity of Hatikote Reserve Forests in Mayurbhanj district, Orissa. Forest Resource Management and Conservation. pp. 55-63 (ed. S.P. Rath and P.K. Mohapatra); PGCES, Dept. of Botany, Utkal University, Bhubaneswar, India.

Rout, S.D. and A.K. Pandey (2007). Some Wild Edible and other useful plants of Similipal Biosphere Reserve, Orissa. In: Advances in Ethnobotany (Eds: A.P. Das and A.K. Pandey), pp. 61-72. Bishen Singh Mahendra Pal Singh, Dehera Dun.

Rout, S.D. and A.K. Pandey (2007). Ethnomedicobiology of Similipal Biosphere Reserve, Orissa. In: Advances in Ethnobotany (eds: A.P. Das and A.K. Pandey) pp. 247-252. Bishen Singh Mahendra Pal Singh, Dehera Dun.

Rout, S.D. (2007). Medicinal Plants of Similipal Biosphere Reserve and our Health Care System. Medicinal Plants (eds: Dr. R.C. Rout and J.K. Behera) pp. 25-31. Principal, S.R. Mahavidyalaya, Baliapal, Balasore, Orissa.

Rout, S.D. (2007): Ethnobotany and its role in the Conservation of Biodiversity. *'SABUJIMA' 2008*. Plant Lovers' Association. Kalinga House, Rasulgarh, Bhubaneswar 16: 30-32.

Rout, S.D. and Pandey, A.K. (2007). Ethnomedicobiology of Similipal Biosphere Reserve, Orissa. In: Das, A.P. and Pandey A.K. eds. Advances of in Ethnobotany. Bishen Singh Mahendra Pal Singh. Dehra Dun, pp. 247-252.

Ricardo Ramos Mendonça-Filho. (2006). Bioactive Phytocompounds: New Approaches in the Phytosciences. In Modern Phytomedicine. Turning Medicinal Plants into Drugs. Eds.

Ahmad I., Aqil F., and Owais M. WILEY-VCH Verlag GmbH & Co. KGaA, Weinheim. pp. 1-24. (ISBN: 3-527-31530-6).

Singh, M.P. and Panda Hemadri 2005. Medicinal Herbs with their Formulations. Daya Publishing House, Delhi.

Satapathy,K.B., Nanda, G.C. and Chand, P.K. (2003). Plants for Diabetic. Divya Prakashanee, Bhubaneswar.

Satpathy, K.B., and Panda, P.C. (1992). Medicinal uses of some plants among the Tribals of Sundargarh district. J. Economic and Tax. Bot. Addl. Ser. 10 pp. 241-249.

Saxena, H.O. and M. Brahmam (1983). Grasses of Orissa. *Proc.* 8th Ann. Conf. Orissa. Bot. Soc. 29.

Saxena, H.O., M. Brahmam and P.K. Dutta (1988). Ethnobotanical Studies in Similipahar Forests of Mayurbhanj District (Orissa). *Bull. Bot. Surv. India*. Vol. 10, Nos, 1-4: pp 83-89.

Saxena,H.O. and M. Brahmam (1989). The Flora of Similipahar (Similipal), Orissa. With particular reference to the potential economic plants. Regional Research Laboratory, Bhubaneswar.

Sarangi, N., and Sahu, R.K. (2004). Ethomedicinal plants used in venereal and gynecological disorders in Kalahandi, Orissa. *Ethobotany*, 16:16-20

Sen, S.K. and Behera L.M. (2003). Ethnomedicinal plants used against skin diseases in Bargarh districts in Orissa. *Ethobotany*, 15:90-96.

Thatoi, H.N., Panda, S.K., Rath, S.K. and Dutta, S.K. (2008). Antimicrobial Activity and Ethomedicinal uses of some medicinal plants from Similipal Biosphere Reserve, Orissa, Asian Journal of Plant Science.

Verma, S.K., Sriwastawa, D.K. and Pandey A.K. (1999). Ethnobotany of Santhal Pargana. Narendra Publishing House, Delhi.

Warrior, P.K. (1997). Indian Medicinal Plants–A compendium of 500 species. Vol. 1-5. Orient Longman Limited. Hyderabad (A.P.). India.

Table 1 : Antimicrobial activity of aqueous extracts of collected ethnomedicinal plants from Similipal Biosphere reserve

Sl.No.	Scientific name	Local name	Family	Parts used	*Zone of inhibition (crude extract) in mm*				
					S1	*S2*	*S3*	*S4*	*S5*
1.	*Acorus calamus L.*	Bacha	Araceae	Stem	-	-	-	-	ND
2.	*Adhatoda vasica* Nees	Basanga	Acanthaceae	Leaf	16	18	14	16	16
3.	*Agave sisalena* Perr.	Nalimurga	Agavaceae	Leaf	-	20	-	-	-
4.	*Andrographis paniculata* (Burm.f.) Nees	Bhuin nimba	Acanthaceae	Stem	14	15	ND	ND	13
				Leaf	ND	ND	ND	ND	12
5.	*Argyreia speciosa* Sweet	Budhadaraka	Convolvulaceae	Stem	-	ND	ND	-	-
6.	*Asparagus racemosus* Willd.	Satabari	Asparagaceae	Root	-	-	-	-	-
7.	*Buchnania lanzan* Spreng.	Chara	Anacardiaceae	Leaf	-	-	15	-	-
				Bark	-	-	15	-	-
8.	*Careya arborea* Roxb.	Kumbhi	Lecythidaceae	Bark	-	-	-	-	-
9.	*Cassia fistula* Linn.	Sonari	Caesalpiniaceae	Leaf	-	-	-	-	-
10.	*Centella asiatica* Linn.	Thalkudi	Apiaceae	Root	ND	12	ND	ND	ND
				Leaf	12	16	ND	ND	ND
11.	*Cissampelos pareira* L.	Akanbindu	Menispermaceae	Root	-	-	-	-	-
12.	*Cissus quandrangularis L.*	Hadajoda	Vitaceae	Leaf	-	-	-	-	-
				Stem	-	-	-	-	-
13.	*Clausena excavata* Burm.f.	Agnijhal	Rutaceae	Leaf	-	-	-	20	-
				Root	15	15	13	14	16
14.	*Coccinia grandis* (L.) Voigt	Bana kunduri	Cucurbitaceae	Leaf	ND	_	_	ND	ND

15.	*Croton roxburghii* Balak.	Putuli	Euphorbiaceae	Leaf	-	-	-	15	-
				Bark	14	17	20	15	-
16.	*Curcuma angustifolia* Roxb.	Palua	Zingiberaceae	Rhizome	-	-	ND	-	-
17.	*Diospyros melanoxylon* Roxb.	Kendu	Ebenaceae	Leaf	15	14	13	-	-
				Bark	-	16	17	16	-
18.	*Enydra fluctuans* Lour.	Hidmicha	Asteraceae	Leaf	17	-	20	-	15
19.	*Eryngium foetidum* L.	Banadhania	Apiaceae	Stem	12	15	ND	ND	16
				Leaf	14	14	ND	ND	14
20.	*Flemingia nana* Roxb	Sabalabhanga	Fabaceae	Root	27	-	18	19	22
				Leaf	-	-	-	-	-
21.	*Glycyrrhiza glabra* (L.)	Jyestha madhu	Fabaceae	Seed	-	-	-	-	-
				Bark	-	-	-	-	18
				Leaf	-	-	-	-	-
				Fruit	23	18	22	17	31
22.	*Grewia elastica* Royle	Mirgchara	Tilliaceae	Leaf	-		-	-	13 -
				Root	-	-	25	22	28
23.	*Hemidesmus indicus* (L.) Schult	Anaantamula	Asclepiadaceae	Stem	-	ND	ND	ND	-
				Leaf	12	ND	ND	ND	13
24.	*Holarrhena antidysenterica* Wall.	Kuluchi	Apocynaceaea	Leaf	-	ND	ND	-	-
25.	*Ichnocarpus frutescens* (L.) R.Br.	Badadudhi, Swanlata	Apocyanacea	Stem	ND	-	-	ND	ND
				Leaf	-	-	-	-	-
26.	*Kaempferia rotunda* L.	Bhuin Champa	Zingiberaceae	Root	-	14	-	19	-
				Leaf	-	11	-	-	-

27.	*Limnophila heterophylla* (Roxb.) Benth.	Ambuja	Scrophulariaceae	Leaf	-	-	-	-	-
28.	*Litsea monopetala* (Roxb.) Pers.	Pojo	Lauraceae	Bark	14	-	-	16	-
29.	*Melastoma malabathricum* L.	Koroli	Melastomataceae	Leaf	-	-	-	21	20
				Bark	16	-	-	16	20
30.	*Nyctanthes arbortristis* L.	Gangasiuli	Oleaceae	Leaf	22	18	ND	ND	13
				Bark	14	15	ND	ND	18
31.	*Opeculina turpethum* Silva.	Tihudi	Convolvulaceae	Leaf	-	ND	-	-	ND
				Stem	-	ND	-	-	ND
32.	*Oroxylum indicum* Vent.	Phenphenia	Bignoniaceae	Bark	-	20	-	-	-
33.	*Pergularia daemia* Chiov.	Uturuchi	Asclepiadaceae	Root	-	ND	-	-	ND
				Leaf	-	ND	-	-	ND
34.	*Pongamia glabra* Vent.	Karanja	Fabaceae	Leaf	ND	-	-	ND	ND
35.	*Pterospermum acerifolium* (L.) Willd.	Muchukunda	Sterculiaceae	Leaf	11	19	21	-	-
36.	*Strychnos nux-vomica* L.	Kochilakhai	Loganiaceae	Seed	-	-	ND	-	-
37.	*Tinospora cordifolia* Miers.	Guluchi	Menispermaceae	Stem	-	-	-	-	-
38.	*Urginea indica* Kunth	Bana Piaja	Liliaceae	Bulb	25	22	26	24	23
39.	*Vitex negundo* L.	Begunia	Verbenaceae	Leaf	16	18	-	-	14
				Bark	13	12	17	17	16
40.	*Woodfordia fruticosa* kurz.	Dhatiki	Lythaceae	Root	-	-	-	-	-

LIST OF TOTAL FAMILIES (105-FAMILIES) TOTAL 315 SPECIES LISTED IN THIS BOOK

Name of the family	*Total No. of species*
Acanthaceae	11
Adiantaceae	1
Alangiaceae	1
Amaranthaceae	4
Amaryllidaceae	2
Anacardiaceae	5
Angiopteridaceae	1
Annonaceae	3
Apiaceae	2
Apocynaceae	6
Araceae	4
Aristolochiaceae	1
Asclepiadaceae	2
Aspidiaceae	1
Aspleniaceae	2
Asteraceae	21
Athyriaceae	1
Barringtoniaceae	1
Bignoniaceae	1
Bixaceae	1
Blechenaceae	1
Boraginaceae	1
Caesalpiniaceae	8
Capparidaceae	1
Caricaceae1	
Celastraceae	1

Clusiaceae1	
Cochlospermaceae	1
Combretaceae	8
Commelinaceae	2
Convolvulaceae	6
Crassulaceae	1
Cucurbitaceae	2
Cyperaceae	1
Dioscoreaceae	1
Dipterocarpaceae	1
Droseraceae	1
Drynariaceae	1
Ebenaceae	2
Equisetaceae	1
Euphorbiaceae	14
Fabaceae	23
Flacourtiaceae	2
Gentianaceae	2
Hemionitidaceae	1
Hymenophyllaceae	1
Hypericaceae	1
Labiatae	1
Lamiaceae6	
Lauraceae	3
Liliaceae	5
Linaceae	1
Lindsaeaceae	1
Loranthaceae	1
Lygodiaceae	2
Lythraceae	6
Magnoliaceae	1
Malpighiaceae	1
Malvaceae	5
Marsileaceae	1

Meliaceae	4
Menispermaceae	1
Mimosaceae	3
Moraceae	2
Myrsinaceae	2
Myrtaceae	4
Nyctaginaceae	1
Olacaceae	5
Onagraceae	1
Ophioglossaceae	1
Orchidaceae	2
Oxalidaceae	1
Papaveraceae	1
Pedaliaceae	1
Periplocaceae	1
Piperaceae2	
Plumbaginaceae	1
Poaceae	7
Polygonaceae	2
Pteridaceae	2
Punicaceae	1
Ranunculaceae	1
Rhamnaceae	3
Rosaceae	1
Rubiaceae	14
Rutaceae	7
Salicaceae	1
Santalaceae	1
Sapindaceae	6
Sapotaceae	2
Scrophulariaceae	4
Selaginellaceae	1
Smilacaceae	1
Solanaceae	5

Sterculiaceae	2
Strychnaceae	2
Symplocaceae	1
Theaceae	1
Thelypteridaceae	1
Tiliaceae	3
Trapaceae	1
Ulmaceae	2
Verbenaceae	10
Vitaceae	4
Zingiberaceae	5

INDEX TO VERNACULAR NAMES

Dhatuki
Dhatura
Dhatura
Dhau
Dhaura
Dhaura
Dhava
Dhava
Dhela
Dhelakanta
Dheniani
Dhera
Dhola chitaparu
Dholasmudra
Dholasmudrika
Dhulda
Dhyamakha
Dikamali
Dirghapatrika
Dodhali
Dodhari
Dolsingh
Donka bejji
Dorabohok
Drakappa
Dubopatli
Dudhi
Dudhi
Dudhi
Dudhilata
Dudura
Dudura
Dugdhika
Dugdugia
Duk
Dukhuri
Dukipotum
Dumbojoda
Dundi
Dunguri
Durga phulo
Durkuri
Eksira
Etka
Etke
Euturudi
Gab
Gaigobra
Gaisani
Gaisiro
Gaiya
Gajapipal
Gajapippali
Gajapippali
Galgal
Gambhari
Gambhari
Gambhari
Gandhabel
Gandhali
Ganga tulsi
Gangaseoli
Gantha khelika
Gara Boi
Gara Hatana
Gara sindur
Gara tiril
Garadhola
Garakode
Garu puru
Gasar
Ghoda languid
Ghorabach
Gileri

Kareta
Karhar
Kari
Kari
Kariyar tharani
Karlitulia
Karra
Karuna
Karwa
Kasarda
Kasinda
Kasma
Kasmar
Kasmari
Kasondi
Kata thohar
Katahi
Katako
Katangai
Kateera
Kath siju
Kathakoli
Katkana
Katnim
Katta pangu
Kaunc
Kaura sago
Kausum
Kaya
Kayaputi
Kayim
Kedar nari
Kena
Kenchua
Kendu
Keralata
Kero
Keu
Keukand
Khairwal
Khajri
Khami khondo
Kharenta
Kharkas
Kharkharia
Khasa
Khatta
Khelopapada
Kher
Kherwa
Khet papra
Khiromula
Kila kerua
Kirata
Kiri
Kiryat
Klmara
Kochila
Kodo
Kodra
Kodravah
Koelekha
Kogue
Kohumu
Koiad
Koim
Kokilaksha
Kokkarai
Kokola
Kokundia
Kola Kendu
Konaka
Kondai
Kongora

Latkan
Ledha chhali
Lendia
Lichi
Lichu
Lishi
Lobanga
Lodh
Lodho
Lodhra
Lohagasi
Lohajanghia
Lohajharia
Longa baguli
Lopong
Ludum
Luila
Lupurg
Luvani
Madar
Madayantika
Madhavi
Madhobi
Madhukah
Madhumalati
Madhumalati
Madhvi
Magha latenga
Mahanim
Mahanimba
Mahula
Mahva
Maida
Maida
Mainphal
Majith
Makirla
Makoi
Malghan
Maljan
Malkamni
Malkungi
Malpi
Mamsarohini
Mandargam
Mandukaparni
Manjeet
Manjuati
Manjur
Mankara Kendu
Marang atkir
Marang gindung
Mardang
Marsinga
Masa
Mashaparni
Mashoni
Mashparui
Maska
Masud
Masundi
Matka
Matsyaksi
Mauwa
Mayur chandrika
Mayur chulia
Meda
Mehndi
Menda
Menhga koli
Merantua sanga
Merle
Mirchai
Mirsinga

Tinpatiya
Tiril
Tisi
Titar
Tobu
Topa
Tripadi
Tuar
Tumri
Tun
Tundpora
Tut
Tutkuli
Udal
Uli
Ulpalasariba
Ulu
Unchi
Unga
Urak
Usangid-ba
Utaran
Utrali
Uttar
Vajri
Vana bhenda
Vanacchedi
Vanaharidra
Vanaraja
Vasak
Vasaka
Vasika
Verenda
Viddari kand
Visalya
Vishamandala
Vriddadaru
Vriddha tulasi
Wilayati tulsi
Zakham-haiyal
Zard kunel

INDEX TO SCIENTIFIC NAMES

Cassia fistula
Cassia occidentalis
Cassia tora
Catharanthus roseus
Catharanthus roseus
Catunaregam spinosa
Catunaregam spinosa
Celastrus paniculatus
Celosia argentea
Celosia argentea
Centella asiatica
Centella asiatica
Centipeda minima
Chlorophytum arundinaceum
Chrysanthemum indicum
Cissus quadrangularis
Citrus aurantium
Citrus medica
Clausena excavata
Cleome viscose
Clerodendrum indicum
Clerodendrum serratum
Clerodendrum viscosum
Clitoria ternatea
Coccinia grandis
Cochlospermum religiosum
Combretum roxburghii
Commelina benghalensis
Costus speciosus
Crinum defxum
Croton roxburghii
Curculigo orchioides
Curcuma amada
Curcuma aromatica
Cyathocline purpurea
Cymbopogon martini
Cynodon dactylon
Cyperus rotundus

D

Dalbergia lanceolaria
Dalbergia latifolia
Datura metel
Dendrophthoe falcate
Desmodium gangeticum
Desmodium oojeinensis
Desmodium triflorum
Dioscorea pentaphylla
Diospyros malabarica
Diospyros melanoxylon
Drosera indica

E

Eclipta prostrata
Elephantopus scaber
Embelia tsjeriam-cottam
Enydra fluctuans
Erioglossum rubiginosum
Erycibe paniculata
Euphorbia hirta
Euphorbia hirta
Euphorbia nivulia
Exacum bicolor

F

Flacourtia indica
Flacourtia jangomas
Flemingia strobilifera
Floscopa scandens

G

Gardenia gummifera
Glochidion lanceolarium
Gloriosa superba
Gmelina arborea
Grewia hirsuta
Grewia tilifolia